# Football Medicine

# Football Medicine

## Edited by

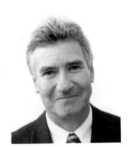

**Jan Ekstrand** MD PhD

Professor of Sports Medicine

University of Linköping

Linköping, Sweden


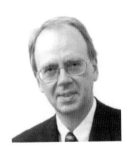

**Jon Karlsson** MD PhD

Professor of Sports Traumatology

Department of Orthopaedics

University of Gothenburg

Gothenburg, Sweden


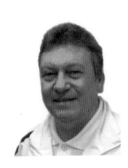

**Alan Hodson** MA DipRG/RT DipTP

CertEd MCSP SRP

Head, Medical and Exercise Science Department

The Football Association

Lilleshall National Sports Centre

Shropshire, UK

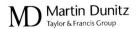

© 2003 Martin Dunitz, an imprint of the Taylor & Francis Group
First published in Sweden in 1998 by Svenska FotbollFörlaget AB

Revised edition published in 2003
by Martin Dunitz, an imprint of the Taylor & Francis Group plc, 11 New Fetter Lane, London
EC4P 4EE,

Tel.:        +44 (0) 20 7583 9855
Fax.:        +44 (0) 20 7842 2298
E-mail:      info@dunitz.co.uk
Website:     http://www.dunitz.co.uk

Although every effort has been made to ensure that all owners of copyright material have been acknowledged in this publication, we would be glad to acknowledge in subsequent reprints or editions any omissions brought to our attention.
A CIP record for this book is available from the British Library.

ISBN 1 84184 164 1

Distributed in the USA by
Fulfilment Center
Taylor & Francis
10650 Tobben Drive
Independence, KY 41051, USA
Toll Free Tel.:   +1 800 634 7064
E-mail:           taylorandfrancis@thomsonlearning.com

Distributed in Canada by
Taylor & Francis
74 Rolark Drive
Scarborough, Ontario M1R 4G2, Canada
Toll Free Tel.:   +1 877 226 2237
E-mail:           tal_fran@istar.ca

Distributed in the rest of the world by
Thomson Publishing Services
Cheriton House
North Way
Andover, Hampshire SP10 5BE, UK
Tel.:             +44 (0)1264 332424
E-mail:           salesorder.tandf@thomsonpublishingservices.co.uk

Printed and bound in Spain by Grafos S.A. Arte Sobre Papel

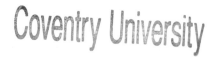

# Contents

Contributors     vii

Foreword by Lennart Johansson     xi

Foreword by Sven-Göran Eriksson     xii

Preface     xiii

1    **The risk of injury and injury distribution** *Jan Ekstrand* .................. 1

2    **Football medicine in the team**
*Roger Gustafsson and Alan Hodson* ........................................ 11

3    **Preventing injury** *Jan Ekstrand* ................................................ 39

4    **The biomechanics of football** *Pekka Luhtanen* ....................... 121

5    **The physiology of football** *Björn Ekblom* ................................. 139

6    **Nutrition and football** *Björn Ekblom* ....................................... 163

7    **The use of nutritional supplements in football**
*Ronald J Maughan* ....................................................................... 173

8    **First aid** *Åke Andrén-Sandberg and Alan Hodson* ............... 197

9    **Muscle injuries** *Per Renström* .................................................. 217

10    **Head injuries** *Yelverton Tegner* ............................................... 229

11    **Injuries to the upper extremities** *Jon Karlsson* ........................ 241

12    **Back injuries** *Leif Swärd* ......................................................... 267

13  **Chest, abdominal and skin injuries** *Anders Falk* ...................... 281

14  **Groin injuries** *Jan Ekstrand* ................................................. 289

15  **Knee injuries** *Jon Karlsson* ................................................. 307

16  **Lower leg injuries** *Jon Karlsson* ......................................... 343

17  **Ankle injuries** *Jon Karlsson* .............................................. 361

18  **Injuries to the foot** *Jon Karlsson* ....................................... 381

19  **Post-injury functional testing for return to competitive play**
    *Alan Hodson* ............................................................. 395

20  **Football-specific injury rehabilitation** *Stenove Ringborg* .......... 415

21  **Disease and medication** *Mats Börjesson* ............................... 443

22  **Late sequelae of football – osteoarthrosis** *Harald Roos* ........... 463

23  **Children and football** *Åke Andrén-Sandberg* ........................ 475

24  **Specific aspects of women's football**
    *Peter Adolfsson, Harald Roos and Anna Östenberg* ............. 493

25  **The role of the referee** *Lars-Åke Björck and Jan Ekstrand* ...... 509

26  **Travelling abroad with a team** *Jan Ekstrand and John Crane* .. 519

27  **Doping** *Sverker Nilsson* ..................................................... 529

Bibliography                                                              537
Index                                                                     551

# Contributors

**Peter Adolfsson MD PhD**

Paediatrician, University of Gothenburg, Gothenburg, Sweden

**Åke Andrén-Sandberg MD PhD**

Professor of General Surgery, University of Gothenburg, Gothenburg, Sweden

**Lars-Åke Björck**

Member, UEFA Referees' Committee, Gotherburg, Sweden

**Mats Börjesson MD PhD**

Specialist in Internal Medicine, University of Gothenburg, Gothenburg, Sweden

**John Crane MB ChB**

Club Doctor, Arsenal Football Club, London, UK

**Björn Ekblom MD PhD**

Professor of Physiology, Karolinska Institute and, Chairman, Medical Committee Swedish Football Association, Stockholm, Sweden

**Jan Ekstrand MD PhD**

Professor of Sports Medicine, University of Linköping and Director, Sports Medicine Clinic, Linköping, Sweden

**Anders Falk MD PhD**

Associate Professor of General Surgery, University of Gothenburg, Gothenburg, Sweden

**Roger Gustafsson**
Head Coach, IFK Gothenburg, Gothenburg, Sweden

**Alan Hodson MA DipRG/RT DipTP CertEd MCSP SRP**
Head, Medical and Exercise Science Department, The Football
Association, Lilleshall National Sports Centre, Shropshire, UK

**Jon Karlsson MD PhD**
Professor of Sports Traumatology, Department of Orthopaedics,
University of Gothenburg, Gothenburg, Sweden

**Pekka Luhtanen MD PhD**
Professor, University of Jyväskylä, Jyväskylä, Finland

**Ronald J Maughan MD PhD**
Professor, School of Sport & Exercise Sciences, Loughborough
University, Loughborough, UK

**Sverker Nilsson MD**
General Practitioner, Falkenberg, Sweden

**Per Renström MD PhD**
Professor, Section of Sports Medicine, Department of Orthopedics,
Karolinska Hospital, Stockholm, Sweden

**Stenove Ringborg PT**
Past Physiotherapist, Swedish Football Team

**Harald Roos MD PhD**
Associate Professor of Orthopaedics and Director, Orthopaedic
Department, Helsingborg, Sweden

**Leif Swärd MD PhD**

Associate Professor of Orthopaedics, University of Gothenburg, Gothenburg, Sweden and Team Physician, England Football Team

**Yelverton Tegner MD PhD**

Associate Professor of Sports Medicine, Institution of Health Sciences, Luleå University of Technology, Boden, Sweden

**Anna Östenberg PT PhD**

Physiotherapist, Helsingborg, Sweden

# Foreword I

Although medical experts have worked for many years to prevent injuries in football and implement new methods for treating injuries, when they do occur the situation seems to have worsened in recent years.

The governing bodies in football are fully aware of the problem but the intensity of the modern game and the frequency of top level matches has created a difficult situation for everyone involved in the game.

One therefore hopes that this book will not only increase the knowledge but also the understanding of the importance of taking preventive measures and help give players adequate treatment when an injury occurs.

Lennart Johansson

# Foreword II

Football is the most popular sport in the world, played by young and old, men and women alike and gives joy to many millions of people. The World Cup is watched by hundreds of millions of people and is the world's single biggest sporting event. Unfortunately, there is a downside concerning the increasing number of injuries and other health-related problems. These can be either short-term, such as cruciate ligament injuries, or long-term sequele, such as osteoartritis of the knee leading to pain and inflammation years after a footballer's playing days are over.

*Football Medicine* is concerned not only with the treatment of football-related injuries, but also covers how they can be prevented. Written by international specialists who have worked closely together with football teams at the highest national and international level for many years, *Football Medicine* provides the reader with the most recent scientific information about football-related injuries.

Today, it is more important than ever to take good care of a player's health. This timely book enables all health professionals involved in the game to identify and diagnose football injuries. *Football Medicine* should be in every therapists' bag and should also be read by players and coaches in order to reduce the incidence and seriousness of all football-related injuries.

I warmly recommend this book.

Sven-Göran Eriksson

# Preface

Football is the world's most popular sport, played and watched by millions of people every week.

Although injuries have always traditionally been part and parcel of football, the changing nature of the game itself and the ever-pressing demands on the players have led to increased awareness of this important issue and interest in preventing and treating medical problems. The injuries are very varied and complex, and good, all-round knowledge of the game is necessary for their successful management and treatment.

*Football Medicine* gives a broad and detailed description of many of the injuries that occur in this increasingly fast-moving sport. Injuries to all parts of the body are covered in depth, and specialist areas such as children's and women's football are also included. To reflect the importance of diet, two chapters are devoted to nutrition and the use of nutritional supplements, while a chapter on doping deals with the other end of the scale. Finally, some of the important but often forgotten areas are discussed in chapters on returning to play, travelling abroad with a team and the role of the referee.

It is our hope that this book will be helpful to all those involved with the game – players, coaches and medical staff – for many years to come.

Jan Ekstrand, Jon Karlsson and Alan Hodson

2003

# 1. The risk of injury and injury distribution

Jan Ekstrand

Football is a popular sport played throughout the world with many participants, which is important to bear in mind as a background to discussions about the occurrence of football injuries in different situations. According to the Federation of International Football Associations (FIFA) there are around 200 million licensed players today in a total of 186 countries. Within the Union of European Football Associations (UEFA) there are 51 countries represented by over 22 million players (nearly 21 million men and over 1.3 million women).

## How is the concept 'injury' defined?

Many studies have been carried out on the risk of injury in the game of football. In order to be able to compare the results from these studies, the injuries have to be defined in a similar way.

In many cases, insurance statistics or hospital records have been used. These studies provide us with an idea of the more serious injuries and the pressure they represent on the resources of the community, but they only record the number of players injured, and not the number exposed to the risk of injury. A high percentage of football injuries in these studies reflects the popularity of football and the great numbers of participants in the game rather than the risk of injury to the individual player.

In recent years, an injury has been defined as any injury a player has incurred in any football-related activity which has caused absence from training or from a match. These studies provide us with an idea of the risk of injury to the individual player and for the team, since they take into consideration the exposure to football and record injuries per 1000 hours of football activity which also provides valuable background information for preventative measures.

### How great is the exposure to football at different levels of play?

Table 1.1 shows the results of a survey carried out to study the differences between the different divisions as far as exposure and injuries are concerned (training sessions, matches etc).

Table 1.1 Football activity and injuries over a 1-year period. The results from the study of the Swedish Super League, Division I, Division IV and Division VI. Each team is represented by an A-team of 15 players (men at senior level)

|  | Swedish Super League | Div I | Div IV | Div VI |
|---|---|---|---|---|
| • Number of training sessions/team | 141 | 129 | 95 | 65 |
| • Training attendance (%) | 84 | 81 | 66 | 60 |
| • Number of hours training/player | 171 | 153 | 95 | 54 |
| • Number of matches/team | 48 | 37 | 36 | 34 |
| • Number of football activity hours/player | 215 | 179 | 139 | 85 |
| • Number of injuries/team | 29 | 24 | 21 | 14 |
| • Number of training sessions/match | 3 | 4 | 3 | 2 |

From Table 1.1 we can see that the exposure to football increases with the increase in the level of play. Training is more frequent in the Swedish Super League, there is better attendance at training and more matches are played than in Division I and so on. The number of injuries also increases the higher the level of play.

### How great is the risk of injury in football?

Table 1.2 illustrates the result of studies where similar definitions and a similar data collation process have been used to record the risk of injury.

**Table 1.2** The risk of injury per 1000 hours of football activity (Sweden)

| Men (senior) | Training | Match | Training camp |
| --- | --- | --- | --- |
| National A-team (1990–97) | 6.5 | 30 | 16 |
| Swedish Super League (1982) | 4.6 | 21.8 | |
| Div II (1982) | 5.1 | 18.7 | |
| Div IV (1981) | 7.6 | 16.9 | 21 |
| Div VI (1982) | 6.1 | 14.6 | |
| Div IV (1996) | 5.6 | 11.2 | |

| Women (senior) | Training | Match | Training camp |
| --- | --- | --- | --- |
| Div III (1991) | 2.1 | 6.5 | |

## FACTS ABOUT THE RISK OF INJURY

- The risk of injury during training is approximately the same regardless of the level of play.
- The risk of injury increases during training camps compared with regular training.
- The risk of being injured during a match is greater than during training.
- In men's football the risk of being injured during a match is greater the higher the level of play.

**Has the risk of injury in football increased or decreased?**
In order to examine whether the risk of injury has increased or decreased in Swedish football, the same Division IV series was followed for 2 separate years, 1980 and 1996. The exposure to football, i.e., the number of training sessions and matches, was unchanged during this 16-year period. In both 1980 and 1996, the teams trained on average 90–95 times and played 34–35 matches per year. The attendance at training sessions was on average 66 per cent during both years. The risk of injury was lower, however, both for training and matches in 1996 compared with 1980.

The results of this study suggest that the risk of injury may have decreased in men's senior football in Sweden possibly as a result of the injury prevention work carried out by the clubs.

**Which injuries are most common?**
In Tables 1.3 and 1.4 we can see the distribution between various types of football injury and the degree of seriousness.

**Table 1.3** Different types of injury in football (men Division IV)

|  | Total (%) | Slight (%) | Medium (%) | Serious (%) |
|---|---|---|---|---|
| Ligament injuries | 29 | 16 | 7 | 5 |
| Musculoskeletal strain | 23 | 17 | 5 | 2 |
| Contusion (collision/crush) | 20 | 15 | 5 | 0 |
| Tendon/muscle injuries | 18 | 9 | 7 | 2 |
| Fractures | 4 | 1 | 1 | 2 |
| Dislocation | 2 | 0 | 2 | 0 |
| Other injuries | 4 | 4 | 0 | 0 |
|  | 100 | 62 | 27 | 11 |

The degree of seriousness of the injury:
Slight = At most 1 week's absence from training or matches.
Medium = Absence of between 1 week and 1 month.
Serious = Absence of more than 1 month.

**Table 1.4** Localization of the injuries. (See Table 1.3 for explanation of degrees of seriousness)

|  | Total (%) | Slight (%) | Medium (%) | Serious (%) |
|---|---|---|---|---|
| Foot | 12 | 10 | 2 | 0 |
| Ankle | 17 | 11 | 5 | 2 |
| Lower leg | 12 | 6 | 4 | 2 |
| Knee | 20 | 11 | 5 | 4 |
| Thigh | 14 | 6 | 5 | 2 |
| Groin | 13 | 9 | 3 | 1 |
| Back | 5 | 4 | 1 | 0 |
| Other | 7 | 5 | 2 | 0 |
| | 100 | 62 | 27 | 11 |

Among outdoor players of football, 60–90 per cent of all injuries are to the leg (the lower extremity). Ankle injuries and knee injuries are most common among senior players while collision or compression injuries (contusions) to the lower leg are most common among junior players. Goalkeepers are, however, more often affected by injuries to the upper body, such as finger injuries, wrist injuries and shoulder injuries.

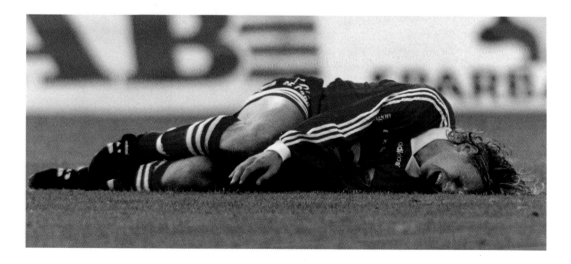

## How great is the risk of an injury
## to the anterior cruciate ligament?

Injuries to the anterior cruciate ligament are one of the most common types of injury a football player can encounter. It is also the injury where the risk of future problems is greatest (see Chapter 22).

The risk of a male senior player incurring an anterior cruciate ligament injury has been estimated at 0.1 per cent/1000 h of football activity. If one takes into account the exposure times in Table 1.2, the risk of a cruciate ligament injury for the individual player is low (on average one injury every 46th year for a player in the Swedish Super League). A team with a 15-man squad can expect statistically to encounter one cruciate ligament injury in the squad every third year in the Swedish Super League, every fourth year in Division I, every fifth year in Division IV and every eighth year in

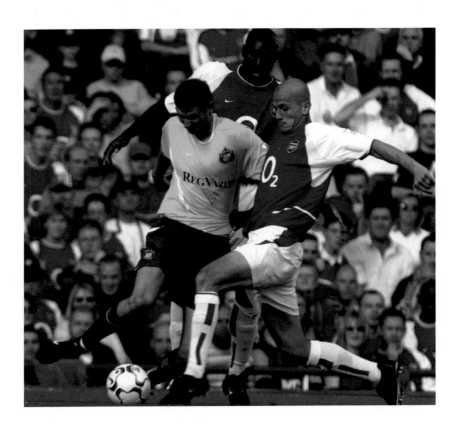

Division VI. If we look at an entire season we might statistically expect four anterior cruciate ligament injuries per year in the Swedish Super League, three per year in Division I, two per year in Division IV and one per year in Division VI.

The risk of incurring an anterior cruciate ligament injury is higher for women than for men. In senior women's football, the risk of injury has been reported at three per 1000 hours of football activity, in other words, a risk of injury three times higher than for male senior players. Women also have a lower average age for when the injury occurs. In junior football, the risk of an anterior cruciate ligament injury is reported to be 4–5 times higher for girls than for boys.

**How are injuries distributed over the football season?**
Figure 1.1 shows the distribution of injuries over the months of the year. The survey was done for a Swedish Division IV season for men in 1996. From this we can see that most injuries occurred during the first part of the year with a peak in March, the month before the start of the season's play.

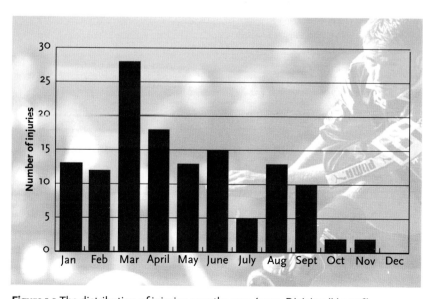

**Figure 1.1** The distribution of injuries over the year (men, Division IV, 1996).

In Figure 1.2 a distinction has been made between injuries due to accidents and overuse injuries. During the months of January, February and March overuse injuries are predominant. When the season's matches are played injuries due to accidents are most common.

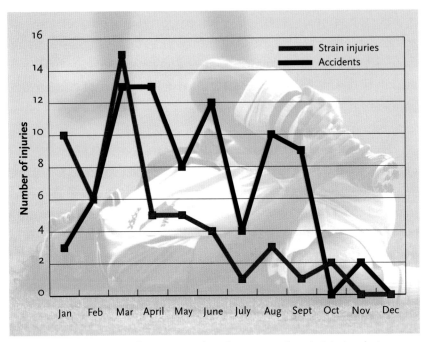

**Figure 1.2** The distribution between accidental injuries and strain injuries during a 1-year period (men, Division IV, 1996).

## Is there any difference between the risk of injury in a match won and a match lost?

In a study of the risk of injury in a national A-team football during the years 1990–1996, it was noted that the risk of injury was higher during matches lost (56 injuries/1000 h played) than matches won or matches ending in a draw (22 injuries/1000 h played). No difference in the risk of injury was noted between home and away matches or matches on neutral grounds.

Possible explanations for the risk of injury being greater during matches lost are shown in the following fact box.

## WHY IS THE RISK OF INJURY GREATER DURING A MATCH LOST?

- **Injuries have a direct impact on the match result**
  The best team is selected to play. The team is weakened if anyone is injured.
- **Injuries have an indirect impact on the result through the match plan**
  The best team plays and the team's tactics are planned according to the starting. If anyone in the 'first team' is substituted, the match plan is disrupted.
- **The result influences the injury profile**
  A substitute may be just as good as the player injured. The substitute may also be very familiar with the tactical plan for the team. In this case it may be the result itself that can lead to an increase in the risk of injuries since players who are losing take greater risks, or that the risk of injury increases through the negative mental impact of the result.

# 2. Football medicine in the team

Roger Gustafsson and Alan Hodson

The finances of the club are decisive for the level at which it is possible to have medical service in a team. This may vary from having an entire football medicine team in the form of doctors, masseurs and various physiotherapists to a contact network of people with the equivalent expertise.

The most efficient way of reducing the cost of medical service in the team is to instruct coaches and players in preventive, acute and rehabilitation measures. Players are often an unexploited resource in this context. It is a question of getting the players to take greater responsibility for their own training and health.

The level of the medical service is based on the views the coach, players and the club have concerning football medicine and the significance of the players' health — both as active sportsmen and women and in general, with, hopefully, a long and healthy life after their football career. The club and club leadership have, therefore, considerable responsibility for the players, which is greater the younger the players are. The club should be active in keeping the players healthy, both during and after their football careers.

This chapter is divided into three main areas:

1. Measures for the prevention of injuries and illness.
2. Acute measures in the event of injuries and illness.
3. Measures for rehabilitation and return to the sport after an injury or illness.

We will not be going into the details but will describe instead the general measures that can be taken, whether the team has access to a football medicine team or whether it organizes a contact network of football medicine experts.

In conclusion we will also describe how the football medicine team can cooperate with coaches, players and other organizers in a team to create a 'team behind the team'.

# Measures for preventing injury and illness

It is obvious that players and coaches want to avoid injuries and illnesses by taking preventative measures. Therefore, both the coaches and players have an obligation to follow the advice and recommendations provided by the medical staff responsible. The medical staff should, in turn, be prepared to keep up to date with the latest research results, be scrupulous with regard to ethics and moral issues and update their familiarity with current doping regulations.

Both coaches and medical personnel must act in an ethically correct way, morally and in accordance with the rules, in all situations; first and foremost, the future health of the players must never be compromised — there should be no doubt about this.

### Awareness of the players' state of health

The coaches and medical personnel have joint responsibility for the players' health. In order to take this responsibility, it is important to be aware of a players' background for example, regarding previous injuries, illness, medication or if there are after-effects from previous illnesses and injuries such as a distended ligament in the ankle etc.

It is also important to be aware of the players' general state of health to be able to help a player quickly, and to be able to adapt the training to the individual at certain times. Are there cases of allergies, asthma, high blood pressure or diabetes among the squad? The simplest way of obtaining such background information is by questionnaires, individual interviews, medical examinations and well warranted medical tests.

In this context, it is important to bear in mind that a team doctor has the same responsibility for his or her players as a hospital doctor for his or her patients. Professional confidentiality applies regarding for example the different levels of medical service, along with the task of keeping medical records of injuries and illnesses. The personnel with medical responsibility may not, for instance, inform journalists of the medical condition, injury or operations involved without the consent of a player.

In cases where no medical help is available within the team, the coach should find out about injuries and illnesses which may be significant for the football game itself or which may present a possible health risk.

The medical details considered to be significant should be selected to create a personal medical register for all players. This register should be kept up to date with any new injuries, illnesses, tests, etc. Remember to report any injuries which may affect the future state of health to the insurance company. The register should be kept under lock and key in the manner of medical records. Players who leave the club should take their register with them.

## Training

Since the coach is responsible for the health of the players, it is important to be aware of the effects of the training. The coach should therefore be aware of this, and perhaps ask for the advice of the medical personnel, to be able to assess what training is appropriate. This may relate to the planning of weight training, suppleness or agility training and stamina training for the entire team or within individual training programmes.

Regular doses of training do not normally cause any problems. Expertise at this level can be obtained during regular courses for coaches and in medical literature. In cases where greater exertion is required, the coach should contact medical specialists for the approval of the training programme.

If the team plans to train more intensively during a certain period, it is essential to know what the consequences of this will be. Will the players be able to cope with the amount of training and will they have time to recover their strength between the training sessions? The basic idea is never to attempt to get more out of a player physically than their strength and capacity allows.

Players are also responsible for getting to know their bodies and capacity at the same time as the instructor has to listen when a player says that they feel tired, finds it difficult to maintain the tempo of the training, or that they are experiencing pain in their joints and muscles. The risk of injuries due to wear and tear arise during hard monotonous training and during training on difficult surfacing, especially after a break in training.

It is also important to find out whether a player feels tired and run down which may be cause for a medical examination.

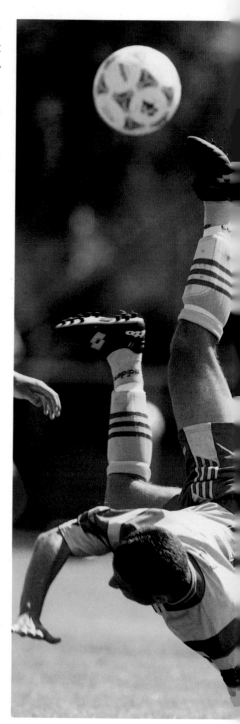

## Warming up and cooling down

Warming up before training and matches is important and the same applies for cooling down after an activity. The correct equipment, hygiene and the environment, for example, the correct boots, clean clothes and clean leg pads along with clean changing rooms, a good surface for training and access to fluids at training sessions and matches — all these details are significant for the prevention of injuries and illness. For instance, check that there is always access to a telephone, that there are stretchers at the training or sports arena and that the team always has a fully equipped first aid bag.

It is important that the players are focused and relaxed in connection with training and matches. This means that they concentrate on the task in hand and have more relaxed muscles which is likely to have the effect of preventing injuries.

It is also important that the players play according to the rules at training sessions and matches. In this way it is possible to avoid unnecessary injuries resulting from foul play. To play and play hard is not the same as dirty and unfair play.

## Discuss injury prevention with the team

To ensure that coaches and players are at the same level and to allow them to take joint responsibility for these issues, detailed information and discussion are recommended at the start of each season.

Information about what is expected, for example, during training camps overseas is also important. There should be clear rules about what food and drink should be avoided. A camp overseas is often costly and the money may be wasted if half the squad have stomach ailments and can neither train nor play. It is, therefore, also important to find out whether any specific protection against infection is required for the destination in question.

# An audit of injuries in professional football

*Background information and research project outline*

Professional football in England and Wales is governed by a very demanding playing programme and this holds true especially when comparisons are made with other footballing nations. The competitive season commences in August, following 4–8 weeks of pre-season training. By the end of the season in May, having competed in their respective leagues and two domestic cup competitions, the majority of teams will have played between 50 and 60 competitive games on top of the numerous matches played during pre-season. Furthermore, with the ever-increasing European club commitments, the elite clubs can be expected to play in excess of 70 games in a season. In addition to this, several players will have international playing commitments throughout the season and will be involved in prestigious summer tournaments such as the European Championships and the World Cup. In the light of the demanding playing programme, the inherent need for players to remain injury free is paramount.

From the start of the pre-season training for the 1997/1998 playing season through to the end of the 1998/1999 playing season, clubs in the Premiership and Nationwide Leagues have completed a comprehensive questionnaire detailing each injury that has kept a player out of match action or training for in excess of 48 h. It is important to note that the figures relate only to football-related injuries and not to training time or matches missed through illness. Details of the sample studied are shown in Table 2.1.

*Injury audit analysis*

During the 1997/1998 and 1998/1999 competitive seasons, 6030 injuries resulting from training and/or competition were documented, approximately 75 per cent of players sustaining at least one injury, the average injury rate over the seasons equalling 1.3 injuries per player per season. Approximately one-third of the injuries

**Table 2.1** Demographics displaying division, playing position and age distribution of the cohort at the commencement of the study

| Division | No. | % | Playing position | No. | % | Age distribution | No. | % |
|---|---|---|---|---|---|---|---|---|
| Premier | 618 | 26 | Goalkeeper | 223 | 9 | 17–22 | 970 | 41 |
| 1st | 712 | 30 | Defender | 817 | 34 | 23–28 | 817 | 34 |
| 2nd | 550 | 23 | Midfielder | 739 | 31 | 29–34 | 508 | 21 |
| 3rd | 496 | 21 | Forward | 597 | 25 | 35+ | 81 | 3 |
| **Total\*** | **2376** | **100** | | **2376** | **99** | | **2376** | **99** |

\*Percentage totals may be subject to rounding errors associated with individual components.

were sustained during training and two-thirds occurred during competition (Figure 2.1).

Figure 2.2 displays the severity of all the injuries, 78 per cent being classified as either slight (2 to 3 days absent), minor (less than 1 week absent) or moderate (1 week to 1 month absent), with a further 22 per cent being severe, preventing the injured player

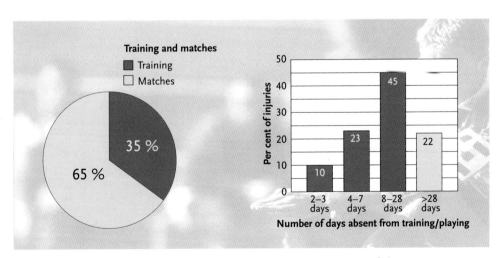

**Figure 2.1** Playing activity at time of injury.

**Figure 2.2** Severity of player injuries.

from training or playing for at least 4 weeks. The total number of days that players were absent over the two full seasons was 145 973 days and a total of 23 876 matches were missed, which equates to an average of 24 days missed per injury including four competitive matches.

Figure 2.3 shows the total number of injuries sustained per month during training and competition. The number of injuries sustained during training gradually decreased throughout the season as did the number of match injuries, the greatest incidence occurring during the month of August.

The nature of the injuries sustained during training and matches are shown in Figure 2.4. Injuries classified as either strains, sprains or contusions represented 69 per cent of all the injuries. The lower extremity was the site of 87 per cent of the injuries reported (Figure 2.5). The majority of the thigh injuries were muscular strains (81 per cent). The incidence of ligament sprains was high, accounting for 67 per cent of ankle injuries and 39 per cent of knee injuries.

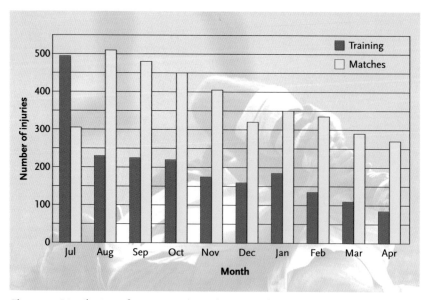

**Figure 2.3** Distribution of training and match injuries throughout the season.

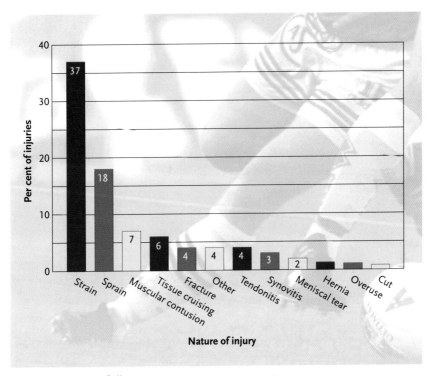

**Figure 2.4** Nature of all injuries.

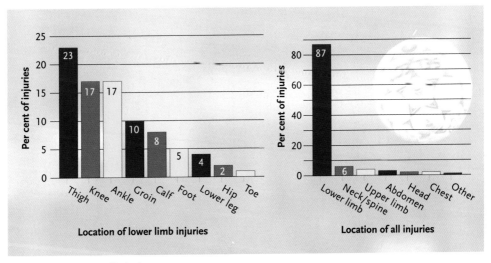

**Figure 2.5** Location of injuries.

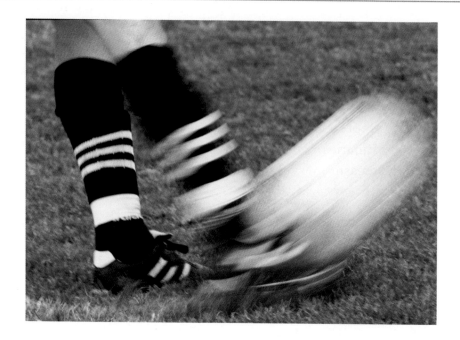

The injury mechanisms are shown in Table 2.2, 38 per cent being classified as resulting from contact with another player or ball and 58 per cent having a non-contact mechanism. Of all the injuries that occured during a training session 26 per cent occurred while

**Table 2.2** Mechanism of injuries

| Mechanism | Number | % | Mechanism | Number | % |
|---|---|---|---|---|---|
| Running | 1114 | 19 | Jumping | 122 | 2 |
| Tackled | 903 | 15 | Other (contact) | 90 | 1 |
| Other (non-contact) | 572 | 9 | Falling | 63 | 1 |
| Tackling | 566 | 9 | Diving | 44 | 1 |
| Twisting/turning | 487 | 8 | Heading | 39 | 1 |
| Collision | 383 | 6 | Use of elbow | 34 | 1 |
| Stretching | 336 | 6 | Hit by ball | 19 | 0 |
| Kicked | 281 | 5 | Dribbling | 8 | 0 |
| Shooting | 257 | 4 | Throwing | 6 | 0 |
| Landing | 227 | 4 | Not specified | 237 | 4 |
| Passing | 213 | 4 | **Total** | **6030** | **100** |

the player was performing some type of running. Over 75 per cent of the training injuries were a consequence of a non-contact mechanism.

The distribution of the competitive match injuries with respect to time is represented in Figure 2.6. Players sustained a greater number of injuries in the second half, with the likelihood of getting injured increasing towards the end of the match.

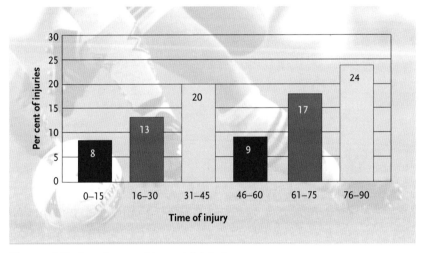

**Figure 2.6** Timing of competitive match injuries.

Re-injuries were accountable for 7 per cent of all the injuries sustained during the study period. Of the 420 re-injuries that were documented, 48 per cent were strains and 18 per cent sprains. Re-injuries within the same season were found to be more severe than the previous injury, the number of missed training days averaging 25 compared to 19 days for the initial injury.

*Injury audit recommendations*

The impact of an injury on the fortunes of a club can be considered in relation to its severity and the number of potential competitive matches missed. There was an average of four matches missed per injury with 78 per cent of the injuries leading to a minimum of one match missed. The average number of days lost per injury was 24 and based on the incidence of injuries per month. The average number of injuries per club season was 39.

In football, injury 'costs' may involve medical fees, increased insurance premiums and reduced income from lower match attendances and diminished prize money received as a result of the final league position. Few clubs have the mechanism or resources to identify the losses separately and examine them systematically. In professional football, especially at the highest level, the financial consequences of injuries to clubs is expected to be proportionately more than in industry as the relative number of injuries in football greatly overshadows industrial figures. To identify the full cost of injuries to a professional football club accurately would require an indepth investigation, however, it is envisaged that the cost to English professional clubs would be substantial with the value of Premiership players alone being £425 million and their wages for the 1998/1999 season being estimated at £241 million. The annual wage bill for all professional footballers was approximately £400 million in the 1998/1999 season, and since, on average, 10 per cent of a squad is unavailable to train each week, the projected financial loss of output due to injury can be estimated to be at least £40 million per year.

Given that players are assets to a club it is important that comprehensive assessments of a player's health are conducted prior to their signing for the club. This need highlights the necessity of having high quality medical staff and centres for this purpose. The transfer of players in 1998/1999 resulted in £316.9 million changing hands, of which £142.2 million was spent on overseas players.

It is suggested that applying aspects of risk management policies used in industry, the risk of injuries in professional football could be reduced. There are four main principles commonly contained in a risk management policy that could be applied to professional football.

The importance of players to professional football clubs

Players are the most important assets to the success of profession-al football clubs. Policies concerned with the prevention of injury, optimal training regimes, player education in terms of health pro-motion and injury prevention and prophylactic programmes are of paramount importance.

The risk of injury can be minimized through optimal fitness and condition of players and preventative policies applied during the closed season, pre-season and in-season. The ultimate aim is a football club in which injuries and ill-health are minimized. If achieved, benefits to the club would surely accrue due to players be-ing satisfied with their physical and mental well-being. Clearly, positive benefits accrue from a fully fit, athletic, enthusiastic and committed team. The needs of the players and the prosperity of the club go hand in hand.

Avoiding injury — the total loss approach

Injuries to players can have a significant effect on the performance, results and morale of a team which also impacts on the financial state of the club. Examination of the causes of all injuries, and potential injuries, can provide valuable insight into inadequacies in risk control and action which could prevent further injuries. For ex-ample, if a player does not wear protective shinpads when training, unnecessary injury may result which could be in the form of bruis-ing, resulting in 4 or 5 days of missed training or a more serious in-jury. Effective prevention and loss control must focus on the cause of injury, not its results.

Optimizing protection of the assets (players) is key factor in the total loss approach principle. Learning from injury incidents achieves effective control. The emphasis is on preventing accidents by identifying risks and the sources of potential injury.

*Injuries caused by absence of adequate management control*

Although the immediate cause of an injury involves a player, the event may arise from failings within the football club. Injury prevention policies should place a heavy emphasis on effectively controlling players. It is suggested that all players have different training needs in order to optimize their physiological and physical states, both of which are major preventative factors.

Players have their own strengths and weaknesses, the majority of which are amenable to modification or enhancement through training and experience and can be identified through player assessments. This requires qualified fitness and conditioning staff who understand the demands of the game. This may be a specialist who works closely with the club coaching staff and players or a member of the coaching staff who has gained the necessary qualifications.

*The role of management and coaches*

The club management has a major influence on the behaviour of players, especially in the design of training programmes and the safety culture it promotes, for example specific strength training and nutritional strategies, flexibility sessions, correct implementation of warm-ups, cool-down and recovery strategies, ensuring player involvement and commitment at all levels. Deviation from set standards should be unacceptable.

The employment/involvement of qualified specialist staff in the field of fitness and conditioning is extremely important and the need for coaches to understand key aspects is vital. The coach's role together with the fitness and conditioning staff is to develop the skills of their players, challenging them, pushing them to their full potential. This includes educating players and developing them technically, physically and mentally, with the knowledge that the fitness programme will not compromise the player and result in unnecessary injury.

*The team approach — the importance of organizational factors*

Effective control of players' medical welfare is achieved through co-operative effort at all levels in the organization. A positive health culture is crucial. This can only happen through the active and continued commitment of the management. They should effectively communicate their beliefs to players and coaches and actively support medical officers, physiotherapist(s) and fitness and conditioning support staff. The whole club is required to share the management's perception and beliefs about the importance of player health and the need to achieve the policy objectives.

The importance of an integrated approach between coaches, medical staff (doctors and physiotherapists) and fitness/conditioning support staff together with the players themselves cannot be overstated (Figure 2.7).

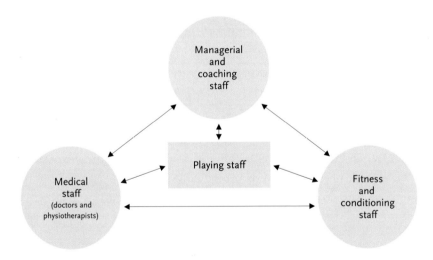

**Figure 2.7** An integrated approach between players and staff.

*Qualification of training needs, facilities and equipment*

The medical and fitness and conditioning staff must be of high quality and be required to attend relevant training courses to maintain their continual professional development. Injuries that do occur must be met with quality assessment, treatment and rehabilitation in modern quality facilities offering all modalities of treatment.

## Medication, doping, alcohol and smoking

In the context of the medical information, it is also appropriate to discuss doping regulations — partly so that no one will be tempted to use doping in any form, and partly to prevent doping by mistake by a player using the wrong pain relief or nasal spray. One important rule is that the players should consult the club's medical personnel before any new product or medication is used. Never take a chance! The medication may contain substances classified as doping. In this context it is also important to consider which rules apply regarding alcohol, narcotics and tobacco. Of course, it is to be assumed that no players use narcotics or drugs in any form. The information should therefore be provided from case to case as deemed necessary.

The restrictions for smoking are general in the community these days. The club premises should be designated no smoking areas, nor should smoking be permitted in connection with training or matches — this should be self-evident, but will certainly create debate. Happily, few footballers smoke. Brief information may be appropriate about the damaging effects of smoking and its role in reducing performance.

Alcohol should be discussed thoroughly. The coach should make his/her position clear to the players and explain the rules that apply. The rules should be preceded by the necessary information about the impact of alcohol, both for the players' football activities and also for their lives outside the sport and after their football careers.

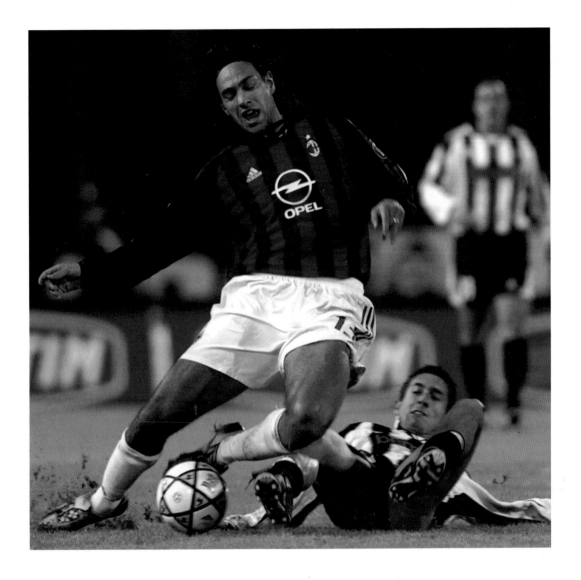

**Food and food supplements (see also Chapters 6 and 7)**

As far as diet is concerned, it is valuable to be able to offer players, who are interested, in a diet intake analysis whereby they can compare their energy intake with their energy consumption. They will then find out their energy balance along with what measures they can take to attain the correct energy balance. A player who might be suspected of eating unhealthily could be offered a diet analysis.

It is advisable to be careful in proposing this, especially with regard to young players, since they often feel that they need to lose weight, in other words eat less, which in the worst case may provoke eating disorders.

Discussions concerning the need for sportsmen and women to take various food supplements have been underway for some time. Within football it has been established that a *regular diet in the correct quantities is fully adequate*. It has been shown that, in general, footballers do not require any form of food supplementation. The most important thing is to maintain a balanced intake of nutrition which is best achieved by eating regular food in the correct quantities.

### Some simple rules

Information about common illnesses is important. What should a player consider if he or she suffers from an upset stomach or has a cold, with regard to both him/herself and the other players? Is there any risk of infection? Should that player stay at home instead of attending training? One tip is that the players should automatically ring and inform the club of their state of health in good time. If they turn up ill at the training session, they could spread the infection.

Taking the pulse can often be an efficient way of checking the state of health. If the players get used to taking their pulse in the morning (pulse while at rest) at the same time every day, they can ascertain at an early stage whether they are 'going down with something'. They run less risk of training or playing a match with reduced resistance and avoid infecting their team mates. Sometimes an infection and illness which does not manifest itself in an increase in temperature or other symptoms can be discovered by an increase in the pulse while at rest.

In order to prevent infection spreading, hand hygiene is especially important. For the same reason, fruit should be washed or wiped before it is eaten.

# Emergency measures in the event of injury or illness

However efficient the preventative work is at a club, players will, sooner or later, be injured or fall ill. Such is the reality of the situation. It is then essential for both coaches and players to take the correct measures. The first thing is to ensure that there is a fully equipped first aid bag to hand and that the contents can be applied in the correct way.

The level of medical service is important. The assessment of the injury or illness and its treatment should be carried out at the highest level possible. If a doctor or other medical personnel are available, they should be called in — if not, the coach should take responsibility. It is therefore also important that the coach has had some medical instruction. This is often a case of being able to help a player with basic problems such as blisters, abrasions, slight cases of bleeding and so on. The coach should also be familiar with the first aid measures to be taken in the event of injury to the soft parts of the body, such as applying pressure and cooling to bleeding in a muscle, and should also be able to stop bleeding.

It is also important to be able to act quickly in the event of serious injuries when a player has to be taken to hospital for treatment. All team personnel should be able to provide first aid in cases where breathing and/or the heartbeat are impeded. This includes removing a player who may have been unconscious or concussed from the game without hesitation, and applying cautionary measures whenever anyone receives an injury to the head. An injured player may not, for example, be left alone and should be examined by a doctor if there is the slightest risk of serious internal damage.

Of course, it is never advisable to take a chance and allow an injured player to continue playing. Only a doctor is qualified, with the player's consent, to permit a slightly injured player to play on, and then only if this implies no danger whatsoever of problems in the future. This is more relevant in the context of top level sport and should never apply to juniors — it may be a case of a slightly sprained foot ligament that can be taped so that the player can play the match to the end.

### Risk of infection

When a player is ill, it is safest to remove him or her from activities, partly for the player's own sake and partly to avoid exposing his or her team mates to the risk of infection. The players should also feel a sense of responsibility in such a situation. If there is a risk of infection, this may involve having a room to oneself at a training camp, not using the same toilet as the other players in the case of an upset stomach, not touching hands, not drinking out of the same bottle or sharing the same bag of sweets.

The spread of stomach infections and colds can be considerably reduced if these simple rules are followed. Players should be informed of all these points and learn to accept them.

## Measures for rehabilitation and return after an injury or illness

After an injury or illness the player should be completely recovered and should return to training and matches as quickly as possible without risk to his or her health. In order for this to be feasible, the medical team should be fully informed about the injury or illness to be able to recommend the correct treatment and rehabilitation measures.

*The player should be completely recovered before he or she plays a match.* This is where coaches and players probably make the biggest mistake — coaches are too ambitious and players are too keen to play which makes it difficult to wait until the player is fully rehabilitated. It is therefore not unusual that an injured player, who returns to activities too soon, is injured once again, sometimes in the form of a new injury, sometimes a recurrence of the old one.

## Training after an injury

Complete rest is usually wrong for an injured player. Correctly planned training and gradually intensifying rehabilitation during the healing period is generally an important part of the recovery process.

Rehabilitation, and even after a longer absence due to illness, can be effected in the form of an individual training programme. The player should also take responsibility for him or herself and realize the importance of correct rehabilitation, but should also be told why and how the rehabilitation is to be planned. The individual training programme should include football practice before the player returns to regular training.

An example of shared responsibility is when both the coach and player can learn to tape a sprained ankle. It simplifies matters if all players are able to do this.

Before an injured player can be approved to return to training and matches, the appropriate tests should be carried out. These may include, for instance, a strength test of the muscles which have been trained during rehabilitation. It may also involve taking the temperature after a cold and checking that the player has been healthy for a recommended period of time before returning to training.

## The team behind the team

There is quite a lot to do for coaches, club personnel and the medical personnel — and the players in themselves are an important resource of course. Information and training in medical issues increases the possibility of achieving a well functioning football medicine service in the team. It is a question of organizing a team that can help the players and deal with the medical requirements within the team.

The club's resources decide which model and what personnel can be employed but if everyone has agreed that the club should take medical responsibility for its players, the requirements must be provided for in one way or another. The tasks can be divided up between the personnel available to the team and some of the requirements can be provided via a network of contacts with people outside the team. A checklist on Page 33 shows all the medical tasks involved around a team. The numbering system is not intended to indicate priority.

## WE IN THE TEAM AGREE THAT

- The health of the players is more important than anything else.
- The number of injuries and incidents of illness should be minimized.
- We should act in an ethically and morally correct way, in accordance with the rules and with the latest doping regulations.
- The advice and recommendations of the person responsible for medical issues should be followed.

## MEDICAL CHECK LIST

### PREVENTIVE MEASURES

**P1**  The players' medical background and condition should be recorded and continually updated.

**P2**  Serious injuries should be reported to the insurance company.

**P3**  The planning and content of training should be approved on medical grounds.

**P4**  Listen to the players and be observant of their behaviour and condition in terms of health.

**P5**  Use the correct equipment and material — make checklists for the various aspects of club activities.

**P6**  Be meticulous about hygiene and the environment in the context of training and matches.

**P7**  Help the players to concentrate in connection with training and matches.

**P8**  Encourage play according to the rules in training and at matches.

**P9**  Provide players and personnel with the appropriate medical information and training courses before each season.

**P10**  Be meticulous about diet, fluid intake and sleep. Provide the opportunity for players to do individual diet analyses.

**P11**  Take up a position on the possible use of approved food supplements.

**P12**  Follow the doping regulations and set up rules for the use of medication.

**P13**  Discuss and set up rules for alcohol, tobacco and narcotics.

**P14**  Set up and follow medical recommendations concerning food, drink and protection against infection for trips overseas.

**P15**  Follow the agreements in cases of stomach infections and colds, partly for one's own health and partly for preventing the risk of spreading the infection.

**P16**  Coaches, personnel and players must take responsibility for their own health and also be considerate of each other's health.

# MEDICAL CHECK LIST

## EMERGENCY MEASURES

**E1**  Drill players/personnel in the measures to be taken in the event of injury and illness.

**E2**  Always have access to a fully equipped first aid bag.

**E3**  Teach everyone how the contents in the first aid bag should be used.

**E4**  Coaches/personnel should be able to treat less serious injuries.

**E5**  Coaches/personnel should be familiar with the first measures to be taken for injuries to the soft parts of the body and be able to stop external bleeding.

**E6**  Take measures quickly in the event of serious injuries when a player has to be taken to hospital.

**E7**  Coaches/personnel should be familiar with resuscitation techniques in the event of respiratory/cardiac arrest.

**E8**  Exercise caution if unconsciousness is suspected.

**E9**  Coaches/personnel should be familiar with the measures to be taken if internal bleeding in the head or abdomen is suspected.

**E10**  Never move a player with a suspected neck/back injury.

**E11**  Never take a chance with an injured or ill player.

**E12**  Take cautionary measures in the event of illness, both for the ill person and to prevent infection spreading.

## REHABILITATION MEASURES

**R1**  Obtain detailed knowledge of the injury/illness.

**R2**  Take the correct medical measures to provide treatment.

**R3**  Set up an individual training programme.

**R4**  Inform the player about how the rehabilitation has been worked out.

**R5**  Help the player to carry out the rehabilitation programme. The coach's support and interest are important.

**R6**  Obtain medical approval that the player is fully recovered.

**R7**  Help the player after the conclusion of treatment, for example, by taping the ankle.

# Plan of action

Start by formulating general objectives for football medicine within the team and then distribute the measures to be taken. Coaches, club personnel as well as medical personnel should give themselves plenty of time to discuss an appropriate organization of the medical activities. A suggested division of responsibilities is presented in the box on Page 37. Each person is assigned responsibility for seeing that a measure is carried out but should, at the same time, obtain any assistance they may require in implementing the measure. Some of the measures may demand that responsibility is shared by several people.

The team leadership should come to an agreement about when those responsible for medical services should be available. In the example presented the team has access to a doctor who is available in his/her free time for one training per week, at home matches and at important away matches. The doctor should be accessible by phone as often as possible and would be able, if necessary, to examine a player on further occasions and to conduct information sessions and courses for players and personnel. The doctor can, if required, attend training camps and possibly accompany the team when it travels abroad.

The club has a therapist (masseur/physiotherapist) who attends all training sessions, matches, training camps and accompanies the team on all journeys. It is possible for the club to employ further physiotherapists for rehabilitation in special circumstances such as after surgery, when highly specialized expertise may be required. Another combination of coach and medical personnel in a club may demand that their responsibilities are distributed according to other principles.

It should also be agreed how the players' visits to the injury therapist and doctor should be organized. When and where should the doctor and masseur be accessible? Should there be an appoint-

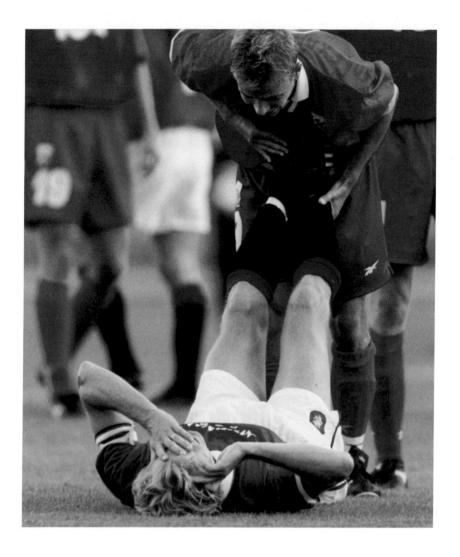

ments system? Who contacts whom in different situations? How should things be organized before training sessions and matches — when should players who are going to train and play receive any treatment planned and when should players who are ill or injured be examined and treated? Who should receive priority? It is particularly important to be well organized with regard to visits to the injury therapists before training sessions. If several players turn up at the same time this will create chaos and will not work.

It may also be a good idea to decide who should make statements concerning medical issues, especially if there is mass media interest in club activities. It is essential to bear in mind the confidentiality which exists here between patient and doctor.

It is clear from the suggested distribution of responsibilities that the coach must show respect for the players' health. As far as training and individual training activities are concerned where there is considerable pressure (approaching the limit of the players' strength and capacity) it may be valuable to discuss the risk of strain with the medical team. One should never, under any circumstances, take a risk with injured or ill players. As a coach there is a lot that can be done to minimize the degree of injury and illness in a team through preventative measures.

Divide up the responsibilities between the coach and medical personnel in time before the start of the season. Information to and courses for the players are probably the best way of ensuring that the football medicine activities will work as well as possible within the team.

### EXAMPLE OF HOW RESPONSIBILITY FOR FOOTBALL MEDICINE CAN BE DISTRIBUTED IN A TEAM

| | |
|---|---|
| Coach 1: | P3, P7, P8, P13, P16, E3–E12. |
| Coach 2: | P5, P6, P16, E3–E12, R5, R7. |
| Doctor: | P1, P2, P9, P11, P12, P14, P16, E1, E3–E12 (E6–E10), R1, R2, R6. |
| Injury therapist: | P4, P10, P15, P16, E2–E5, E11, E12, R3–R5, R7. |

Everyone in the team should be able to carry out E6–E10. Treatment should be carried out at the highest possible level of competence.

# 3. Preventing injury

Jan Ekstrand

Injury in the context of football is a problem for both players as well as for coaches and the club as a whole. We are, unfortunately, forced to accept injuries as part of the game of football. However, injuries do not occur at random. There are explanations for why they occur, in other words, various injury mechanisms, and it is also possible to reduce the number of injuries and the degree of seriousness by means of various injury prevention measures.

Several scientific studies have shown that the risk of injury can be reduced considerably. By using an injury prevention programme which includes the assistance of a doctor and a physiotherapist, as much as 75 per cent of injuries can be avoided. Not every team has access to a doctor and physiotherapist, however, but they are still able to achieve a good effect by means of the preventative work that can be led by the team coach. It has been shown that coaches who have attended a theoretical and practical course on injury prevention can reduce injuries by around 50 per cent in their teams.

The prevention of injuries can also provide a financial saving both for the club as well as for the community. In a study carried out on Division IV players in Sweden (1982), it was shown that injuries sustained over 1 year cost € 90 000 for the whole division or about 8000/team. This cost included both direct expenses for hospital care and the expense of the loss in production, or sick leave. By means of injury prevention measures, the costs could be reduced by € 13 000 altogether for the whole division or around € 1100/team.

Both expertise and investment in the form of time and other resources are required if injury prevention measures are to have any effect. It is obvious for a coach to analyse tactical dispositions and to spend time and resources on training to improve the game itself. The same reasoning should apply to injuries. The coach should make an analysis of the team's injury profile and the mechanisms behind the injuries as well as spend time during and in connection with training sessions for preventative measures. The significance of the coach in injury situations is considerable.

It has been possible to show that injuries within a team are connected with the coach's football education and experience. In this chapter, different risk factors are described for football injuries and their possible interaction with each other, after which the various injury prevention measures will be considered. The chapter is concluded with examples of ways in which injury prevention work can be carried out in practice.

# RISK FACTORS

There are two types of sports injury — accidental and overuse injuries. In football, accidental injuries are most common, constituting approximately two-thirds of all injuries.

Accidental injuries are caused by the pressure on one specific occasion (for instance, during a tackle or a burst of speed) exceeding the maximum durability of a tissue such as a ligament, a bone or a muscle tendon. In football and other contact sports, the risk of accidental injury is apparent since contact between the players, such as during a tackle, releases considerable force. It should be remembered, however, that in football the body can be subjected to a high degree of strain even in other situations in the game which do not involve a tackle or contact with an opponent.

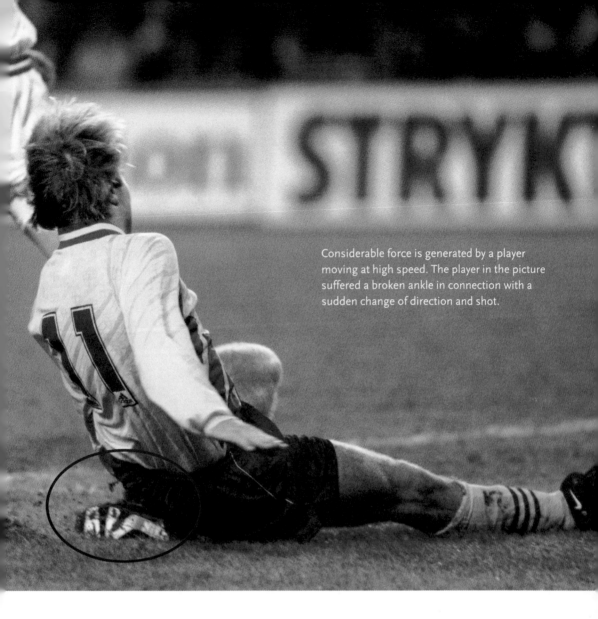

Considerable force is generated by a player moving at high speed. The player in the picture suffered a broken ankle in connection with a sudden change of direction and shot.

**Overuse injuries,** such as runner's or jumper's knee, are caused by repeated strain. This type of injury often arises during heavy pre-season training or during a training camp.

The mechanism behind an injury is often complicated and there are a number of risk factors involved. A football injury is the result of the complex interplay between different risk factors. Examples of the risk factors that could be connected with the risk of injury in football are summarized on the Page 42.

## FACTORS THAT CAN INFLUENCE RISK OF INJURY IN FOOTBALL

| INTERNAL (PERSON-RELATED) | EXTERNAL (ENVIRONMENT-RELATED) |
|---|---|
| **General** | **Strain/overuse** |
| Age | Playing level |
| Gender | Training dose |
| Bodily constitution | Number of matches |
| Health | Recovery |
| | Training camps |
| | Combination of sports |
| **Football factors** | |
| Skill/technique | **Equipment** |
| Training situation | Shin pads |
| | Shoes/boots |
| **Anatomical factors** | |
| Anatomical defects | **Surface/arena/climate** |
| Stability of joints | Artificial grass |
| Agility | |
| Strength | |
| Coordination | |
| Status after previous injury | **Football factors** |
| | Playing tactics |
| **Mental factors** | Referee |
| Personality | Coach |
| Goals | Medical service |
| Susceptibility to risks | |
| Stress tolerance | |
| Motivation | |
| Self-esteem | |

A musculoskeletal overuse injury such as runner's knee, may be caused by continual repetition of running movements, for example, during a training camp where the training is increased compared to previous regimes. Overuse is probably also affected by other factors, such as a change in the surface or cold weather (external causes) or by muscle tension or poor running technique (internal factors).

An injury to the anterior cruciate ligament (ACL) is an example of an accidental injury. An anterior cruciate ligament injury usually occurs in a tackle. For example, during a tackle, the considerable force involved places great strain on the knee joints. If the strain exceeds the durability of the ligament, the ligament snaps. Any player can incur an injury to the anterior cruciate ligament if the violence released by the tackle is sufficiently extensive. A well-trained player can, however, withstand greater strain and, therefore, more forceful tackles.

The force involved and the strain placed on the ligament is therefore the greatest injury risk factor in a tackle. Other factors, both internal and external, can affect the impact. The risk of injury increases if the player is not fit or has not undergone adequate rehabilitation after an earlier injury. In such cases, the durability of the ligament is impaired and even slight force, such as a milder tackle, could result in a ligament injury. The same amount of force would perhaps not have resulted in an injury for a player who was fit.

The player may have experienced a lack of physical control at the moment of the tackle after having lost his or her footing on the pitch (external factors). This can result in the ligament being subjected to much greater strain during the tackle since the player had not had time to activate the muscles which protect the knee joints.

The player is not a passive object of strain. Strain can vary and its impact can be influenced. The internal factors or those related to the person constitute the player's capacity while the external factors (related to the environment) can be classified as strain. Strain

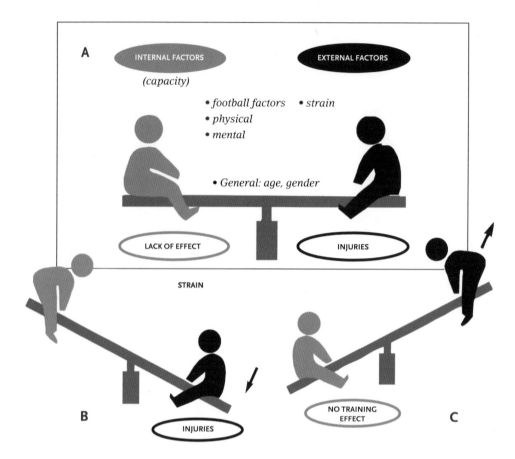

**Figure 3.1** Strain and capacity have to be balanced (A). If the strain is too great in relation to the player's capacity, an injury occurs (B). If the strain is too little, training is not having the optimal effect (C).

and capacity have to be in balance. Injury prevention measures aim to decrease strain. Capacity can be increased by influencing one or more of the person-related factors. Technique training, agility training or rehabilitation are examples of measures which can increase a player's capacity and thereby reduce the risk of injury.

Strain can be reduced by playing fewer matches, extending the rest periods between training sessions, improving the health care within the club, using shin pads etc.

# Internal factors

## General

### *Age*

Children and young people run less risk of being injured at football than adults. This is because the players weigh less, move at lower speeds and play less aggressively. Taken together, these factors mean that the body is subject to less strain. Injuries to children and young people are often less serious and different in character compared with adults.

With children and young people who have not finished growing, injuries can occur in the so-called growth zones (see Chapter 23). Coordination and balance are not as well developed either and this leads to a greater risk of falling resulting in broken bones in arms or hands.

The risk and seriousness of injury increase with age. In puberty the body's volume and amount of muscle increases. Increasing age is accompanied by more aggressive play and greater risk-taking which means that greater forces are developed in playing football.

Older players are more at risk of being injured that players between 18 and 30 years. Increasing age leads to less elasticity and strength in tissues which means that they can withstand less strain and are more readily damaged. Older players also sometimes overestimate their abilities in relation to their actual fitness. Further, they have often been subjected to injury during a long career and this can have led to lingering weakness in, for example, muscles and ligaments and this increases the risk of new injuries. Above all, the risk of suffering torn muscles and strains increases with older players.

### *Gender*

Older studies showed a greater risk of injury in women's football as compared with the men's game while more recent studies have shown the reverse. The reason for this change may be related to football. Today's players begin playing football at a younger age and they have more experience of football and, in general, better technical skills and a greater understanding of the game than earlier generations.

Damage to knee ligaments are more common in women's football and often arise in situations where there has been no bodily contact. The reason for this is unknown, but a high risk of injury to knee ligaments has also been noted in other women's sports, for example basketball and handball. The reason for these differences in injury risk and in location of the injuries between women's and men's football may be entirely to do with the game itself. It may be a matter of different ways of playing (less tackling and fewer infringements of rules in women's football) or age (lower average age in women's football). The differences may also depend on mental factors (personality, susceptibility to risk) or hormonal factors. Women subject to pre-menstrual tension (PMT) suffer an increased risk of injury during the period of tension.

Strain is also relatively more common in women's football. Women have a weaker musculoskeletal system with about 25 per cent less muscle/kg, their bones are less dense, their pelvises are wider and their joints more mobile than in men. These factors can increase the risk of serious strain.

### Bodily constitution and state of health

The relationship between bodily constitution and susceptibility to injury has not been exhaustively investigated. One study shows, however, that tall, thin boys aged 16–17 years suffer more injuries than boys who are short and muscular. Obesity in older players may increase the risk of injury by interacting with other factors such as poor training, muscular weakness, etc.

A poor state of health may also mean an increased risk of injury. Poor health leads both to reduced tissue strength and to poorer coordination. These changes are partly caused by the worsened state of health itself but also indirectly in that poor health also prevents effective training. For example, in connection with influenza, the condition of body tissues is worsened and for a period during the illness, the player cannot undertake fitness training which further reduces the quality of body tissues.

# Football factors

### Skill/technique
The more skilled and technically proficient the player is, the less risk there is of injury. In a study of young players aged 11–17 years, a correlation was established between football technique and injuries. The better the result of the technique test, the lower the risk of injury.

A technically skilled player is less subject to tackling and bodily contact with opposing players since the technical player gains control of the ball and can pass it before an opponent has time to tackle him.

### Training
A well-trained player runs less risk of being injured and this has been shown in several football studies. Lack of training is a common cause of injury, especially in the lower divisions. Football under the auspices of company sports is an example of this. The risk of injury in company sports' football is much greater than in series football which is mainly due to the company sports' players being less well trained. With better training, football skills and technique can be improved. At the same time, the training also leads to an improvement in internal factors, for example the tone of body tissue is improved as are strength, agility, fitness and coordination.

Mental factors such as self-confidence, ability to withstand stress, etc. are probably also positively affected by increased training. The fitness and stamina of players also influences the injury picture (see Chapter 5). Players who are less fit tire more quickly and their playing technique and agility are reduced which can lead to greater risk of injury.

# Anatomical factors

### Anatomical postural abnormalities

Congenital postural abnormalities and abnormal biomechanics (mechanical functions) can lead to increased or one-sided strain in tissues. Such postural defects can therefore increase susceptibility to injury. Flat-footedness (falling of the arch of the foot), exaggerated pronation, high arches, knocked-knees, different lengths of leg, etc. are examples of conditions that are considered to increase the player's risk of muscle strain.

Flat-footedness can reduce the body's ability to absorb shock when placing the feet on the ground and can thus increase the risk of strain injury to the foot, ankle, lower leg, knee and back. A high foot arch can also lead to problems since it is often overly rigid and thus less able to absorb shock.

The most common postural defect in connection with running is considered to be increased pronation. Pronation, which is a natural movement in the lower leg, foot and ankle when running or walking, involves turning the lower leg inwards and lower-

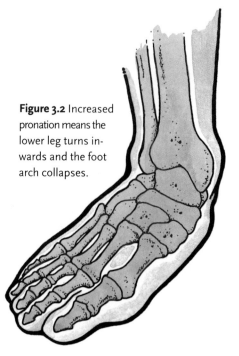

**Figure 3.2** Increased pronation means the lower leg turns inwards and the foot arch collapses.

ing the longitudinal arch of the foot when weight is put on the foot. Exaggerated pronation is considered to be linked with an increased risk of inflammation of the sole of the foot, periostitis, damage to the Achilles tendon, pain in the front of the knee and stress fractures.

Differences in leg length can create problems. A difference in length of up to 15 mm is normally not troublesome for people taking physical exercise but a difference of 5–10 mm can give rise to overuse injuries in active sportsmen and women. These anatomical defects are not related in a predictable manner with specific injuries. This factor is probably less significant in determining susceptibility to injury than many other factors, for example degree of strain and fitness.

A football player with an anatomical defect, for example flatfeet or legs of different length, can probably completely eliminate the extra risk of injury that results from the defect. The postural defect can be compensated by other factors, for example the gradual and successive hardening of the tissues which makes them better able to withstand strain.

Congenital excessive mobility in joints is another example of a factor that may be linked to increased risk of injury. For outfield players it is commonly excessive mobility in foot or knee joints that can cause problems. For a goalkeeper, excessive mobility in the back and shoulders are of importance. Excessive mobility can, to a degree, be compensated by other factors, for example by building up muscles and by training coordination.

It may be that the fact that excessive mobility of joints is uncommon among football players is an indication of a natural selection of players. Football requires stable joints and players with excessive joint mobility perhaps do not manage the game as well and therefore choose other sports rather than football. Another possibility is that players with excessive mobility suffer more injuries to their joints and therefore choose, or are forced, to give up football.

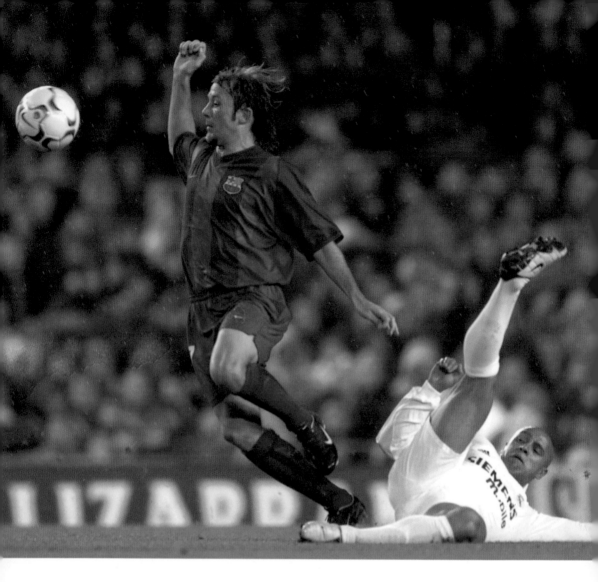

### Joint stability

The most common injuries in football are damaged ligaments in the ankle and knee. Three out of four ankle injuries are preceded by sprained ankles. It is also a known fact that a sprained ankle often gives rise to a lengthening of one or more ligaments in the ankle. This instability, in turn, increases the risk of new injuries.

Even injuries to knee ligaments can lead to permanent instability of the knee. Players who have suffered a damaged ligament in the knee and who have a permanent instability following the injury also run an increased risk of new injuries.

## Mobility

Football players often have taut leg muscles and reduced mobility in their ankles, knees and hips. It has been thought that this tautness was the result of earlier damage to the muscles with resulting growth of scar tissue but this has not been confirmed by scientific studies. It has, on the other hand, been possible to show that it would seem to be playing football which causes muscle tautness among players. A single hard training session can lead to stiffness in thigh and calf muscles which can reduce mobility in hips, knees and ankles by up to 10 per cent. This stiffness can remain for 2–3 days. Since football players normally train several times a week it is conceivable that the player will be subjected to a new dose of training within this period leading to further stiffness. The muscular tautness to be found in football players may depend on the accumulation of stiffness from training and matches.

Muscular stiffness and reduced mobility increase the risk of muscle damage. When the same trial was conducted with the introduction of light jogging and stretching after the training session, it was found that there was no stiffness and that mobility increased by 4–5 per cent. A better warm-up with stretching and cooling down after training and matches led to a reduction in muscular stiffness among football players and thereby a reduction in the risk of injury.

## Strength

A popular claim in the world of sport is that stronger sportsmen perform better and are less prone to injury; a claim that has been difficult to substantiate in scientific studies.

There are still inadequacies in our ability to measure muscle strength. Nowadays muscle strength is measured using isokinetic measuring apparatus. Examples of such apparatus are Cybex and Kin-Com. Measurements taken using isokinetic techniques mean that speed is identical throughout the whole course of movement. This is, of course, different from how we normally use muscles but

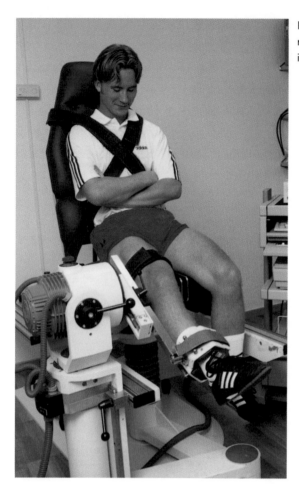

**Figure 3.3** Measuring thigh muscle strength using isokinetic equipment.

many studies have revealed a close relationship between isokinetic muscle strength and performance in sports requiring explosive muscle strength.

Measurements are taken at movement speeds of between 30°/sec and 300°/sec.

We know that football players have stronger thigh muscles than people of the same age who do not play football. It has also been shown that players in the higher divisions have stronger thigh muscles. No difference has been found in muscle strength between right and left legs or between the shooting leg and the supporting one.

Male footballers were measured for thigh muscle strength in a pre-season test. The players were then monitored for a year to determine whether there was any correlation between strength of thigh muscles and knee ligament injuries. For players who damaged ligaments in contact situations, for example in tackles, there was no correlation with muscle strength. This means that any player can suffer this type of injury regardless of thigh muscle strength, if the impact is sufficiently great.

On the other hand, it was shown that players who injured ligaments when stopping, turning, dodging or in other situations not involving contact with a player from the opposing side, had less muscle strength at the pre-season test, i.e. prior to the injury. This may be an example of inadequate rehabilitation after an earlier injury.

It has been claimed that an imbalance in muscle strength, for example between right and left or between flexors and tensors would increase the risk of injury. A football player with a difference of more than 10 per cent between right and left legs or who has muscle strength in the rear of the thigh less than 60 per cent of that in the front muscles of the thigh would be more prone to knee injury on the weaker side. But these studies are not free from objection. Muscle strength is normally expressed as 'peak torque', i.e. the maximum measured strength. What one is really measuring is the torque, which is expressed in Newton metres (Nm).

When measuring the HQ quotient, that is the quotient of muscle strength between the hamstrings (H) and the quadriceps (Q), problems arise in the measurement technique. If one measures the quotient between peak torque for the quadriceps and hamstrings, the peaks are at different angles for the knee. If one wants to measure the same angle, which angle is it to be? In addition, the measuring situation is hardly like real football. When measuring by machine, players are strapped down and movement reaches a maximum velocity of 300°/sec whereas a football kick can reach a velocity of 900°/sec i.e. three times as fast or more.

It is quite possible that muscle strength in the thigh is significant in protecting against injury to the knee joint but the methods
of measuring are insufficient to demonstrate this.

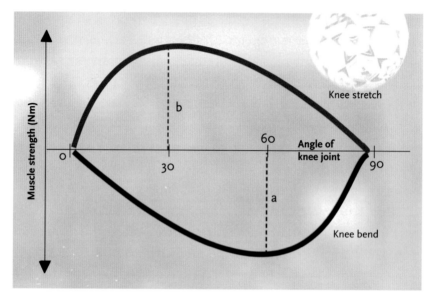

**Figure 3.4** Measuring thigh muscle strength using isokinetic technique. Muscle
strength is expressed as torque in Newton metres (Nm). The top curve represents a
knee stretch from a 90° angle to an outstretched knee. It reflects anterior thigh muscle
strength (quadriceps). The bottom curve shows a knee bend from an outstretched knee
to a 90° angle and indicates posterior thigh muscle strength (hamstring). The so-called
HQ quotient, i.e. the quotient between anterior and posterior thigh muscle strength,
is obtained by dividing the measured peak torque for the posterior thigh muscles (a) by
the measured peak torque for the anterior thigh muscles (b).

## Coordination

Coordination, the ability to activate the muscular system and to
coordinate movements is important in all sporting activities. With
regard to muscle strength and risk of injury, it may be that actual
muscle strength is less important and activation and coordination
are of greater importance in preventing accidents. There is much to
suggest that coordination training is an important factor in preventing many types of injuries.

## Status after earlier injury

As many as 15–30 per cent of all football injuries are recurrent. The reason is often inadequate treatment of the original injury.

An example is injury to the ligaments of the foot. As many as 75 per cent of ligament injuries to the foot affect players who have already suffered the same type of injury and who have an instability remaining in the ankle joint. If a ligament injury is treated in accordance with the methods described in Chapter 18, there is greater possibility of the ankle being completely cured and repetitive injuries can be avoided.

Another reason for repetitive injuries may be insufficient time for healing which is common in connection with torn muscles. Such injuries are often underestimated. Players start training and playing matches too early and the injury recurs.

### AVOIDING REPETITIVE INJURIES

- Treat all injuries intensively.
- Do not ignore minor injuries, they can lead to more serious injury.
- Allow injuries sufficient time to heal.
- Provide adequate rehabilitation.

It is also important to treat minor injuries. It has transpired that 20 per cent of all minor injuries lead to larger and more serious injuries within 2 months. These more serious injuries may either be an aggravation of the original injury or a completely new injury. In the latter case, it is believed that the minor injury has led to a disturbance in coordination and balance leading to the more serious injury.

Probably the most common reason for recurring accidents is lack of rehabilitation. An injury causes weakening of the tissues. Adequate rehabilitation aims to restore the strength and function of the tissues and if this is not achieved then there is an increased risk of recurrence of injuries.

# Mental factors

Mental factors such as personality, goals, self-confidence, motivation, ability to withstand stress and susceptibility to risk determine a player's performance in footballing situations. Mental training is sometimes used to improve the performance of individual players or the whole team. The connection between mental factors and risk of injury is seldom discussed and the area has been subject to little scientific study.

In recent years psychological tests — Profile of Mood States (POMS, see form on Page 115) — have been used in sport. The tests measure the moods of sportsmen and are used to reveal so-called over-training. These tests have also been used to study the connection between mental factors and injuries. It has transpired that characteristics that are linked with high performance are also linked to a reduced risk of injury and more rapid rehabilitation following injury.

It has been claimed that positive thinking, powerful concentration on the task, adequate self-confidence, high level of motivation and a good ability to cope with stress reduces the risk of injury. On the other hand, mental factors like poor concentration, low motivation, negative thinking, lack of self-confidence and lowered ability to deal with stress increase the risk of injury. POMS tests have also shown that players who suffer injuries are also influenced mentally. In connection with more serious accidents, a reduction in mental well-being, almost a tendency to depression, is not uncommon. This is thought to retard rehabilitation and can possibly increase the risk of new injuries as the player enters a psychological 'vicious circle'.

The physical rehabilitation of an injured player should be monitored carefully to check that physical qualities such as strength, agility and coordination are restored to reduce the risk of further injury. A similar argument can be made for treating mental well-being in the same way.

The association between injuries and mental factors applies to accidental injuries. It has not been possible, on the other hand, to demonstrate any correlation between mental factors and strain injuries.

The connection between injuries and susceptibility to risk has been discussed. One speaks of 'accident-prone people', meaning that they are greater 'risk takers'. They are more disposed to taking risks and therefore more readily find themselves involved in accidents. There has been speculation as to how the same phenomenon might be found in sport, that is, that there are players who are inclined to take risks and who therefore take greater chances and are often injured. 'Accident-susceptibility' is, however, not a constant characteristic of a person but can vary during certain periods. Stress due to changed circumstances of life can, for example, make the player less focused, thereby increasing the risk of injury.

# External factors

### Strain

Severe strain that exceeds the strength of the body's tissues is the fundamental factor underlying most injuries. Other external and internal factors can modify the strain but analysing the strain factor in itself is important. The strength of tissue can be exceeded (and an injury arise) at specific moments of increased strain (for example when tackling) or through constantly repeated minor strain (for example when running). The relationship between strain and the number of repetitions and the risk of accident is illustrated in Figure 3.5.

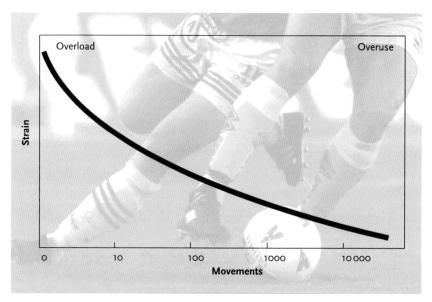

**Figure 3.5** Correlation between strain and occasions of strain. The red line shows the strength of bodily tissues. If the degree of strain exceeds the strength of body tissues, the tissues are damaged.

For a football player, it is important to know that tissues are dynamic, that is, that the quality of the tissues changes depending on the strain that is involved. This means that if tissues are stimu-

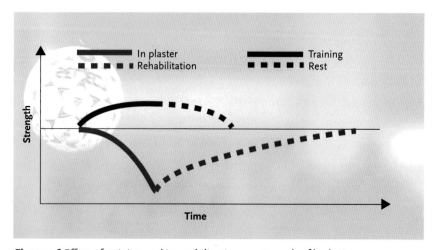

**Figure 3.6** Effect of training and immobilization on strength of body tissues.

lated by strain — during training — their strength increases and the player then can withstand more training without suffering injury. The opposite can also apply. In a period of inactivity, when absent from training, wearing a plaster-cast and other situations where training, i.e. stimulation of the tissues, is absent, the strength of body tissues is reduced (Figure 3.6).

All body tissues can be trained, even ligaments and tendons. Different tissues have different blood circulations and metabolisms which means that the time required to build up strength and firmness varies between different types of tissue.

**Table 3.1** Time for training effect for different tissues

| Tissue | Time (months) |
|--------|---------------|
| Muscles | 1–2 |
| Bones | 2–3 |
| Ligaments | 3–6 |
| Tendons | 6–12 |

In Table 3.1 a rough estimate is shown of the time required for training to have an effect (increased strength, firmness) on different tissues.

Muscle strength and tone are relatively easily trained. The reason is that muscle training rapidly affects the circulation of the blood in the muscle tissue and metabolism is rapid. This means that improvements can be noted after a mere 4–6 weeks.

The ability of the skeleton, connective tissue and tendons to withstand strain takes much longer to improve since these tissues have a lower metabolic rate. It takes 6–12 months to improve the condition of an Achilles tendon, for example.

It is not the amount of training per se that causes injury but rapid changes in training. Strain injuries are, therefore, more common among football players during preliminary training and training camps.

These injuries are the result of changing the amount and intensity of training too rapidly. Too much, too soon is often the explanation.

It is important to remember that all basic training is time-consuming and that the amount of training should be increased very gradually. A simple rule of thumb is that the amount of training should not be increased by more than 10–15 per cent/year. The amount of training should not be subject to large variation during a short period.

Football is a team sport. If all training is undertaken collectively, there is a risk that it is only the best possible training for certain players. For others, the amount of training may be too little. Tissues are not sufficiently stimulated and the training of these players is ineffective. The reverse is true for other players — their training is overly intensive. Strain on tissues is greater than they can withstand and injuries occur. For the coach, it is a matter of individualizing basic training by gaining an understanding of the level of strain appropriate for different players and adjusting training accordingly. Imbalance in the degree of training can arise, for example, if a player is absent from training for a period on account of injury, etc.

There is a special problem with young players moving up from junior teams or lower divisions. These players are often subjected to a radical increase in the amount of training leading to overuse injuries. Players moving up from junior teams or lower divisions want to establish their position and are probably unwilling to complain. Coaches therefore need to be especially vigilant in observing signs of strain in such players.

## Level of play

The playing level is also a significant factor in the risk of injury. In the Swedish system the total risk of injury does not alter much between divisions. But the distribution between injuries incurred during matches and during training does vary. The higher the level of play, the greater the risk of injury in connection with a match which probably depends on several factors. The matches are more important — the players are willing to take greater risks and the football is faster with greater power released and greater strain on tissues. The risk of injury during training, on the other hand, increases at a lower level of play. This can be explained by less well-trained players, by the fact that coaches and referees are less proficient, by poorer preparation, fewer good players, etc.

## Determining the training dose

### Increased training brings success

In a study of male players from the fourth division, the relationship between the team's total amount of training in relation to injuries and successes was analysed. It was shown that there is a clear correlation between how much the team trained and how many points the team won in the series. The more the training, the greater the degree of success.

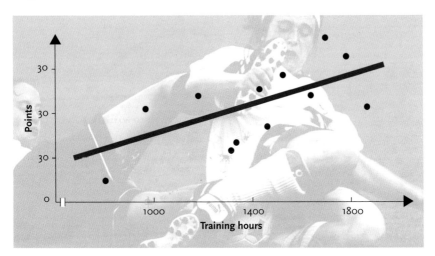

**Figure 3.7** This figure illustrates the correlation between training and success. Each point represents a team of 15 players. The amount of training for each team is expressed as the number of training sessions multiplied by attendance. Success is expressed by the number of points gained by the team in the league.

## A well-trained player suffers fewer injuries

The same study also showed a clear correlation between the team's amount of training and injuries. The average number of training hours for teams was 1500, representing an average of 90–95 hours of training for individual players in the 15-man teams. Teams with a less than average amount of training (i.e. 1400 hours) suffered more injuries with an increased training dose. This can be explained by the greater exposure, i.e. the amount of time that the players risk injury goes up with increased training. Teams that trained for longer than average suffered fewer injuries per unit of time in spite of the greater amount of training. This means that the risk of injury per unit of time was lower. The study can therefore be said to support the claim that a well-trained player is less prone to injury.

An analysis of the injuries showed that it was accidental injuries that varied most with the amount of training while the risk of strain injuries was not influenced. That accidental injuries decreased with increased training may be explained in several ways:

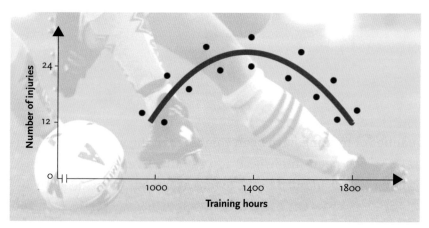

**Figure 3.8** A well-trained player is less prone to injury. The figure shows the correlation between amount of training and accidents. Each point represents a team of 15 players. The amount of training for each team is expressed as the number of training sessions multiplied by attendance. Teams that trained less suffered more injuries when the training dose was increased. Teams that trained more than average, on the other hand, suffered fewer injuries when the training dose was increased. The study supports the claim that a well-trained player is less prone to injury.

improved coordination, greater fitness and increased muscle strength. That strain injuries did not vary with the amount of training may suggest that it is not merely the quantity of training but also the quality that is important.

### Optimal training requires highly developed intuition

Training is generally beneficial. A well-trained player is less prone to injury. Teams that train more are more successful and have fewer injuries. But this is dependent on the organiszation of the training — quality and quantity. The wrong sort of training increases the risk of injury and too much training or too rapid an alteration of the training intensity can lead to over-training. The training dose requires highly developed intuition on the part of the coach.

### Over-training

Over-training is caused by intense physical activity and means that it is not possible to benefit from and react to the training stimuli. Over-training leads to a reduction in performance and a loss of form.

A whole team can suffer from over-training if the team's training is too hard or one-sided, if the content has been changed or the intensity has been increased too rapidly. From this, it is evident that over-training is not just a matter of too much training. It can also mean that training has been too intense, or that different qualities of training have been combined in the wrong way or that training has been intensified too rapidly. Even if the collective training is well adapted to the team's average training needs, individual players may find themselves in the risk zone for over-training. This is especially the case with players who have been absent from training on account of injury as well as new players in the team.

At the early stages of over-training, body symptoms are dominant. Most common are pain, stiffness in the working muscles as well as irritation, inflammation and tenderness in muscle and tendon attachments. The symptoms are reminiscent of 'stiffness'.

Players find that they perform less well — they suffer a loss of form. Both players and coaches often react by increasing the training dose which can lead to a negative spiral. If the training dose and its intensity are reduced or if gentler types of training — swimming or cycling — are introduced at this point, symptoms often disappear of their own accord.

An over-trained player is highly motivated to train. If the training dose is retained or increased, the condition gets worse and the player may then suffer from generalized symptoms such as increased fatigue, disturbed sleep and psychological symptoms in the form of irritability, poor concentration and dejection. The over-training syndrome can then lead to a burn-out which is more difficult to treat.

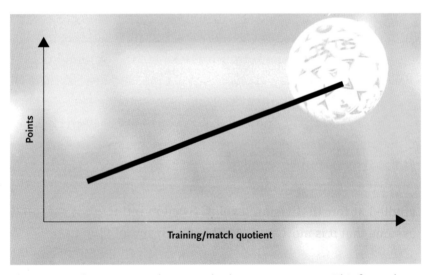

**Figure 3.9** High training/match quotient leads to greater success. This figure shows the relationship between success and the training/match quotient. The training/match quotient is the quotient between the number of training sessions that teams had during a season in relation to the number of matches that the team played. Success is expressed as the number of points that respective teams gained in the league.

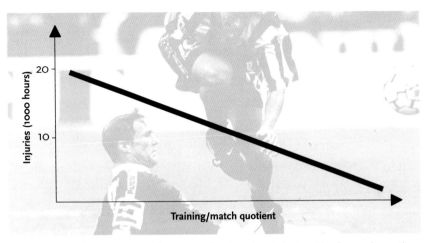

**Figure 3.10** High training/match quotient leads to less injuries. The figure shows the correlation between training/match quotient and injuries.

### Frequency of matches

The way in which the season is planned is also important from the point of view of injuries. The relationship between training and matches, the training/match quotient, affects both chances of success and risk of injury.

A high training/match quotient, that is, many training sessions in relation to the number of matches gives more success and fewer injuries. Simply put, one can say that training sessions are beneficial while matches are destructive. The relationship has only been studied at fourth division level in Sweden but there is reason to assume that it is more marked at higher levels of play.

### 'Over-matching'

Too much or the wrong sort of training can lead to over-training which is manifested as physical tiredness, a sort of pronounced stiffness. Too many matches can lead to 'over-matching' which leads to mental problems, a form of mental burn-out. Quite simply, players are no longer able to gear themselves up for matches and training sessions, their powers of concentration decline and this can affect their coordination. A decline in coordination theoretically means that a player performs less well and is more susceptible to injury. It is not the 90 minutes of football during a match that is the major stress factor and thus the most destructive aspect. Rather, it is the mental preparation for matches, travel and possible adaptation to changes of time and climate.

It is known from other sports that competing too much can result in burn-out and poorer performance. A runner rations his or her races during a season and there is good reason to discuss whether this should not be applied to football, too. Players at top international level are obliged to play numerous matches during a season. Besides the normal league matches, successful teams have numerous national and international matches. And they play for their countries.

In Europe, there is a considerable difference in the number of matches in the various leagues. British teams play a large number of league matches compared with the Italian and German teams. It would be interesting to study the susceptibility to injury and the types of injuriy in the different countries and compare countries which play many league matches with those playing fewer matches.

For young players, this training/match quotient is very important since the beneficial effects of training are very evident at these ages. Unfortunately, a number of youth teams are run by very ambitious coaches who match their teams too assiduously with short-term success as their goal. UEFA recommend a training/match quotient of three for young players, that is, three training sessions qualify for one match. The match quotient can be too high for good players who play in several teams.

## TRAINING/MATCH QUOTIENT

Should be $\geq 3/1$ i.e. three training sessions qualify for one match.

## Recovery

Body tissues follow the principle of biological adaptation to training. During a training session or a match, the tissues tire. During periods of rest, the body recovers. If training sessions and matches are suitably spaced out, body tissues are built up successively and grow stronger and develop endurance. If training sessions and matches are too close in time, the tissues do not have time to recover and suffer a destructive effect instead.

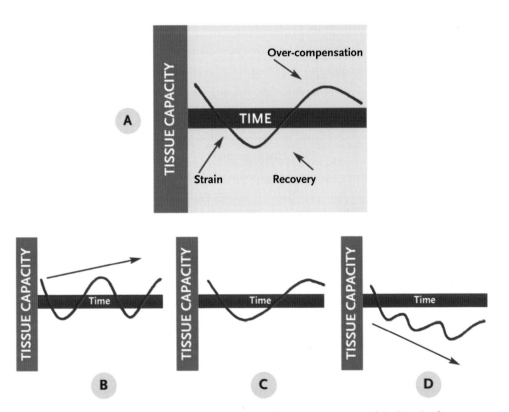

**Figure 3.11** The principle of how body tissues adapt to training (A). If the length of time between training sessions is about right, the sessions have a building-up effect (B). If the time between the sessions is too long, there will be no build-up, the current level will be maintained (C). Too short a time between sessions has a breaking-down effect (D). Diagram from Jon Karlsson, *Motions- & Idrottsskador och deras rehabilitering*, 1997 (in Swedish).

## Training camps

The risk of injury at training camps is 2–3 times greater than at normal training sessions. This fact has been demonstrated both among players at lower levels and at national team level. The reason for the increased number of injuries is normally an overly rapid change in strain and playing surface.

Many teams normally train 2–3 times per week. During the winter and spring, training often takes place on a hard surface.

Training camps are often held in places where a grass pitch is available and the surface may be different from that on which players have been training immediately prior to the camp. The amount of training also often increases, two sessions per day not being unusual. This severe increase can give rise to all sorts of strain injuries. Frequently, these injuries do not heal during the ensuing season and the players are unable to train and play efficiently.

## Combining sports

Specialization at ever younger ages means that it is unusual for people to compete in several different sports these days. In lower divisions, however, footballers also devote themselves to winter sports such as ice-hockey.

For children up to the age of 12 years, it can be advantageous to participate in several different sports. The body develops all-round fitness and it is conceivable that this lessens the risk of injury as an adult player. For adults, combining football with other competitive sports may be disadvantageous.

It the player combines football and ice-hockey, for example, the seasons overlap. If the player continues with ice-hockey until the end of the season, he or she will have missed most of the basic pre-season football training which is so important. If, after the ice-hockey season, the player joins the football training sessions, he or she will be more susceptible to strain since muscles are used differently in the two sports.

# Equipment

### Shin pads

Shin pads are intended for protection of the lower leg. It has been shown that the risk of injury to the lower leg is five times as great in players who do not use shin pads as in those who do. FIFA has decided that the use of shin pads will be obligatory in football. The Swedish Football Association decided in 1994 that only approved shin pads may be used in matches.

Since obligatory marking of shin pads was introduced, the pads have improved. So far, it has not been possible to produce shin pads that can prevent bone fractures under all circumstances. Shin pads must protect, must fit well and be reasonably comfortable. Approved pads are therefore tested both from technical and practical points of view.

---

**SHIN PADS**

- Shin pads are to be worn by all players.
- Shin pads used by players over the age of 15 years should have been approved by the Football Association and shall carry their mark of approval.
- Alterations to shin pads or other attempts to get round the rules pertaining to obligatory use of shin pads are forbidden.

*Source: Rules of football*

---

### Shoes and boots

When the foot is lowered on to the ground, the tissues of the lower leg, the pelvis and the back are subjected to pressure. In walking, this pressure is just about the same as the weight of the body. In running the load increases to 3–5 times body weight. A burst of speed or landing after a jump can increase the load to 4–6 times body weight. A player puts his foot down from 10 000 to 15 000 times in each training session or match and the total load on body tissue is, therefore, large. Tissues are easily subjected to overuse and players suffer strain injuries.

Shock absorption varies between different types of shoes. A jogging shoe generally has a thick and relatively soft outer sole as well as an inner sole formed to support the arch of the foot. These shoes are excellent shock absorbers. The risk of strain injuries is reduced.

With football boots, priority is given to other aspects. Players want a light and stable boot. The outer sole of a football boot is generally thin. The inner sole is also thin and, usually, completely flat with no arch support. These boots have very little shock absorption. The risk of strain injury is therefore greater with football boots than with jogging shoes.

The uppers of a football boot are made of thin, malleable, leather material so that the player has the best possible ball-feeling. The thin upper of a football boot provides very little protection from the forces to which the foot is exposed when kicking or trapping the ball. An ankle shot, for example, or trapping the ball involves severe forces. Filming with a high-speed camera that takes several thousand frames per second, has shown that the ball is kicked with an initial speed of 120 km/h. At the moment of shooting, the foot is violently angled and the tissues of the foot are put under severe strain. This violence can lead to permanent injury.

It has been found that 90 per cent of all elite football players suffer from osteophytes and calcification of the ankle, visible on radiographs (see Chapter 17).

The number of studs, their design, position and the material of which they are made are also important from the point of view of injury. In studded boots there is a concentration of the load where the studs are positioned. The fewer the studs, the greater the risk of

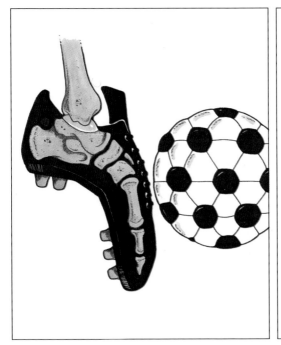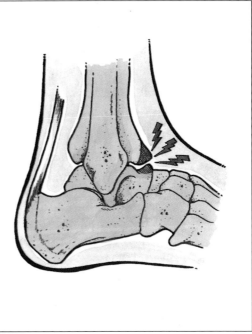

**Figure 3.12** An ankle shot involves severe forces. Both the foot and the ball are deformed and foot tissues are subjected to heavy strain. It has been found that 90 per cent of all elite players suffer from osteophytes and calcification in the foot and ankle as the result of years of playing football.

'tramping through' which can cause pain in the ball or heel of the foot.

Screw studs absorb less shock than rubber studs and should only be used when the pitch is soft and damp. If screw studs are used when the pitch is hard, the risk of overuse injuries increases.

The length of studs is also significant. Long screw studs provide a better grip since friction between foot and ground is increased. If the foot is firmly fixed to the ground, twisting forces are released in the knee and the risk of damaged knee ligaments increases. Most serious knee injuries, for example injuries to the various ligaments of the knee, occur when the player's supporting leg gets stuck and therefore suffers an abnormal twisting of the knee joint.

It has been shown in American football that the length and number of studs influence the risk of knee and ankle injuries. Players who used boots with a small number of long studs suffered more injuries to knees and ankles than players who used boots with more and shorter studs. It has not been possible to prove such a correlation in European football. There are differences between European and American football in the way the players move and in the pitches. American football is an impact sport with a great deal of body contact and many tackles. These 'collisions' are independent of the surface.

In European football, the connection between foot and surface is of much greater importance. A good grip (high friction) between boot and the ground creates large twisting forces in the knee. The risk of knee injuries increases accordingly. However, a good grip between foot and ground is necessary if the player is to be able to change direction rapidly, start, stop and jerk as is required in good football. If one lessens the friction between the foot and the ground by removing the studs or by using shoes with very short studs, the player's grip is reduced and he or she slips. This not only means that the player is less proficient but the risk of injury may also increase.

*Friction between foot and ground must always be carefully considered. Too much friction increases the risk of injury and too little friction lessens proficiency.*

## Playing surface – arena – climate

In the international rules of football drawn up by FIFA, there are regulations concerning the size of pitches acceptable as match arenas. There is also a general rule allowing the referee to cancel or abandon a match if the weather or lack of light should require this. Football should not be played if there is a lightning storm, for example. The risk of lightning striking the players is great. On an open pitch, the players act as lightning conductors and have been struck. Driving rain can also be a reason for cancelling or abandoning a football match. On a water-logged pitch, play is difficult and the risk of injury is increased since the players easily slip. Poor visibility also increases the risk of injury.

The actual playing surface is also of great importance. It has been found that between 20 and 25 per cent of all football injuries may be linked to the playing surface or to the combination of boots and playing surface. Two factors principally influence the correlation between playing surface and risk of injury: the hardness of the surface and the friction or grip between boot and surface. The friction between boot and surface has already been discussed in the previous section. The hardness of the pitch is significant for the risk of strain injuries. The reason for this is that the foot lands less elastically and the strain on body tissues increases on a hard pitch whereas on a soft pitch the foot lands more gently. The foot 'sinks into the ground' and the load on the foot can be spread over a longer time period. The strain on tissues is reduced.

It is normal for the playing surface to change, particularly during the training periods of winter and spring. Because of the weather and for practical reasons, training one day may be indoors on a hard surface, the next day on gravel and the following day on artificial grass. These changes between different surfaces increase the risk of strain injuries. Different muscles are activated differently depending on the playing surface. One can adjust to a new surface but this can take five or six training sessions to achieve satisfactory adaptation.

When artificial grass was introduced, it rapidly became popular for many different sports. Many people saw advantages with artificial grass; a wide range of uses, hard-wearing and low maintenance costs. In football, too, there were high expectations of artificial grass as a playing surface. The possibility of playing all the year round regardless of the weather was envisaged. The expectation that artificial grass would be suited to a wide range of uses, that is, for football, as well as other sports, exhibitions, etc. proved to be unrealistic. The early types of artificial grass meant for a wide range of uses proved to be unsuitable for football. The character of the game was changed and the risk of injury increased. Players often suffered burns on account of the high level of friction. The new types of artificial grass with sand and rubber pellets are very similar to natural grass. This means that playing on them is like playing on grass. If artificial grass is like natural grass then the risks of injury will be similar. The risk of skin damage (superficial burns) is hardly greater than with natural grass.

Playing indoors on a hard surface has also become increasingly common. An increased risk of injury has been reported from indoor play and the reasons for this are probably the hard surface and the small playing area.

# Other factors

### Playing tactics

Most injuries in football arise from contact during matches. Since each individual player only has contact with the ball for 2–4 min/match, the risk of injury is particularly great while in possession of the ball. The risk of injury can thus change with the style of playing both for the individual player and for the team.

Certain teams have an aggressive style of play with the emphasis on physical strength. Other teams have a more technical style. Teams that play technical football with fast, direct passes, little kicking of the ball and, therefore, brief possession of the ball run less risk of injury. Since their style of play means that each player's contact with the ball is very brief on each occasion, contact with their opponents is minimized and there is less risk of contact injury. When the opposite applies, i.e. when the players have lengthy contact with the ball, there is a greater risk of injury as the opponents come in to bodily contact with the player holding the ball (tackling etc.).

### Referees

The referee can influence the risk of injury by the ways he or she interprets the regulations, that is by 'setting the right level' for the match (see Chapter 25).

### Coaches

The coach has great significance for a team's injury risk. His or her significance lies on several levels. A highly professional coach, through his or her understanding of football medicine, can minimize injury. It is the coach who decides how the team will play and thereby affects the risk of contact injury. The coach's attitude to injuries, rehabilitation and preventive action is also of importance.

### Medical service

Medical service at a club is important in this context. A club must have good contacts with doctors, physiotherapists, osteopaths or other medical experts.

Medical service can be on various levels. The basic level consists of dealing with injuries. If injuries are correctly diagnosed and promptly treated, there is a greater possibility of more rapid healing and of the player's quicker return to active football. Both player and club benefit. If the club wishes to have medical service on this level, it should establish contact with a doctor or physiotherapist to whom the players can be sent for diagnosis and treatment. One makes use of the medical staff's general professional capabilities.

The next level of medical service consists of the medical professionals not only treating injuries that have arisen but also deciding on methods of rehabilitation and injury prevention. Every fifth football injury is a recurrent injury which means that the rehabilitation of the original injury was insufficient. If the doctor, coach and player collaborate on organizing rehabilitation, the risk of a recurrence is lessened. Work at this level places greater demands on the medical professional. She or he must be interested in and be knowledgeable about football as a sport and must also possess knowledge of sports medicine.

There is yet another level of medical service. At this level, the medical professionals collaborate with the team coach to improve performance of the team. There are many medical aspects of football training for example, planning the season, preparing for matches, nutrition, liquids, travel, training camps, etc. This places great demands on the medical staff's knowledge of football if their collaboration at this level is to be of value to the coach and the team.

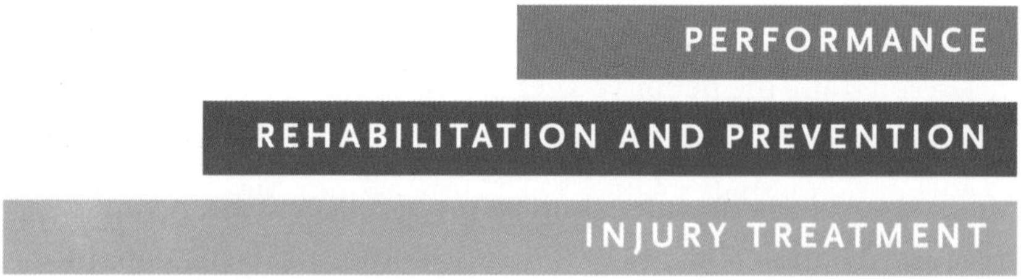

PERFORMANCE

REHABILITATION AND PREVENTION

INJURY TREATMENT

**Figure 3.13** Football medicine services.

# INJURY PREVENTION METHODS

## Basic training

In general, it has been established that the best way of preventing injury is to maintain a high level of physical fitness. Training improves many qualities that are important from an injury prevention point of view. Tissue strength increases and protective reflexes improve. It has been proven that fit teams (those that take part in frequent, high-quality training sessions at which there is a high level of attendance) have fewer injuries. The relation between training intensity and injury is also applicable to individuals. Poor training routines, i.e. low attendance at sessions or a long absence from training, make players more susceptible to injury.

In general, the basic principle of specificity applies, i.e. 'the more you train, the better you get'. There is, therefore, a good reason to imitate match situations in training sessions and try to make all the training football related. For young people, however, there is a risk associated with starting specific training at too early a stage. One-sided pressure on a growing skeleton can damage it. It is generally believed that players who have participated in many different sports when growing up, and who are therefore generally fit, are less susceptible to injury than older players.

## Planning for the season

It has previously been established that the way in which a season is planned is significant both for the success of the team and for the amount of injuries sustained. The correct amount of training and matches is important.

### Avoiding over-training

The early symptoms of over-training are pain in the working muscles, tenderness and perhaps pain while resting in the tendons and muscular attachments that have been put under particular strain. Over-training is especially common in connection with training camps or with intensive pre-season training. Players who come from youth teams or from a lower division run a greater risk, because the amount of training and its intensity in the new team can be greater than what the player is accustomed to.

Both players and coaches should be aware that persistent pain and tenderness after putting the body through training could be a sign of overdoing it. Certain types of aches and pains are normal after a tough training session. Intense pain, especially pain that persists until the next day, can be a sign of over-training.

### Assessing pain using the visual analogue scale

People experience pain differently. A Visual Analogue Scale can be used to classify pain. On the VAS, there are 10 grades of pain where 0 is 'no pain at all' and 10 means 'unbearable pain'. After a tough training session, aches and pains up to grade 2 on the scale are deemed normal and harmless. Pain between grades 2 and 5 means the body has perhaps been put under too much strain and a grade of over 5 means that it is likely that the body's tissues have been overstrained.

*No pain*                                                    *Unbearable pain*

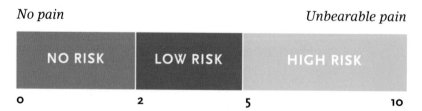

**Figure 3.14** The VAS classifies pain between 0 and 10 to measure pain both during and after activity. Pain between 2 and 5 means the body may have been overexerted, pain over 5 on the scale should be avoided.

A player must 'listen to the body's signals', and learn what his or her training threshold is. The coach must also watch for signs of overexertion in players. It could be useful for everyone if the coach or another member of the medical team talks to the players about planning for the season and the dangers associated with training too hard. In connection with this, it is important for the coach to encourage players to talk about any signs they have of overexertion. It is particularly important for the team to get help from medical personnel at training camps, where the problem is more common.

If individual players or perhaps even the whole team show signs of over-training, this can be remedied by rest or alternative training methods. Suitable alternatives include cycling, pool training or more playful footballing activities, such as football tennis. Other options which place much less strain on the body, but which are nevertheless closely associated with football, are individual skill training, precision training, tactical training and the training of set pieces are other examples of alternative training that place less strain on the body. If the symptoms of over-training are dealt with early enough, it is sufficient to replace the odd training session with some kind of alternative activity.

### Avoiding too many matches

Players may show signs of burn-out if they play too many matches in too short a period of time or too many matches in comparison to how often they train. Since this is mostly a psychological problem, the coach should be alert to signs such as apathy, lack of motivation, fatigue, anger and low spirits.

Sometimes it may be as simple as asking the question: 'Are you having fun?' Good communication with players and empathy are important qualities in a coach especially during intensive periods when many matches are being played. At the same time, the coach must be careful not to burn-out him or herself. American studies have shown that a coach with a specific style of leadership is more susceptible to burn-out, especially one who is more socially oriented. Such coaches always give 110 per cent and the risk of burn-out is much higher.

Players often try to keep such symptoms to themselves. It is therefore important for the coach to create an atmosphere that allows feelings to be aired. For players, it is important to be able to expressive negative feelings, disappointment and frustration.

If there is a suspicion that too many matches are being played, the number should obviously be reduced. This can be done in different ways. One way is to have a large squad of players, which allows individual players to be rested for some of the matches. Another way is to have fewer pre-season friendlies.

## Rehabilitation after injury

It has been claimed that recurrent injury is the most common type of injury in football. It is unfortunately all too common that an injured player returns to training and starts playing matches far too quickly and the old injury flares up. Designing a good rehabilitation programme as well as deciding when the injured player can return to training and has reached match fitness are difficult tasks for the medical team. In many clubs, there is no medical team and it is then up to the injured player themselves, in consultation with the coach, who decides when she is fit enough to return.

Rehabilitation starts as soon as the injury has occurred and how emergency treatment is administered is important. Its aim is to minimize the after-effects and symptoms of an injury. The correct treatment of soft body parts will minimize haemorrhaging and swelling. At this stage, it is important to relieve the pressure on the damaged tissue.

Rehabilitation obviously depends on the type and seriousness of the injury. In general, there is a basic principle for all rehabilitation:

**Rehabilitation should consist of gradually increasing the load on the damaged tissue and at the same time avoiding pain and swelling.**

Pain and swelling are the body's warning signals and should be respected. The gradual increase in load strengthens the tissue and increases its resistance.

Figure 3.15 shows an example of a rehabilitation programme where the load is gradually increased after an ankle injury.

Rehabilitation begins at the scene of the injury with emergency treatment. When the player can walk without limping, the load can be gradually increased. The first stage is jogging straight ahead. The next stage is jogging in figures of eight, to begin with slowly in large figures, then faster in smaller figures. All training should be free from pain (less than 2 on the VAS scale, see Page 78). If pain or swelling occur, go back a stage and train on a painless level for a few days before increasing the load again.

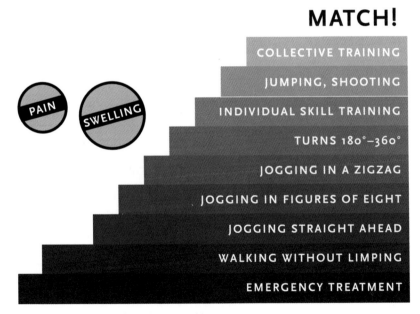

**Figure 3.15** Rehabilitation following an ankle injury.

When the player can turn 360° at full speed in both directions, individual skill training with a ball can be introduced. The next stage is more explosive individual exercise such as jumping, shooting and fast acceleration. When the player can carry out these exercises without experiencing pain, full training can be resumed. Tackling is now introduced. If a player can participate in full-scale training without any problems, he or she can be said to be match fit.

When it is a question of more serious injuries, rehabilitation is normally a matter for the doctor and physiotherapist who are treating the injury. The aim of physiotherapy is to help the tissue heal and strengthen so that it can tolerate the load placed on it in everyday and work situations. For a footballer, the tissues must also be able to tolerate strain during training and matches. This phase should be football-specific and demands cooperation between the player, the medical team and the team coach.

Rehabilitation means normalization, i.e. restoring the function. The aim of rehabilitation is not just to heal the damaged tissue but also to increase strength. In addition to strength, other functions must be 'normalized', i.e. mobility, muscle strength and coordination.

For coaches, it is important not to forget the mental factor, since it has been shown that players are affected psychologically by injury. Low spirits and a tendency towards social isolation are common mental symptoms in a badly injured player. This can lead to

## THE KEY TO SUCCESSFUL REHABILITATION

- Know what load is exerted by different forms of training.
- Exert the right amount of load.
- Build up the load gradually.
- 'Listen to the body's signals' and adjust the training accordingly.

*Level of rehabilitation*

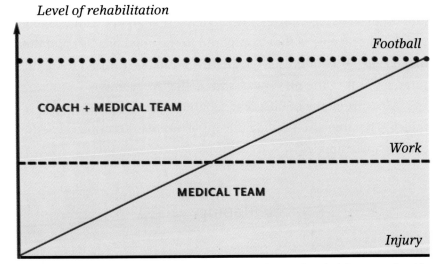

**Figure 3.16** Football rehabilitation. A footballer needs specific rehabilitation to be able to return to training and match fitness. At this stage, the key word is cooperation – between the player, coach and the medical team.

reduced motivation, which in turn can prolong the rehabilitation period.

It is therefore important for the coach to support the injured player and show interest and commitment during the rehabilitation phase and encourage participation in training sessions and other activities despite the injury. Players often are unable to participate in collective training at the beginning but can (at the same time as the others are training) follow his or her own specific rehabilitation programme and in this way feel the sense of camaraderie which football brings.

If the coach shows interest and commitment in the rehabilitation of a player, the chances of an early return to full-scale training will be increased. It is therefore often beneficial to put the rehabilitation programme in writing. Footballers are often very competitive and a well-defined rehabilitation programme will stimulate their competitive instinct.

During the rehabilitation period, it is worth performing measurements of different qualities, such as mobility, muscle strength and fitness. For leg injuries you can usually compare with the good leg. A general rule is that, compared to the good leg, full mobility and 80–90 per cent muscle strength should be restored to the injured leg before the player can start collective training.

Measurements of different rehabilitation qualities whilst the injury is healing also provide the opportunity to scrutinize and adjust the programme.

# Taping

Tape is tearable, non-elastic sticking bandage. The aim of taping is to support a weakened part of the body without restricting its function. When taping an ankle, for example, the tape bandage supports the lateral ligament and prevents it from being put under strain on the outside, whilst the vertical movement of the foot is not affected. A correctly applied tape bandage does not therefore reduce the performance capacity of the player. Practical advice on taping and examples of different types of tape bandages that can be useful for footballers are found in Chapter 20.

Tape can be used both to prevent injury and during rehabilitation. For acute injuries, however, taping should be avoided as a rule until the swelling has died down. A non-elastic tape bandage applied to a damaged area where there is haemorrhaging and swelling can cause circulation problems. For acute injuries, a compression bandage with elastic tape should be used.

## Taping to prevent injury

Preventative taping of a previously injured ankle reduces the risk of the injury recurring. There are, however, no studies that have shown that taping a healthy ankle is beneficial, even if it is done extensively.

There are various theories concerning why taping the ankle acts as prophylaxis against an injury. One theory is that a tape bandage gives rise to a mechanical improvement in ankle stability. It has been shown, however, that the tape gradually loosens during physical activity, while still restricting the ankle's movement outwards. Another theory is that the tape bandage irritates the skin causing a reflex in which the muscles surrounding the ankle tighten which has a stabilizing effect.

There are several different techniques for applying a tape bandage. Unfortunately, there are no studies that have evaluated whether there is any difference in the effectiveness of these techniques or whether the combination of non-elastic tape and elastic sticking plaster has the same effect. Neither do we know with any degree of certainty whether there is any difference in effectiveness between a tape bandage applied by a player him or herself or by someone else (experienced or inexperienced).

**Taping during rehabilitation**

Taping is probably most useful during rehabilitation after an injury. Acute injuries, however, should be treated in accordance with the principles described for the treatment of acute soft part injuries in Chapter 8.

When the swelling has gone down, taping can be useful. If base tape (a first layer of tape) is used, the tape bandage itself can be left on for several days. Base tape reduces skin irritation without lessening the effect of the tape. A correctly applied tape bandage can mean that a player can return to training and playing matches more quickly.

# Supports (protectors)

### Ankle protectors

Several studies have shown that footballers who have previously sprained their ankle can reduce the risk of recurrent injury considerably by using an ankle protector, such as the Aircast (see Figure 3.17). It has not been proven, however, that different ankle protectors reduce the risk of injury in previously uninjured ankles. The risk of knee injury does not increase with the use of an ankle protector or if the ankle is taped.

An ankle protector has the same effect as a tape bandage, i.e. it reduces the outward movement without affecting performance capacity. There are both advantages and disadvantages of using an ankle protector as opposed to tape. The advantage is that ankle protectors are both cheaper and easier to use than tape. The disadvantage is that they can often feel somewhat cumbersome.

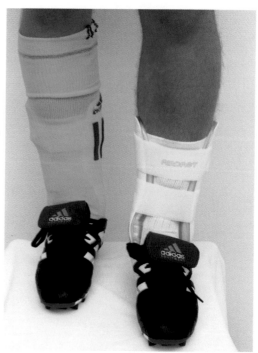

**Figure 3.17** Ankle orthosis (Aircast). Ankle protectors can be used to prevent ankle injuries or as a rehabilitation aid after a sprained ankle. The protector consists of an outer part made of rigid plastic and an air-cushioned inner part. The air cushions can be inflated to give the best fit and optimum stability. To avoid skin irritation, the protector should be used with a stocking bandage underneath.

The player's right leg shows what the protector looks like with a football sock over it.

### Knee protectors

There is no evidence that using some kind of knee protector reduces the risk of knee injury in football. Knee protectors of different types are used frequently in other sports, but seldom in football, since many feel they are a hindrance when playing. Using a protector that contains metal parts during a match must have the approval of the referee.

# Coordination training

Training on a balancing board and other types of coordination training are not only useful as an injury prevention measure but also during post-injury rehabilitation. After having sprained his or her ankle, a player often has reduced positional sense in the foot and experiences weakness and instability in the ankle. This phenomenon is probably caused both by a weakening in the calf muscles and reduced reflex activation. The result is a reduced capacity to position the ankle correctly when it comes in contact with the ground or floor, which increases the risk of further sprain.

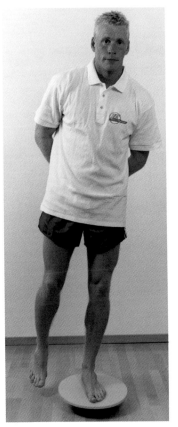

It has been shown that if a footballer trains on a balancing board for 5 min/day/foot for 2 to 3 months, his or her calf muscles will gain extra strength and have quicker reflex activation. Training of this nature reduces the risk of recurrent ankle sprain at the same time as the player's foot feels stronger and more stable.

**Figure 3.18** Training on a balancing board.

# Agility training/stretching

Over the last few years, most football teams have started using agility training and stretching. The risk of muscle rupture is thereby reduced. Warming up and stretching increase the temperature in the muscles and connective tissue. Elasticity and range of movement increase as does muscle and muscle attachment strength.

For purely practical reasons, one should differentiate between warming up and limbering up which includes stretching. The aim of warming up is to prepare the body for playing football. During a warm-up, the temperature of the whole body increases and a large proportion of blood is redirected to the working muscles. Co-ordination also improves, i.e. nerve and muscle function, which is important in a technical sport like football. Warming up also fulfils a mental function as it reduces any tension.

The general warm-up should last for at least 5–10 min and include the large muscle groups. The most common form of warm-up has previously been some light jogging, but a better and more specific form in football is 'the square' or other exercises with a ball. Explosive exercises, for example shooting, fast acceleration and jumping should be left until the end of the warm-up, since they increase the risk of muscle rupture. Only when the muscles are well warmed up should agility training and stretching begin. The most common form of stretching, so-called passive stretching, involves gently stretching the muscles laterally. The stretched position is then held for about 30 sec. Each movement is repeated 3–5 times. It is important not to sway while in the stretched position.

From an injury prevention point of view, it is important to prioritize the muscles which are most susceptible to injury. For outfield players, this means the anterior and posterior thigh muscles, the groin and the calf muscles. Practical details of special stretching exercises for football are given in Chapter 20.

After a training session or match, players should cool down. This can take the form of some light jogging or stretching the leg muscles with the aim of softening up the muscles after a tough training session or match, which reduces the risk of stiffness and tightness. Stiff and tight muscles reduce performance capacity and increase the risk of muscle injury in subsequent training sessions or matches. It is equally important to stretch after a match than after a tough training session, but sometimes it can be difficult to do on the football field. A tip is to encourage players to stretch in the shower after a game.

Today, agility training and stretching are used by most football teams, but for stretching to be effective, it is important to do it properly. It can be worth getting a physiotherapist to go through the various techniques of agility training and stretching with the players at the beginning of the season. Even if the coach chooses to let the players warm up and stretch individually, it is advisable to do it collectively at regular intervals. The reason for this is both to stress the importance of warming up/stretching/cooling down for the players and to check that they are doing things properly from a technical point of view.

# Equipment

Having the right equipment is an important injury prevention measure in many sports. The most important pieces of equipment for preventing football injuries are shin pads, boots and insoles.

## Shin pads

A coach who wishes to minimize the risk of injury for his or her team should always insist the players wear shin pads even at training sessions. The quality and appearance of shin pads vary.

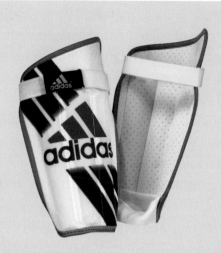

## SHIN PADS SHOULD MEET THE FOLLOWING REQUIREMENTS

- They should cover a large part of the shin.
- To be effective, they should be good shock absorbers. The pad should reduce the peak force in a kick to the shin.
- Approved studs should not puncture the pad.
- They should be a good fit so that the player feels comfortable wearing them.

### Boots

It is also important to use the right boots or shoes for the right occasion. When fitness training on hard surfaces, boots without studs should be worn — normal jogging shoes are better suited for this.

A player who often suffers from overuse injuries in the legs, for example periostitis, can reduce the risk of recurrent injury by using jogging shoes instead of football boots when training on hard surfaces.

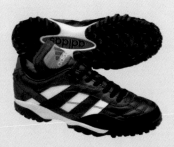

## A GOOD FOOTBALL BOOT SHOULD

- Function as a good shock absorber to prevent straining the leg and lower leg.
- Grip the surface well so that the player has a good foothold when accelerating quickly, stopping and turning.
- Not grip the surface too well so that the foot gets stuck — this increases the risk of ankle and knee ligament damage.
- Be flexible and light.
- Be reasonably priced.

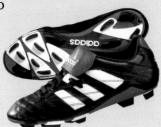

### Insoles

Shock absorption can be increased by putting an insole into the boot. If one is only looking for this quality in an insole, then ready-made ones can be bought in a sports shop that are specially made for football boots.

Some foot problems also need support for the foot arch. The ready-made shock-absorbing insole may therefore be insufficient and an alternative is to get an orthopaedic technician to make one specially.

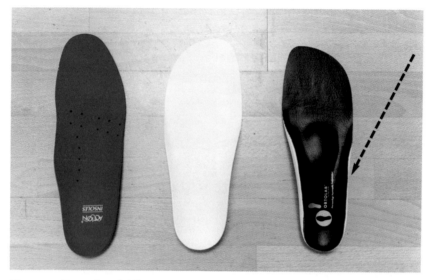

**Figure 3.19** Examples of different types of insole. The insole on the left is pre-fabricated and its primary function is to increase shock absorption. The insole in the middle has been moulded to fit a specific foot. The insole on the right is built up in the middle to give extra support to the foot arch.

# Rules

### Infringements and injuries

About 25–30 per cent of all injuries that happen during a match occur as a result of a foul. In a study of players in the men's fourth division in Sweden, it was found that serious injuries that occurred as a result of a foul were suffered by the player committing the foul. It is possible that players at this level compensate for a lack of technical skill by fouling opponents. For a coach at this level, it is more effective from an injury prevention point of view to encourage players to abide by the rules and refrain from criticizing the referee.

At higher levels, it seems to be a different matter. During the 1994 World Cup in the USA, 44 of the 52 matches played were video-filmed. Analyses showed that the majority, 71 per cent, of injuries did not occur as a result of a rule infringement (according to the referee) and only 29 per cent of the injuries that occurred during a match occurred as a result of unfair play. Of all fouls, only 3 per cent led to injuries that needed some form of treatment. Of the injuries that occurred as a result of unfair play, two out of three were as a result of unfair challenges.

In general it was found that defenders ran a greater risk of injury than other players. There was no difference between the different playing positions when it came to injuries as a result of fouls. Injuries occurring as a result of a foul were suffered by the player who had been fouled in 95 per cent of cases. In only 5 per cent of cases did the player committing the foul suffer injury.

The results suggest that new interpretations of the rules as regards sending players off and a tougher attitude by the referee as regards fouls have reduced the risk of injury. The crowd gets to see the best players and more action.

## Free substitution

In many ball sports, it is permitted to substitute players freely during a game. Free substitution means that as many players as one likes can be substituted at any time during a match. A Danish study found that although free substitution did not lead to reduced injury risk, it did shorten the rehabilitation period for less serious injuries. The reasons for this are probably better assessment and better emergency treatment of injuries. The coaches, players and medical personnel of those teams participating in the study were positive towards free substitution. Free substitution means that an injured player can stop playing immediately and be replaced, while the injury is assessed and treated off the pitch. If the injury is not serious, the player can replace the substitute again.

# Other factors

### Medical service

It is important for a team to have access to medical service both as far as dealing with emergency injuries is concerned and in terms of work done to prevent injuries. Studies have shown that as many as 75 per cent of injuries in a team can be prevented if the team has access to a doctor and a physiotherapist. Since accidental injuries are common in football, it is important that the medical team has a good knowledge of traumatology. We should not forget, however, that many other types of medical problems can arise in a football squad. It is therefore wise to have good general medical expertise. Despite this, problems can always occur which lie outside the competence of the medical team and it is a great asset to the team if its medical support can call on a broad contact network including other fields of medical specialization.

### Fitness training

A well-trained player has less of a propensity for injury than a poorly trained player. Getting into shape is therefore an important injury prevention measure. When a player is not sufficiently fit he or she does not have the energy to maintain the same level of technique and coordination which increases the risk of injury.

### Diet and fluid intake

In Chapter 6, the importance of the diet and fluid intake for optimal performance is underlined but the risk of injury also increases parallel to the decrease in performance due to lack of fluids or unbalanced diet. As with tiredness, technique and coordination are primarily affected. If energy stocks are empty, fluid intake is insufficient and fitness is flagging, these factors can provide the explanation for the findings shown in several surveys where there is an increased risk of injury at the end of matches and training sessions.

## Hormones/the contraceptive pill

It has been found that women players have a higher risk of injury prior to and after their menstrual period. The risk was particularly marked for women who experienced discomfort before and during menstruation. The women who were using the contraceptive pill were affected by fewer accidental injuries compared with players who did not take the pill, which suggests that there is a link between hormonal factors and injuries. The findings are interesting but need to be confirmed and further studies have to be made before we can come to definite conclusions and provide general advice.

## Mental training

There is sound evidence that mental training can influence performance ability positively. It is tempting to believe that mental training could therefore also reduce the risk of injuries although this remains unproven. There is, however, clear evidence that mental training does have some connection with the risk of injury. Players with low self-confidence and impaired concentration and performance under pressure, are more easily injured. It is therefore important to increase the self-confidence of the players — this improves their performance and reduces the risk of injury.

In order to develop the team, the coach should analyse each player's individual needs. Regular development interviews might be one way of creating a picture of what each player needs to progress further. If every player developed into a better (and injury free) player, the whole team will improve.

It is not only football factors that affect the players, factors external to football also play a part. For example, it has been shown that a player who is affected by adverse events in his or her life, such as family problems or problems at work, is injured more easily. This is probably because of the increased risk that the player is 'thinking about other things' too much and is therefore less focused when playing football. This means that the coach has to have the entire picture concerning a player and should work with them both on and off the pitch. Performance on the pitch is heavily dependent on how one functions off the pitch — harmony and disharmony are reflected both in the team spirit and in the game.

# PREVENTATIVE MEASURES IN PRACTICE — PRE-SEASON MEDICAL EXAMINATION

The ideal opportunity for applying injury prevention measures is at a pre-season check-up, by carrying out a medical examination before the season begins. A pre-season check-up allows the examiner to analyse and correct individual factors which could trigger injuries. If these weaknesses are eliminated by means of various injury prevention methods, the risk of injury during the season will be reduced.

## Why conduct pre-season check-ups?

The pre-season check-up is an ideal opportunity for the medical team to familiarize themselves with the players and establish the players' general health including any injuries that they may have. The check-up will also provide an idea of the player's normal level of mobility in the joints and any instability can be noted from previous injuries. If new injuries should occur during the season, it is important to be aware of the condition of the joint before the injury. If, for instance, looseness in the joint is discovered after a new injury has incurred, it is important to know whether this had been caused earlier or whether it has been caused on this occasion.

## REASONS FOR A PRE-SEASON MEDICAL CHECK-UP/EXAMINATION

- **Security.** It provides a sense of security for the player if the club does everything it can to minimize the risk of injuries.

- **Performance.** Injuries are a negative factor that undermines the overall performance of the team. The coach who manages to maintain his or her team intact and free from injury has a better chance of achieving success in pure football terms. In the division statistics recorded each year, it is often apparent that the teams that are most successful are also the teams who have used fewest players during the year. Conducting a medical examination in the form of a pre-season check-up is an effective method in this context. In addition, the tests carried out can also be of interest from a performance point of view. For example, the functions tested include balance, muscle strength (one leg hop) and agility. All these tests are basic qualities contributing to performance.

- **Finance.** Injury prevention also provides financial advantages. Many clubs set aside funds in their budgets for emergency treatment of acute injuries. An operation on a cruciate ligament injury is very expensive. Furthermore, a player who has had surgery on the cruciate ligament is out of football for at least 6 months. It may also be financially wise to carry out a medical examination on a new player before the contract is signed.

- **Psychology.** A pre-season check-up can be valuable from a psychological point of view. The knowledge that the club does something that other clubs neglect to do is psychologically strengthening.

**Documentation and the protection of confidentiality**

The findings of the examination and results of the tests should be documented in specific test records or medical files. The person responsible for medical service within the team is obliged to keep medical records of any treatment for injuries even if the treatment occurs on the pitch.

All the information in the medical records is confidential and should be handled in accordance with the law concerning professional secrecy. Information from the records of a specific player may not be released to a third party (not even to the coach) without the player first being consulted and giving his or her consent.

# Procedure and content

The pre-season medical examination may include different aspects and may be carried out in various ways taking into consideration the personnel conducting the examination and the equipment used. Here are some examples of medical check-ups which can be practically conducted at a pre-season medical without access to advanced equipment.

The tests recommended have been evaluated and found to be 'reproducible' (repeated measurements provide similar values) and 'valid' (they measure what they are intended to measure).

**Previous injuries or illnesses**

A review of previous injuries and any remaining problems is an important part of a medical check-up. A template should be used at the medical and the results and findings should be noted in a record. Examples of records used for Swedish players both at national and club level are shown in the test records on Page 100.

### Which injuries and illnesses should be included?

When registering new injuries prospectively (forward in time from a given date), it is usual to define an injury as 'any injury the player incurs during football activities and which results in absence from at least one training session or match'. When injuries are registered retrospectively, in other words, injuries which have already happened, it can be difficult to remember less serious injuries which have caused absence from individual training sessions or matches. It is therefore only practical to register more extensive or serious injuries. Injuries and illnesses that have caused at least 2 weeks' absence from training or matches, or injuries and illnesses which have led to surgery or a period in hospital should be noted.

### Medication, diet, allergies, vaccinations

When surveying the players' medical condition it is also important to note some factors of general interest such as the use of medication (check against the doping lists), diet (player X cannot eat certain foods), allergies and vaccinations (football players should be vaccinated against polio and tetanus).

### Shooting leg, take-off leg

It is also useful to note which is the take-off leg and shooting leg. The most common situation is that players are right footed and use their left leg as the take-off leg. Certain types of injury are unevenly distributed between the shooting and the take-off leg:

- Ankle sprains are more common on the shooting leg (right footed players sprain the right ankle).
- Cruciate ligament injuries are more common to the supporting leg.
- Jumper's knee (injury to the knee cap tendon) is more common to the take-off leg.

## EXAMPLE OF A MEDICAL EXAMINATION RECORD

Date of birth: *781012*
Name: *Anders Andersson*
Address: *Alpstigen 1, 111 11 A-town*
Telephone: *0234-12 32 32*
Club: *A-town FC*
Height (cm): *180*  Weight (kg): *72*
Shooting leg: *Right*  Take-off leg: *left*
Playing position: *Left midfield*

Date ...............

Medication: *0*
Diet: *No fish*
Allergy: *Pollen*
Vaccinations: *Havrix 19--*
*Tetanus 19-*
*Polio 19--*

### Previous injuries or illnesses

1. *Left knee. Surgery anterior cruciate ligament 1996. Patellar tendon. Absent 6 months. No current problems.*
2. *Right peroneal fracture 1995. Absent 3 months. No problems.*
3. *Right ankle. Sprain 1998. Injury to peripheral ligaments. X-ray. Absence 4 weeks. Continues 'sense of instability'.*
4. *Shin splints right + left. Frequent problems pre-season on hard surfaces.*
5. *Right groin. Last season, pain during bursts of speed and shots during pre-season training.*
6. *Concussion 1998. Absent 2 weeks. No current problems.*

| Pos | | Pos | | Pos | Comments |
|---|---|---|---|---|---|
| **1.** | **General condition** | 4.2 | Periosteum | 2.2 | *High foot arch R+L. May be linked to periosteum problems.* |
| 1.1 | Heart Pulse 56 | 4.3 | Other | | |
| 1.2 | Lungs | **5.** | **Knee** | | |
| 1.3 | Blood pressure 120/80 | 5.1 | Swelling | 1.2 | *Distended ligament after previous sprain to right ankle.* |
| 1.4 | Pharynx | 5.2 | Thigh muscle *Weaker L* | | |
| 1.5 | Abdomen | 5.3 | Flexibility range 0-140 degrees | | |
| 1.6 | Other | 5.4 | Palpation/soreness | 1.3 | *Poor balance R+L foot. Should train on a balancing board.* |
| **2.** | **Foot** | 5.5 | Kneecap | | |
| 2.1 | Ball | 5.6 | Q-angle 10 degrees | | |
| 2.2 | Arch | 5.7 | Cruciate ligaments | 5.2 | *Weaker thigh muscle, left leg after surgery on cruciate ligament.* |
| | High arches R+L | 5.8 | Collateral ligaments | | |
| 2.3 | Heel | 5.9 | Menisci | | |
| 2.4 | Other | 5.10 | One leg jump | 5.7 | *Slightly increased drawer sign left knee after cruciate ligament surgery. Distinct termination. Pivot shift neg.* |
| **3.** | **Ankle** | | R 201cm, L 185cm | | |
| 3.1 | Ligament | 5.11 | Other | | |
| 3.2 | Stability | **6.** | **Hip/groin** | | |
| | 1+ drawer R | 6.1 | Hips | 5.10 | *Poorer jumping ability left leg due to reduced muscle strength after cruciate ligament surgery. Should train thigh muscle strength.* |
| 3.3 | Solec test | 6.2 | Groin *see comments* | | |
| | R leg 34 secs. | 6.3 | Other | | |
| | L leg 40 secs. | **7.** | **Back** | | |
| 3.4 | Other | **8.** | **Shoulders/elbows/hands** | | |
| **4.** | **Lower leg** | | | 6.2 | *Sore lower area of abdomen, right side. Abdominal weakness when tested.* |
| 4.1 | Heel tendons | **9.** | **Other** | | |

### ADVICE

1. *Soft shoe supports for longitudinal foot arches to compensate stiff arches and reduce risk of periosteum problems.*
2. *Taping of right ankle before training and for matches for 6 months.*
3. *Training using a balancing board, both legs, 5 minutes per leg per day for 3 months. Will receive written programme.*
4. *Thigh muscle training (strength and coordination) left. No rehab after cruciate ligament surgery. Will receive written programme. Rehab to be supervised by physiotherapist. New test with one leg hop in 3 months.*
5. *Weight training programme for lower abdominal muscles to reduce groin problems due to abdominal weakness.*

*Doctor: Jan Ekstrand.*

## Assessment of general condition

Although injuries are common among footballers, we should not overlook the importance of their general condition and this should be checked. A minimum examination includes examination of the heart (bruit, normal rhythm?), blood pressure (high?), lungs (bruit?), pharynx (current infection?) and abdomen (soreness?). If the player has reported previous problems during his/her medical history, further tests may be appropriate before the go-ahead to play is given.

## Examination using a mirror box

A mirror box is a valuable aid in assessing the feet, lower legs, pelvis and back. A mirror box can be easily moved into the changing room or any other location for the examination. When the player is standing on the mirror box with the back turned away from the examiner it is possible to make an assessment of the feet and also look for any anatomical displacement of the back, pelvis or lower legs.

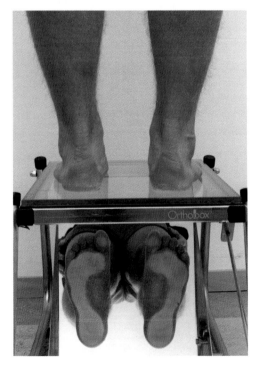

## The spine

When examining the spine any displacements should be noted (see Chapter 12). If the player experiences pain in the lumber area when they bend backwards, this may indicate vertebral displacement. Further examination including a radiograph of the lumber region should be considered.

**Figure 3.20** Examination using a mirror box. A mirror box is a practical aid for examination of the feet and for assessing the lower legs, pelvis and back. It is possible to see how pressure is distributed on the soles of the feet in the mirror along with areas that are not subjected to pressure.

## Muscle weakness

It is also useful to assess whether there are any visible signs of muscle weakness (atrophy) in one or more of the muscle groups after an earlier injury. In the event of a leg injury, the uninjured leg can be used for comparison.

## Foot arch

The foot works as a shock absorber. Well functioning foot arches are important to help absorb shock when pressure is exerted, such as when running and jumping. If the arches are fallen (*pes plano-valgus*, 'flat-feet') or if they are high and inflexible (*pes cavus*, 'high arches'), the shock absorption is impaired and the risk of overuse injuries increases.

If the player stands on a mirror box, the pressure surface of the sole of the foot can be analysed. The player should be asked to balance the pressure equally on both feet. Normally, the ball and heel areas along with the outer half of the middle area bear the pressure. This middle section can be used to assess the pressure on the arches. If the pressure is less than 25 per cent of the total mid-section, the player has a high, inflexible arch. If more than 75 per cent of the total mid-section is subjected to pressure, the arch is fallen.

If there is no mirror box available, a general assessment can be made using the wet foot test. The player dips his/her foot in water and then walks across the floor. The foot print illustrates the pressure distribution.

If the player has fallen or high arches and/or has experienced problems with overuse injuries in the legs, insoles can be recommended to prevent new injuries.

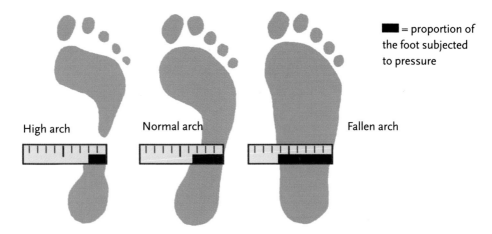

**Figure 3.21** By measuring the width of the mid-section of the foot, the shock absorption function of the foot can be assessed. On the left is a foot with a high arch (the mid-section is less than 25 per cent of the total foot width), the centre foot is normal and the foot on the right shows a fallen arch (the mid-section is more than 75 per cent of the width).

## Examination of the ankle

An ankle sprain often leads to instability which may mean that the ankle is easily injured again. Instability can be mechanical or functional or both.

### Mechanical instability

In cases of mechanical instability, there is distension of one or more of the other ligaments and the mobility of the ankle increases. This type of instability can be diagnosed by using a drawer test (see Chapter 17). New injuries can be avoided if the player uses mechanical protection such as taping or an ankle support.

### Functional instability

Functional instability means that the player has an impaired sense of position of the ankle. The ankle is felt to be weak and unstable despite the fact that there may not be any looseness. A rough assessment of functional instability can be carried out by asking the players if they experience feeling of weakness or instability. The diagnosis of functional instability can then be established more conclusively during a balance test.

New injuries can be best avoided by balance and coordination training.

## The balance test

Coordination and balance can be evaluated in different ways. In a biomechanical laboratory, it is possible to use a stabilometry method to make a data analysis of the body's tendency to lean to one side. Several surveys of football players have shown that a considerable leaning movement during a stabilometry test indicates a functional

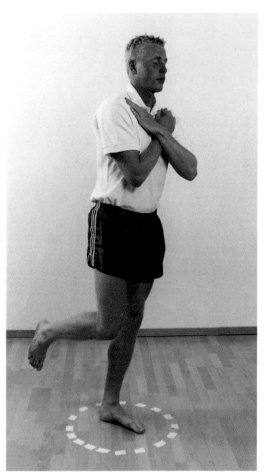

**Figure 3.22** The SOLEC test. The player stands barefoot on one leg in a chalk circle 0.5 m in diameter. The arms should be crossed over the chest. The other leg should be bent 90 degrees at the knee. The player closes his/her eyes and tries to remain standing on one leg for 60 seconds. Movement within the circle is permitted. Three attempts are allowed. The best time is recorded.

It is important to maintain concentration during the test so no other people apart from the examiner and the player should be in the room during the test.

instability and therefore increased risk of injury. If access to a biomechanical lab is not possible, it is simple to conduct a SOLEC test. The SOLEC test (Standing on One Leg Eyes Closed) assesses the player's ability to stand on one leg.

A player who is unable to stand on one leg for 60 sec should be advised to train on a balance board with the aim of preventing injuries. Experience has shown that training for at least 3 months provides positive results. During this period, the player should always train at least 5 min/foot each day. A footballer should always train one foot at a time — standing with both feet on the balance board is often too simple for a trained player.

The training using the balance board can also be varied (see Chapter 20).

## Examination of the knees

Knee ligament injuries and particularly injuries to the anterior cruciate ligament are serious football injuries. An anterior cruciate ligament injury is always a threat to a footballing career. As a rule, it is not possible to play football without a functioning anterior cruciate ligament. A footballer who incurs an anterior cruciate ligament injury has, therefore, in most cases to choose between reconstructive surgery and the subsequent rehabilitation for 6–9 months, or to stop playing football. A player who suffers an injury to a knee ligament also risks suffering from the side-effects long after the end of his or her football career. It is therefore of the utmost importance that knee ligament injuries are prevented.

Two ways of preventing knee injuries have been shown. One involves rehabilitation after previous injuries and the second method involves balance and coordination training.

## Rehabilitation after earlier injuries

Footballers who suffer ligament injuries in the knee often return to the game before they are completely recovered. Players who returned to the game believing themselves to be completely recovered have been shown to have a continued reduction of muscle strength in the injured leg compared with the uninjured leg of on average 15–20 per cent. This indicates that rehabilitation is insufficient. In the examinations carried out, it has been thought sufficient to measure only thigh muscle strength. It is possible that the players have been insufficiently rehabilitated in other areas, such as fitness, coordination, tissue strength etc.

It is possible to analyse which players have suffered earlier ligament injuries (from details about previous injuries in the records) at a pre-season examination and ascertain whether there is continued instability (using stability tests during an examination of the knees), impairment of muscle strength (by measuring the one leg hop) or coordination (by measuring balance). Players with previous injuries and continuing weaknesses can then receive individual training advice for example, in the form of weight and coordination training.

## Coordination training

In a survey of 600 footballers in Italy, it was discovered that an injury prevention programme with balance and coordination training reduced the risk of anterior cruciate ligament injuries. The injury prevention training consisted of 20 min of daily training using a balancing board during one pre-season month. During the season itself, the players underwent balance training three times a week. The risk for anterior cruciate ligament injuries was reduced considerably among the players who did the balance training compared with players in a control group.

A pre-season check-up is an excellent opportunity for informing players about this option for reducing the risk of cruciate ligament injuries. One possibility is to equip each player with a balancing board and formulate individual training programmes.

Many parents are concerned about reports of cruciate ligament injuries in football and the risk of permanent side-effects. A good way of helping to minimize this injury is for parents to buy a balancing board and encourage their children to follow a coordination training programme. Parents can, in this way, contribute to minimizing the risk of serious knee injuries.

Every coach knows that it can be difficult to motivate team players to train individually. It is a pedagogical challenge for the coach to motivate the players to train with a balancing board individually. It is said to be firmly established that coordination training reduces the risk of ankle and knee injuries — possibly other football injuries too — as well as the fact that it also improves the player's football skills.

# Examination of the hip

Early wear in the hip is more common in footballers than in the rest of the population. It is possible to check whether the player has any early signs of wear in the hip along with any other symptoms in the hip joint itself by testing the rotation capacity of the hip joints. If rotation in the hip joints is impaired, the hip should be X-rayed to confirm or eliminate any disease in the hip.

# Examination of the groin

Groin pain can be caused by a number of different conditions. Some of the most common include too much strain on the groin muscles (adductors, which pull the hip inward) or the abdominal muscles. Soreness when pressure is exerted or pain on contracting this group

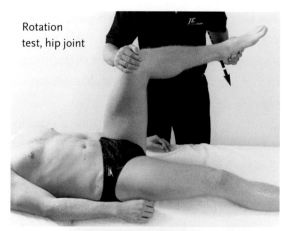

Rotation
test, hip joint

**Figure 3.23** Passive inward and out-ward rotation of the hip joint is an excellent way of evaluating the occurrence of primary hip problems. Inflexibility and impaired rotation are often the first signs of wear and tear in the hip.

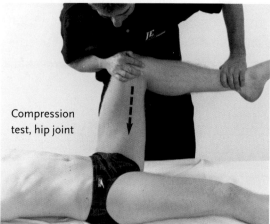

Compression
test, hip joint

**Figure 3.24** Another method of testing the condition of the hip joint is to do what is known as a compression test. By pressing downward from the knee along the thigh, increasing pressure is applied to the hip joint which causes discomfort if there is an injury or disease of the hip joint. The test also causes discomfort if there is a stress fracture of the femoral neak. A radiograph or possibly an iso-topic scan (scintigraphy) will verify or disprove the diagnosis.

of muscles at the pre-season check-up may be a sign of such strain and the cause should be analysed. Two causes are common among football players; relative muscle weakness in the groin and abdominal muscles, or strain in connection with matches and training.

### Relative muscle weakness

Several surveys have shown that footballers have strong thigh muscles. In order to stabilize the pelvis when shooting, stopping and during bursts of speed, a high level of strength is required in the other muscle groups around the pelvis. Some researchers claim that footballers have relatively weaker abdomen and groin muscles in relation to the strength of their thigh muscles and that this imbalance in the strength ratio may lead to strain on the weaker muscle groups, i.e. the abdomen and groin muscles. There is as yet no scientific evidence for this theory but those who advocate it recommend weight training for the abdominal muscles (specific training of the lower region of both the upright and oblique muscles) and of the groin muscles to prevent injuries.

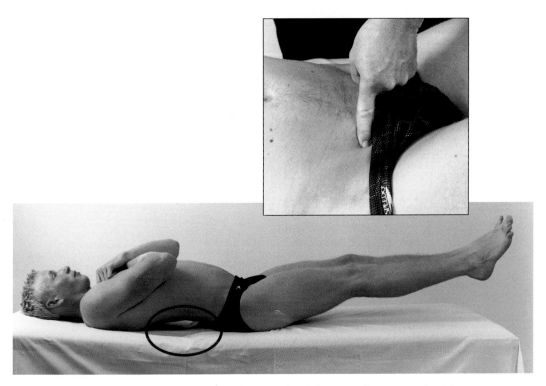

**Figure 3.25** Test of relative muscle weakness in the abdomen and groin muscles. The player lies on an examination couch and lifts his or her legs from the couch keeping them straight. If the player has weak abdominal muscles in relation to the thigh muscles, he or she will not be able to keep the lumber region of the lower back flat against the couch. If the lumber region arches considerably, abdominal weakness should be suspected.

On the occasion of the same test, the lower part of the abdomen should be palpated (the area around the annulus externus, the outer hernia port, see insert picture). If the player experiences pain this can be interpreted as abdominal weakness.

### Strain

Another possible cause of discomfort in the groin and abdominal muscles can be strain, or overuse. The origin/insertion of the muscles in the pelvis is placed under considerable strain during football — pain and soreness in muscles and the muscle root can therefore be an indication of general strain.

If individual players show signs of strained muscles, their pressure points should be analysed. This may be a question of a player who comes from a lower division and who is used to less training or players who have been away from training due to injury or illness etc.

If the pre-season check-up shows that several of the players in the squad suffer from muscle pain, then the coach should analyse the cause. Too many matches? Inappropriate training? Progressing with training too rapidly? Frequent changes of surface?

# Measuring mobility

Muscle tightness and reduced suppleness are associated with muscle injuries. By analysing the suppleness at a pre-season check-up and by recommending stretching and agility training to players with muscle tightness, the risk of muscle injuries later in the season can be minimized. For players who play outdoors, the occurrence of muscle tightness in the legs should be analysed.

The result of a mobility test will be more accurate if the examination is carried out by a physiotherapist or someone familiar with the procedure for such tests.

A rough assessment of whether a player suffers from muscle tightness in the legs can be made by using the Janda test. For example, an analysis of weakness in the muscles using the Janda test only provides a rough idea of whether there is muscle tightness in the leg. If one wishes to make a more accurate assessment or follow the results of agility training and stretching, mobility analysis should be conducted with accurate methods of measurement. Mobility measurements with considerable accuracy (only a 1–2 per cent error margin) can also be conducted at the clubs if standardized methods of measurement are used.

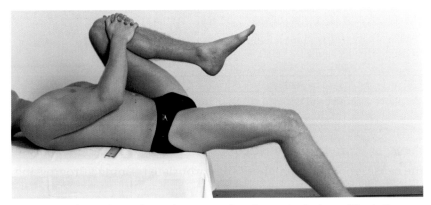

**Figure 3.26** The Janda test for analysing muscle tightness in the legs of footballers. The initial position is with the player lying on the examination couch with the legs over the short end of the couch. When one leg is bent at the hip and knee until the lumber area is flat against the couch, tightness in the muscle of the other leg can be analysed. The person carrying out the examination can check that the leg is bent correctly by placing a ruler between the couch and the lower back. The correct angle has been reached when the ruler is pressed between the lower back and the couch. If there is stiffness in the muscles bending the hip (the iliopsoas), the hip joint will also bend (the thigh cannot be held in position over the edge of the couch). If a 90° angle cannot be maintained in the knee, this indicates stiffness in the anterior thigh muscles. If the thigh is angled outwards (is abducted), this indicates stiffness in the outward angling muscle in the hip (tractus iliotibialis).

**Figure 3.27** Measurement of the outward angling (abduction) of the hip joint. The occurrence of muscle stiffness in the adductor muscles (pulling inward) can be analysed by measuring the outward angling of the hip joint. In order to obtain good results for this measurement, the pelvis should be stabilized. This can be done by having the player lie on his or her back on a couch with the leg which is not to be measured over the edge, with the knee bent at a 90° angle. The measuring device should be placed with one arm along the connecting line of the anterior illiacs (spinae). The other arm should be positioned along the length of the thigh.

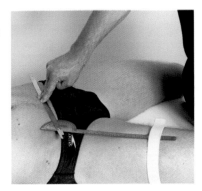

**Figure 3.28** Test to establish the bending capacity in the hip joint. The pelvis and the other leg should be stabilized using a band. The measuring device should be fastened to the outside of the thigh, 5 cm above the kneecap and the lower leg should be placed on the shoulder of the examiner. The player should be asked to relax. The leg is then bent at the hip joint while both of the examiner's hands are held against the player's knee. The measuring device should be read when the player starts to bend the knee joint.

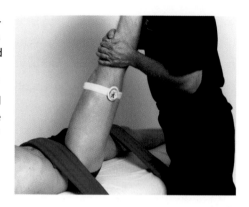

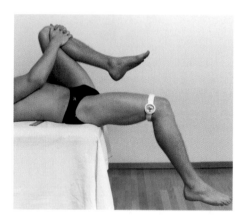

**Figure 3.29** Test to establish the stretching capacity of the hip joint. The measuring device is fastened to the outside of the thigh, 5 cm above the kneecap. The player grips the knee of the other leg and bends it at the hip joint until the lower back is pressed flat against the couch. The player should be asked to relax. The figure recorded on the device should then be read.

**Figure 3.30** Test to establish the bending capacity in the knee joint. The player lies on his/her stomach with the pelvis stabilized by a band. The measuring device is fastened above the outer ankle bone. The examiner bends the player's knee passively. The device is read when the player begins to bend at the hip.

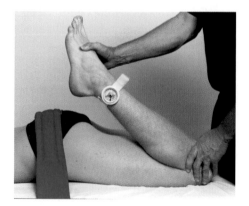

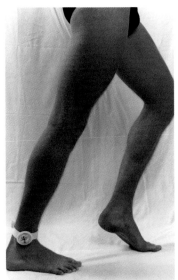

**Figure 3.31** Measurement of bending capacity of the ankle with the knee straight. The measuring device is fastened above the outer ankle bone. The player stands with feet facing forward, leaning against a wall. The player should be asked to continue bending the ankle by leaning more and more towards the wall. The examiner reads the device when the player either lifts the heel off the floor or starts to bend the knee.

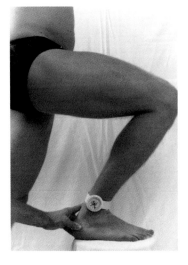

**Figure 3.32** Test to establish the bending capacity of the ankle with bent knee. The measuring device is fastened 5 cm above the outer ankle-bone. The player stands on the floor and places the foot to be measured on a stool. The player continues bending the ankle by bending forward. The device should be read when the player starts lifting the heel off the stool.

**Table 3.2** The normal values (in degrees) when measuring the range of flexibility and limit values for muscle tightness in footballers

|  | Normal value | Muscle tightness |
| --- | --- | --- |
| Outward angling in the hip joint | 37 | <31 |
| Bending of the hip | 78 | <70 |
| Stretching the hip | 74 | <63 |
| Bending the knee | 141 | <132 |
| Upward bending of the ankle, with straight knee | 23 | <18 |
| Upward bending of the ankle, with bent knee | 27 | <22 |

## One leg hop to test thigh muscle strength

As described earlier it is possible to measure thigh muscle strength with considerable accuracy with special advanced apparatus. It has been shown that jumping capacity (long jump and high jump) correlates well with the strength of the anterior thigh musculature. At the clubs, it is therefore possible to measure a player's capacity to jump on one leg to ascertain the strength of the anterior thigh muscles.

Players who have a sideways difference in the length of their jump exceeding 10 per cent (quotient right/left leg <0.9 or >1.10) and those who have the shortest jump in the squad should be given training advice for building up the strength of thigh muscles with the aim of preventing injury. A functional training programme consisting of interval cycling, knee bends on steps and skating jumps could be recommended.

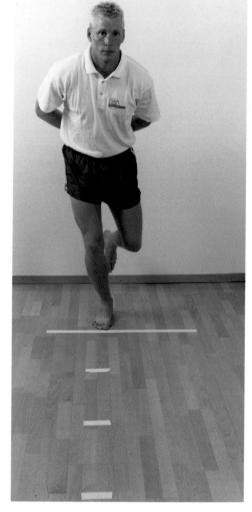

**Figure 3.33** One leg hop. The initial position is with the player standing behind a line marked on the floor. The hands should be held crossed behind the back. The player should then perform three one legged jumps on each leg. The best length for the jumps is recorded. The total length of the jump and the quotient between the right and left leg can be recorded.

# The POMS test

The link between psychological factors and performance and the risk of injury has been discussed earlier. The POMS test is a method for testing the state of mind. It is used in many sports to diagnose over-training at an early stage and is also used to assess mental factors which may be associated with injuries. During a POMS test, the player has to complete a questionnaire with 65 short questions. The questions describe feelings and state of mind and the answers are on a five-grade scale from 'not at all' to 'very much'. On the basis of the answers, six factors can then be established. See Figure 3.35.

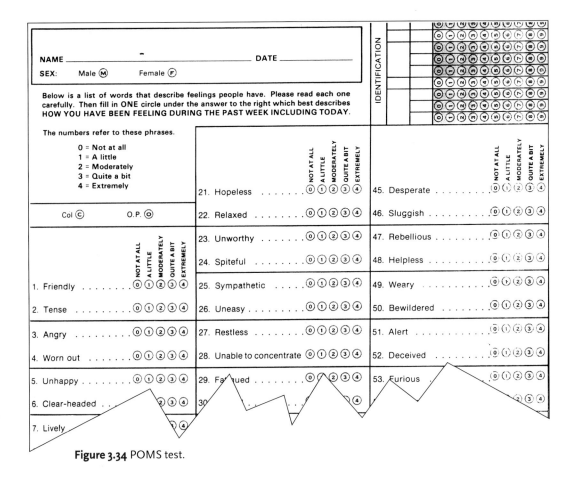

Figure 3.34 POMS test.

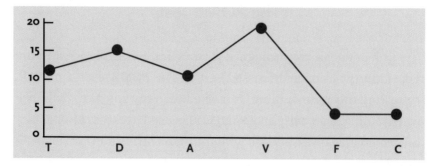

**Figure 3.35** Examples of test results for a POMS test. The scale along the Y-axis shows global POMS = G. T = tension, D = depression, A = anger, V = vigour, F = fatigue and C = confusion.

Sportsmen and women are characterized by a low total POMS result (low G) with more energy and lower levels of tiredness than non-sporting people (known as the iceberg profile). In cases of over-training, POMS is characterized by a high total result (high G), low energy and increased tiredness (reverse iceberg profile).

By allowing the team to take POMS tests regularly, a coach can follow the stress level of the team during the course of the season. Experience has shown that the degree of stress follows the level of mental tension. The POMS test also provides an opportunity to discover signs of over-training early among individual players. When interpreting the test results, one has to consider that the football factor, pressure in the form of training and matches, is only one form of stress. Other stress factors outside football may also affect the result. But general stress can also give rise to the risk of football injuries. It is important to find out how much stress attributable to football factors and to other factors for the POMS test to be of maximum use. A coach should therefore have a good relationship with the players and be sensitive enough to be able to evaluate the different test results.

# Giving advice

### Feedback for the individual player

When the tests have been carried out and analysed by the medical team, the test results should be evaluated and discussed with each player individually. Individual training advice can then be given using the test results as a basis. It is often useful to provide each player with a copy of the record of the tests with written comments and the individual training advice.

The tests done in connection with the medical examination should be seen as an aid to assessing the weaknesses of the individual player — they should not be interpreted as football performance factors on which team selection is based. The test results are intended for individual comparison, that is to say, the player should compare the latest results with his or her earlier results. A piece of advice to the person leading the testing is to inform the players of the test results individually along with, perhaps, an average result for the team as a whole so that the player can place his or her values in relation to an average. The formulation of a best and worst list should be avoided since these are medical test results and not football performance assessments.

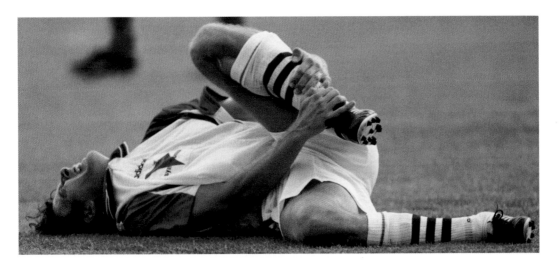

## Feedback for the team

The test results of the individual player and the findings from the medical examination can also be put together to establish a team result. The entire team's joint result should be discussed and analysed by the team personnel responsible, the coach and the medical team. If access to a database is available with earlier results from the same team or other teams, it is interesting to discuss the differences. Please note that the medical results of any individual player may not be made public or discussed without the player's consent. The common findings for the team can lead to changes in training, the planning of the season etc. Here are some examples:

• If the team has a number of players with ankle problems and a tendency to suffer from sprained ankles, it is probably useful to introduce balance training for the ankles during collective training sessions.

• If several players have or have had problems with symptoms of leg strain such as tendonitis or shin splints, it is worth discussing sole inserts for the whole team or analysing the amount of training or the surface.

• If several players suffer from groin problems, the causes can be discussed. If it is felt that the cause is weak abdominal muscles in relation to leg muscles, collective abdominal training can be considered. If the groin trouble is seen as a symptom of too much pressure due to too many matches or too much pressure from training, an analysis of the team's itinerary for the season should be made with a view to possible changes in activities to reduce the pressure of training.

• If the team has been affected by many injuries in connection with training camps, preventative measures can be introduced, for example, by revising the training programme during the camps, having access to medical personnel and by being aware of the early signs of strain/overuse.

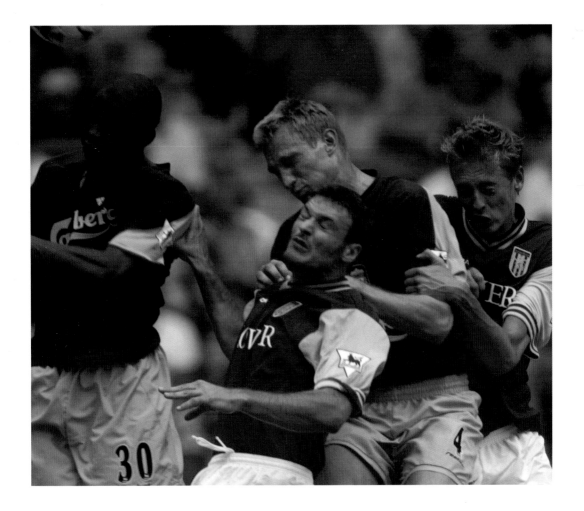

### Follow-up and checks

The results of the pre-season check-ups should been channelled towards a number of measures, partly individual training advice for specific players with weak points and partly possible changes in the collective training and planning of the season for the whole team. It is useful for players who are given individual training advice to have follow-up tests later on in the season so that their weak points can be eliminated. Since footballers often have a highly developed competitive instinct, a player is often encouraged to train hard if he or she can look forward to follow-up tests.

# 4. The biomechanics of football

Pekka Luhtanen

Biomechanical methods can be used to analyse and understand how different patterns of movement can be performed more efficiently with the aim of developing better football.

## Basic movements in football

With the aid of video or film recordings, it is possible to register the patterns of movement and the mobility of the players, their tactical behaviour etc. to study and analyse them in detail.

The following study of 20 professional football players shows that during a specific match they travelled an average of 9 km, with certain players travelling up to 14 km. The mobility, in terms of metres, was distributed as follows:

| | |
|---|---|
| Walking ........ ~ 3020 m | Backwards ..... ~ 875 m |
| Jogging ........ ~ 5140 m | Sideways ......... ~ 215 m |
| Trotting.......... ~ 1500 m | With the ball ... ~ 220 m |
| Burst of speed ~ 660 m | |

A player performed an average of 96 runs which varied between 1.5 and 105 m. One match included around 50 turns and jumps. As can be seen in the Chapter 5, this survey is generally representative of the physical nature of football.

The amount of maximum effort expended and number of completions is low for the average number of players during an entire match. If we assume that the number of matches in one season is 60 and the number of training sessions 220 (an average of five training sessions during 44 weeks) means that the average football player at top level accumulates 3000 km and takes 2.5 million running steps during a season. With these figures as a background we can see how important a factor the playing and training surface and boots are for the players.

Table 4.1 Football activities during matches and training during an entire season

| | Match | | Training | | Whole season | |
|---|---|---|---|---|---|---|
| | 1 match | 1 season | 1 training | 1 season | | |
| Activity | Dist (km) | Dist (km) | Dist (km) | Dist (km) | Dist (km) | No. of steps |
| Walking | 3 | 180 | 2 | 440 | 620 | 890 000 |
| Jogging | 5 | 300 | 4 | 880 | 1180 | 980 000 |
| Trotting | 1.5 | 90 | 3 | 660 | 750 | 290 000 |
| Speed | 0.7 | 42 | 1.5 | 330 | 372 | 130 000 |
| Other | 1 | 60 | 1.5 | 330 | 390 | 400 000 |
| Total | 11.2 | 672 | 12.5 | 2640 | 3312 | 2 690 000 |
| With the ball | 0.2 | 12 | 0.4 | 87.4 | 100 | |

**Number of respective moves during:**

During a top-level football match, there are 900–1000 different actions with the ball, 350 one-touch passes, 150 two-touch passes and the remainder with a greater number of touches or dribbling with the ball. Successful top teams need an average of 16–30 attacks and 7–10 shots to score a goal. An attack which is completed with a goal takes an average of 10–12 sec. The main difference between matches and training is that the training session includes more high intensity play on a smaller playing area with more ball contact, passes and running with the ball, starts, turns, jumps and tackles.

An estimate of the total volume of activities during an entire football year based on the registration of the different activities a player is involved in during matches and training sessions illustrates clearly how great the total load can be on a player during the year.

**Table 4.2** Football actions during matches and training along with the total for one season

| Number of respective actions: | | | | | |
|---|---|---|---|---|---|
| | **During match** | | **During Training** | | **Total** |
| | 1 match | 1 season | 1 training | 1 season | season |
| **Action** | no. | no. | no. | no. | no. |
| Passes | 35 | 2100 | 100 | 22 000 | ~ 24 000 |
| Runs with ball | 7 | 420 | 50 | 11 000 | ~ 11 500 |
| Headers | 6 | 360 | 15 | 3300 | ~ 3700 |
| Shots | 1 | 60 | 10 | 2200 | ~ 2300 |
| Tackles | 7 | 420 | 15 | 3300 | ~ 3800 |
| Jumps | 9 | 540 | 15 | 3300 | ~ 3800 |
| Turns | 7 | 420 | 30 | 6600 | ~ 7000 |

# Individual technique training is important

The contact time between the foot and the ball is on average 1/100 sec. A player has approximately 35 000 incidents of ball contact in 1 year which means that the total time for ball contact is only 35 000 × 0.01 sec = 350 sec = 5 min, 50 sec. This means that the importance of individual skill training is considerable.

## How does technique training work?

In all technique training external and internal feedback is very important. The sensors in the skin provide information about contact with the ball. The sensors in the joints (receptors for joint sensation) control the angle of the joint. The muscle spindles provide information about the length of the muscle and the Golgi apparatus senses the tension in the tendon. These mechanisms are active and interplay when the player carries out finely tuned and accurate movements such as passing, running with the ball, shooting etc.

The work of the muscles is controlled by the nervous system, that is, the brain, the spine and the nerve roots from the spine (Figure 4.1). The movements directed by will start from the cerebral cortex. Electric nerve impulses are sent out from the motor cortex of the cerebral cortex and travel to the nerve pathway in the spine via the central nervous system and reach the motor units (a motor neurone and the muscle fibres supplied with nerves from this neurone are referred to as a motor unit).

In muscles, joints and tendons there are sensors which register changes in the length of muscles and tendons, the angle of joints etc. Nerve impulses from these sensors are passed via nerve fibres to the central nervous system. This information is essential for the muscle activity to adapt rapidly even to minute changes in the mechanical strain. Other information from external sources such as sight and hearing impressions, can also influence this information. From the central nervous system the corrected movement signals are sent out to the muscles at work.

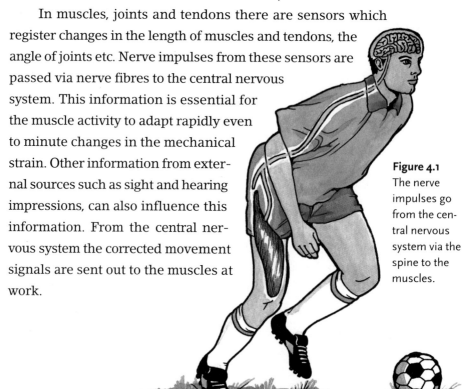

**Figure 4.1**
The nerve impulses go from the central nervous system via the spine to the muscles.

A footballer's basic movements are automated, in other words, they can be said to be pre-programmed in patterns of movement. Both figuratively and literally, most movements occur automatically 'in the stem of the brain'. These patterns of movement are probably both inherited and learned. Our will controls what is to be done while the pattern of movement controls how the task is done.

Patterns of movement, and therefore capacity and skill, can be modified through training. Training means that the player, with the aid of his or her will, adjusts patterns of movement by repeatedly going through the movement and concentrating on certain adjustments. An example of this is free kick training. However, too much control can have a negative impact on a simple movement. A penalty should probably be placed in the way that the coach has directed in advance — if a player attempts to carry out a pattern of movement which is not part of their repertoire there is a greater risk of failure.

The movements of the game of football are carried out with the support of inner feedback. Joint and muscle sense mean that the sensors in the muscles, joints and tendons provide information to the central control system. At central level this information is used in the spine, the cerebellum and in the reconnection stations in the brain. At these levels in the central nervous system the movements are adjusted primarily on the basis of learned patterns of movement and secondly on the basis of, significantly slower, control by the will. When a movement is performed the information is processed centrally and is used to control and modify the movement to achieve the aim. A large number of external and internal sources of information are used for this purpose.

During matches and training sessions the player makes a host of decisions on the basis of what she or he wants to achieve, and has the help of incoming stimuli from various sources. Unimportant information is sorted out and discarded while important data are used, mainly the information which has significance for a strategic decision.

**FEEDBACK**

## Internal feedback

Information about how the body's various parts relate to each other and how the external load will be absorbed by the internal structure.

1. The sensors in the joints (joint receptors) control the angle of the joint.
2. The muscle spindles provide information about the length of the muscle.
3. The Golgi apparatus in the tendon provides information about tension.

## External feedback

Information about how the body relates to the suroundings:

1. Sight
2. Hearing
3. Balance
4. Nerve ends in the skin provide the footballer with information about contact with the surface and with the ball.

In other words the skill of the footballer incorporates all aspects of the human nervous system and the external and internal feedback systems are important for efficient play.

# Biomechanics and skill in football

In both literal and figurative terms skill is the sum of four different biomechanical factors.

**SKILL =**

Force + speed + precision + purpose

A skilfully executed shot or pass means that all these four biomechanical factors have to be activated at the same time and in exactly the right combination.

## Force

The body is influenced by internal and external forces which exist in
equilibrium. By internal force we mean a force which is activated
within the player: 1) muscle/tendon force, 2) joint contact force and

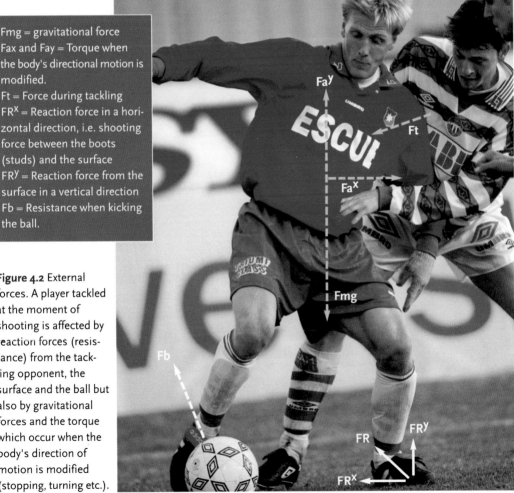

Fmg = gravitational force
Fax and Fay = Torque when
the body's directional motion is
modified.
Ft = Force during tackling
$FR^x$ = Reaction force in a horizontal direction, i.e. shooting
force between the boots
(studs) and the surface
$FR^y$ = Reaction force from the
surface in a vertical direction
Fb = Resistance when kicking
the ball.

**Figure 4.2** External
forces. A player tackled
at the moment of
shooting is affected by
reaction forces (resis-
tance) from the tack-
ling opponent, the
surface and the ball but
also by gravitational
forces and the torque
which occur when the
body's direction of
motion is modified
(stopping, turning etc.).

3) ligament/capsule membrane force. The external forces include: 1) reaction forces from the surroundings (ground, opponent, air, ball), 2) forces of inertia and 3) gravitational force. These internal and external forces balance each other. The sum of external strain (forces and torque) is balanced by the internal forces such as muscle/tendon forces, compression forces in the joints and tension forces in the ligaments and joint capsules etc.

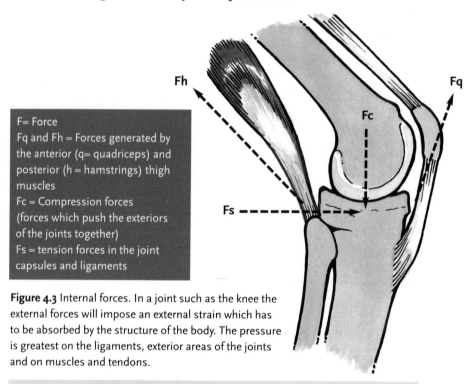

F= Force
Fq and Fh = Forces generated by the anterior (q= quadriceps) and posterior (h = hamstrings) thigh muscles
Fc = Compression forces (forces which push the exteriors of the joints together)
Fs = tension forces in the joint capsules and ligaments

**Figure 4.3** Internal forces. In a joint such as the knee the external forces will impose an external strain which has to be absorbed by the structure of the body. The pressure is greatest on the ligaments, exterior areas of the joints and on muscles and tendons.

## FORCE WHEN KICKING THE BALL DEPENDS ON

- The length and weight of the leg.
- Muscle strength in the leg and hip.
- The speed of the foot at the moment the ball is kicked.
- Muscle coordination (timing).
- Agility of the joints.

### Speed

In the human body, speed is created in the motion of the extremities (foot, hand, head) by means of a system of leverage via the joints. The speed of the body parts is dependent on the length and angle speed of the leverage arm in the joint located above it. The angle speed in each body segment is created by the muscles which function above the joints (the thigh muscles etc.).

### Precision

Precision, or the accuracy of the movement, is an important part of a player's skill.

### Purpose

Purpose means that the ultimate result is what was intended for that specific point in the respective match situation. Most of such points and manoeuvres in a match situation are carried out with sub-maximal force and speed but with high precision and purpose. The most successful actions in the game can be seen when the purpose of an action is unique and precision, speed and the exploitation of force is maximal.

## The biomechanics of the kick

The kick is an important movement for a footballer. When a hard shot is struck, a considerable quantity of movement is conveyed to the ball. The quantity of movement is created by the mass of the leg multiplied by the swinging speed of the leg.

A player with strong legs can shoot harder than a player with thin legs, on condition that both can create the same angle speed (or create the same speed) from the shooting leg. It is not only the weight and speed of the shooting leg, however, that is decisive for how hard the shot will be — it is also important that the shot creates a high impulse at the moment of impact. The impulse is created by the force multiplied by time. The longer the foot is in contact with the ball, the more energy is conveyed from the foot to the ball.

*The more efficiently the player transfers energy from torso to leg, from leg to foot and from foot to ball, the harder will be the shot.*

The role of the arms during a kick is to maintain the balance of the body, increase the moment of inertia in the torso and increase the resistance to rotation along the vertical axis of the body.

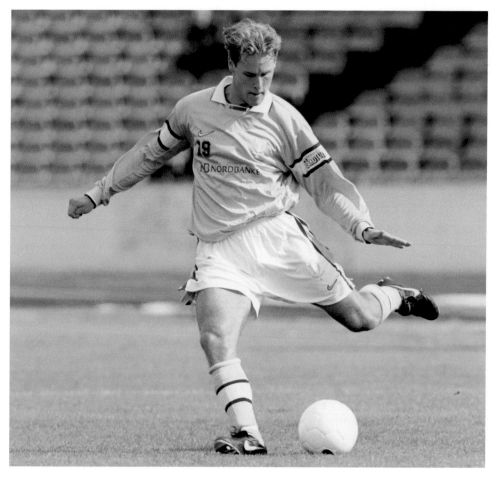

**Figure 4.4** The player shoots and leans away from the ball at the same time to extend the leverage in the shooting leg and thereby create greater force in the shot.

The ankle kick is the kick most often used for maximum force and length, both for shots at goal and for long passes. The force in the long kick is achieved by running up to the ball and from the movement of a maximum number of parts of the body — hip and torso rotation, bending of the hip, stretching the knee and bending the ankle.

A skilful footballer creates high ball speed by maximizing the angle speed of the thigh and lower leg while increasing the time taken for the kick. The longer the foot is in contact with the ball at the moment the ball is kicked, the greater the force conveyed to the ball. Compare the force in a 'toe kick' (short swing = short kick time) with a Brazilian free kick (long swing = long kick time).

Precision in the kick depends mainly on the contact surface between the foot and the ball. The bigger the ball, the greater the precision. Precision has been seen to be greatest when the speed of the ball is around 80 per cent of maximum.

The internal coordination of the movement is important in relation to the impact of the foot on the ball when the speed is maximized at the moment of shooting. Joints with good agility improve shooting capacity.

The greater the distance from the ball's centre to the centre of the active joints in the kick, the longer the leverage effect and speed

## THE SPEED OF THE BALL CAN BE INCREASED WHEN IT LEAVES THE FOOT BY

- Increasing the speed of the foot during the contact phase between the foot and the ball.
- Increasing the kick time (contact time between the foot and the ball).
- Leaning the body away from the ball.
- Balancing the body with the arms stretched out during the shooting motion.

of the kick. By stretching the leg out fully at impact and leaning away from the ball, the player increases the speed of the foot.

### Ball/foot speed in a kick

A good shooter can achieve ball speeds of 17–28 m/sec (60–90 km/h). Top speeds of 32–35 m/sec (115–125 km/h) have been recorded.

### Muscle activity in a football kick

An important aspect of a football kick is how the interplay between different muscle groups works. An agonist is a muscle which interacts with other muscles to achieve a certain movement. An antagonist is a muscle which brakes a movement, or which acts in the opposite direction from another muscle. When, for example, you bend your knee, the posterior thigh muscles act as agonists and the anterior thigh muscles as antagonists. A muscle or group of muscles can work alternatively as agonists (starting or carrying out a movement) or as antagonists (braking the movement).

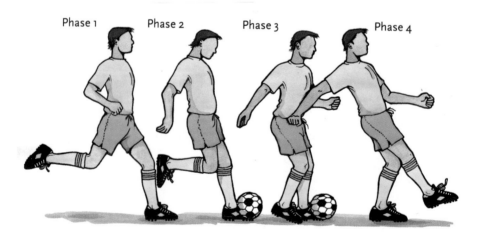

**Figure 4.5** Here we can see the most important active groups of muscles (anterior thigh and hip muscles along with the posterior thigh muscles) and the interplay between them during a football kick.

*Phase 1 – backward swing*

In the first phase of the kick, the backward swing of the leg, the posterior thigh muscles work as agonists. At the termination of the backward swing the movement is braked by an eccentric contraction (the muscle develops tension through being shortened) of the anterior thigh and hip muscles. These muscles function here as antagonists to brake the movement.

*Phase 2 – downward swing*

In the second phase, the downward swing towards the ball, the anterior thigh muscles are the agonists. The swinging movement towards the ball occurs as these muscles contract (develop tension and become shorter). The posterior thigh muscles of a skilful player are relaxed during this phase.

*Phases 3 and 4 – the kick and follow through*

When the ball is kicked and in the follow through movement, in some players the posterior thigh muscles (the hamstrings) dominate leading to the movement of the thigh and the knee being stopped suddenly. At the same time the kick is followed through by the hip bending further.

It is believed that the antagonistic activity of the posterior thigh muscles protects the knee in the same way as the posterior thigh muscles work together in contact with the surface of the joint of the thigh-bone. The posterior thigh muscles pull the shinbone back to stabilize the knee.

By comparing muscle activity in a football kick among skilful and less skilled players, what is important for the quality of the kick can be illustrated. Skilful players have more relaxed antagonistic muscles during the swing phase. Players who shoot hard can also generate more force in the anterior thigh muscles during this phase.

# Risk of injury when heading the ball

The header is unique to the game of football since very few ball games are played with the head. The risk of injury is minimal for adult players with good technique — they have sufficient skill and weight to resist the force of the impact. For children with a less developed heading technique and weaker neck muscles there is some risk of head and neck injuries, especially if the ball is heavy and wet. Children should therefore use smaller and lighter footballs.

The child's head is smaller and weighs less. Therefore, it is exposed to more forceful acceleration during the heading. At the same time the child has weaker neck muscles and, therefore, less strength to resist the damaging acceleration created by the impact.

## Heading technique

The ideal contact surface when heading the ball is the central part of the forehead. This is where the skull is thickest and the risk for pain at the moment of impact least. The forehead is also the flattest part of the skull and should increase precision.

As a player becomes more skilled at heading, other parts of the forehead can be used, or other parts of the head such as the side or the top. For example, a ball directed sideways to the head requires contact with one side of the forehead.

When the footballer jumps up, the movement diminishes as gravity reduces the speed.

At the moment of impact the amount of movement of the head depends on the amount of movement at the jump and at what height contact occurs. If the ball is touched at the same time as one leaves the ground the body will have, largely, the same speed as at the moment of take-off. On the other hand, if the ball is touched at the highest point of the jump, the vertical speed of the body will be zero, which means that the required amount of movement has to be created by the musculature of the torso.

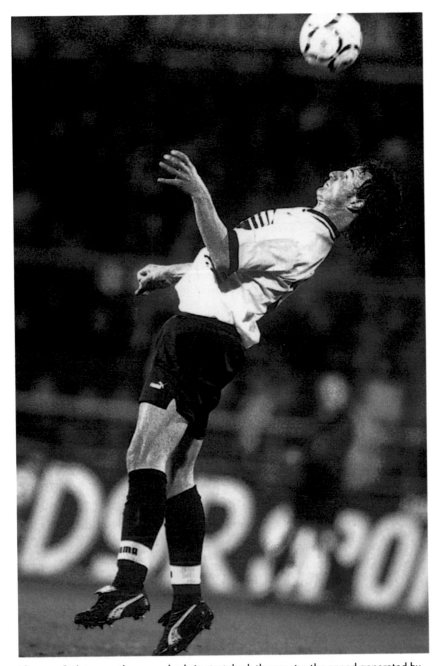

**Figure 4.6** The more the upper body is stretched, the greater the speed generated by the upper body and head in a forward movement. Force is created when the muscles which bend the torso (e.g. the stomach muscles) are contracted just prior  to contact along with the muscles which bend the hip and stretch the knee.

The body's movement when heading has been compared with a catapult where both the upper and lower parts of the body are extended backwards after leaving the ground. The stretch of the torso is probably an important factor in achieving stronger torso musculature in a standing jump and is like a curve.

# The throw-in

Two types of throw-in have been described in biomechanical studies: throw-ins with a short build up and long throws of over 30–40 m.

The long throw-in has been developed into a real offensive weapon in the game of football, especially in the vicinity of the opposing goal, since it is more precise than a corner kick. Many football teams have a player who can throw exceptionally long throw-ins that create opportunities for shots and goals.

The long throw-in demands energy which is created by a long build up or by using the whole body like a spring. The traditional throw-in relies on a rapid bending of the torso in combination with the stretching of the shoulders and elbow and the bending of the wrist to achieve force at the moment of the throw. The backward swing consists of over-stretching the torso, stretching the hip and bending the knee while bending the elbow and over-stretching the wrist. The player leans back and brings the ball as far back as possible. When the torso is propelled forward and stretched, the arms and the ball are placed as far as possible behind the head in relation to the body in the same way as the movement in a baseball throw or baseball strike. When the torso reaches its most forward position, its forward rotation stops and the arms and ball accelerate forwards. The elbows and wrists reach maximum angle speed at the moment the ball leaves the hands.

# Jumping

The ability to jump is important for players and for goalkeepers. A jump can be performed with or without build-up. A jump without build-up can start from the crouching position, the upright position with a downward stoop or with simultaneous movements with the arms. Laboratory tests from a standing position have shown that a footballer can jump around 50–60 cm when jumping using simultaneous arm action. Mechanically, the elastic energy created in the body in combination with the powerful hip and thigh muscles is exploited. A maximal jump does take a long time, however.

During a match the player has to be able to exploit the jump in relation to the situation. The timing of the jump and technical heading ability are important.

When jumping on one leg, the goalkeeper takes a long step on the take-off leg and both arms and the free leg accelerate upwards just before the leg lands. The take-off leg is then stretched forcefully to push the body in an upward direction towards the ball. Goalkeepers and players should be 'two footed', in other words, they should be able to reach maximum height regardless of which foot is used for take-off.

# 5. The physiology of football

Björn Ekblom

## The physical profile of the game of football

Football is a very complicated and exciting sport. It involves many different technical, tactical, psychological and physiological factors which affect the game and the players.

In order to be able to analyse the strain and physiological reactions of a footballer during a match, one needs to know the following:

- How much does the player move about the pitch?
- What sort of movement patterns are involved?
- Are there differences between players in different parts of the team?
- Are there differences between men's and women's football?

Top-level male footballers (with the exception of goalkeepers) walk and run on average around 10–11 km during the 90 min of a match. Central defenders run the shortest distances, then the forwards, and the midfielders run the most along with certain left or right backs. The same players cover approximately the same distances at every match despite different conditions. The greatest distance measured is just less than 14 km in 90 minutes.

Top-level women footballers run distances around 2–3 km shorter, at around 7–8 km, during a match. Male and female junior players (around 18 years old) do not differ significantly from older top-level players in this respect. No significant differences in distance have been noted between male teams in the Swedish Premier League and Divisions I, II and III.

During extreme climate conditions, such as in hot weather, the distances are clearly shorter. This indicates that football is a sport requiring high fitness levels, which are significantly affected by external conditions such as temperature, etc. The distances covered are somewhat shorter during the second half compared with the first. This indicates that tiredness developed during a match affects the patterns of movement.

During a match a player performs many different activities. In all, a player will 'change activity' up to 10–15 times/min, that is go from walking to jogging, from standing still to a rapid sprint, head the ball, receive and control the ball, etc. This movement profile does not differ between divisions or between genders, nor does it differ between younger and older players.

Top-level women footballers and male players from lower divisions make fewer sprints and headers and they also tackle less than top-level male players. The difference between top-level male players and players from lower divisions is, therefore, that the former run significantly faster. The same difference can be seen between women's and men's football at the same level, as well as between junior players and adult players of the same gender.

The physical profile of the game of football is characterized, in other words, by intermittent, non-continuous work with instances of very high intensive effort and interrupted movement patterns such as fast turns, tackling, heading and start and stop movements. The following conclusions can be drawn concerning the physiological profile:

- Match play – regardless of level, gender or age – places high demands on a series of different physiological factors.

## STUDY OF PLAYERS DURING A MATCH

- For more than 50 per cent of the time the player is standing or moving slowly.
- For 35 per cent of the time (around 30 minutes) the player is running or jogging at relatively moderate speed.
- The player sprints or bursts into highest speed for only 7–8 per cent of the time, around 7 minutes.
- The number of short bursts of speed of 2–4 seconds has increased in top-level men's football during the past 10 years from an average of 80–90 to 110–120.
- In addition to this, a player is involved in an average of 10–12 tackles and heads the ball slightly fewer times.

- External and internal influences of various kinds, such as tiredness and a cold or hot climate, affect the players and the game.
- The pattern of movement in different physiological training models need to be as similar to the match situation as possible to have maximum effect.

# Movement

The patterns of movement in football are affected by the impressions generated by the circumstances around the game. The player carries out a series of both (1) automatic and (2) conscious muscle activities.

1. In many commonly occurring situations during the game, the movements are automatic, for example when receiving the ball, feints and short fast movements. Sight and hearing as well as other

impressions affect this but these movements are carried out more or less automatically with considerable precision.

**2.** The conscious part of the footballer's pattern of movements is influenced by tactical considerations, sight impressions from team mates' and opponents' movements along with much else. The pattern of movement is therefore varied.

Top-level players are characterized by a combination of well coordinated automatic and conscious movements. The movements are nevertheless affected by a number of internal (for example, thoughts, feelings, tiredness) and external (for example, the spectators, the heat, the playing conditions) factors which means that the road to top-level play in general involves the young player experiencing many different situations — in other words, gaining experience.

# Muscle strength

Muscle activation is necessary for movements such as running, shooting etc. The muscles are activated via the nervous system. When the nervous system sends out signals via the spine and motor nerves, the muscles contract. The rate of the nerve impulses control the strength of the muscle contraction. The more the signals, the stronger the muscle contraction. Depending on which nerves are activated simultaneously, a movement occurs which can be controlled in the desired way in conjunction with the muscle strength exerted.

The result of the muscle activation depends on the resistance the movement receives. If the resistance is less powerful than the force of the muscle activation the muscle is shortened and concentric muscle activity is seen. If the resistance is overwhelming then it is a static contraction. If the resistance in the muscle is greater than the force in the muscle activation, which means that the muscle is extended despite being activated for contraction, the muscle develops eccentric muscle force.

As an example, the thigh muscle works concentrically in jumping action and eccentrically in braking action, when landing after a jump. When we stop the movement after jumping up, a static muscle contraction is developed. In football almost every movement includes a start and stop action, jumping and shooting — a combination of concentric, static and eccentric muscle movements. Various kinds of muscle strength can be trained separately in weight training but more important is that the patterns of movement that are practised are similar to those which occur during the game of football.

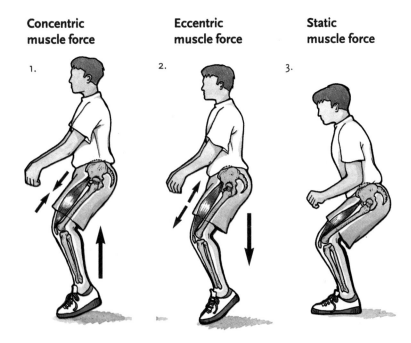

**Concentric muscle force**

**Eccentric muscle force**

**Static muscle force**

**Figure 5.1** The work of the thigh muscle during a jump (1), landing (2) and while standing still (3).

The strength in muscle development is a combination of the coordination of agonists and inhibition (toning down, relaxing) of the antagonists. All of these can be trained, mainly during the formative years. The surface and other factors such as tiredness, injury and other influences can disrupt coordination and strength development, which can then present a risk factor for muscle injuries.

The different movements within football involve a very complicated interplay between the activation of muscle groups and the relevant situation, that is the type of movement, the surface, the relation to the ball etc. The leg goes through a series of different movements involving concentric and eccentric movement during a shot. The jerking action in the muscle activity, especially in rapid movements, is probably a significant factor in the occurrence of certain muscle injuries.

### Fast and slow muscle fibres

A muscle contraction is effected through activity in the elements which make up the muscles, the muscle fibres. The muscle consists of two types of fibres — slow type I fibres and fast type II fibres. Type I fibres are slow and enduring. They can be trained to withstand high degrees of force developed over a long period of time. Type II fibres are generally larger than type I fibres. They are larger in men than in women and larger in people who do weight training than in those who do not.

### DIFFERENT TYPES OF MUSCLE FIBRES

| Properties | Type I | Type IIa | Type IIb |
|---|---|---|---|
| Contraction speed | slow | fast | fast |
| Force development | quite small | great | great |
| Endurance | high | quite high | low |

Type II fibres can be divided up into two sub-groups: type IIa and type IIb. Both permit rapid development of force and are characterized by considerable tendency to tire while type IIa fibres can be trained for greater endurance. With training many type IIb fibres become type IIa fibres which improves the endurance of the whole population of type II fibres at the same time as they retain their capacity of rapid development of force.

These fibres probably have considerable significance for fast movements of different kinds within football. Type IIb fibres function in very rapid corrective movements, such as in the case of wrong footing. If these fibres do not receive the correct information via the incoming (afferent) signals from the receptors in the joints, muscles and tendons, it is possible that no correcting muscle contraction would take place. This is a typically fast reflex-controlled muscle contraction.

During hard training the muscles have a tendency to 'become shorter'. Football places high demands on mobility and flexibility. Inhibited mobility could lead to impaired muscle function, which might increase the risk of muscle injuries since many football situations require large, rapid muscle contractions. Stretching exercises after warming up, matches and training sessions are therefore of great importance in the prevention of injuries.

## Different energy systems

Energy is needed for the body's muscles to be usable. Energy is stored in chemical form in the body as fat and carbohydrates (Figure 5.2). Before a movement can be affected, energy has to be transformed to mechanical energy .

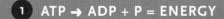
**1  ATP → ADP + P = ENERGY**

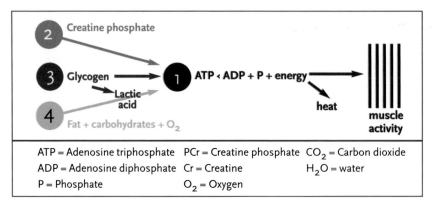

**Figure 5.2** Different energy systems.

The transformation of chemical energy to mechanical energy to be able to perform a movement occurs when the chemically stored energy ATP (adenosine triphosphate) is broken down to ADP (adenosine diphosphate) which releases energy. The speed of this process is very rapid. The amount of ATP in the musculature is small and is only sufficient for a few seconds of hard work.

The concentration of ATP in the musculature is largely the same in well-trained people compared with people who are healthy, but do not train at all. Nor is there any difference between men and women. However, the size of the muscle mass can be increased by weight training, which also increases the total amount of ATP in the musculature. With more ATP and increased muscle strength, the effect (speed and endurance) in fast movements can be improved.

Since the amount of ATP is small in the musculature, it has to be manufactured continuously to enable rapid muscle activity to be maintained. This occurs by energy being transformed by different pathways of the interactive energy system (see Figure 5.2).

### Energy turnover without oxygen (anaerobic function)

A. Creatine phosphate – 'quick charge'

**2  PCr → P + Cr + ENERGY**

The fastest way to recreate ATP is to use the energy obtained by the division of creatine phosphate (PCr) into creatine and phosphate. This process occurs without oxygen. Creatine phosphate is stored in the musculature. Well-trained footballers have a greater total amount of creatine phosphate than untrained people due to their greater muscle mass.

The speed of the division of creatine phosphate can possibly be affected by training. The total amount (but not the concentration) of creatine phosphate can be increased when type II fibres increase in size due to training. In this way the effect increases during activity. Creatine phosphate can be rapidly re-created with energy from other energy systems during repeated bursts of speed.

The diet can affect the concentration of creatine phosphate. Vegetarians have a lower level of creatine phosphate. Taking creatine in tablet form increases the concentration of creatine phosphate in the musculature. It is not clear whether this is an advantage in football since taking creatine increases the body weight. There may be greater disadvantages than advantages in an increased concentration of creatine phosphate. This is probably why several footballers take creatine regularly these days.

### B. An anaerobic breakdown of carbohydrates

### 3 GLYCOGEN → LACTIC ACID = ENERGY

Carbohydrates in food (potatoes, pasta, rice etc) are broken down into glucose (sugar) and stored as glycogen (long glucose chains or sugar molecules). If the sugar is broken down without access to oxygen such as during an explosive burst of speed, lactic acid is formed along with the necessary energy for the movement.

Lactic acid indicates that an anaerobic conversion of energy has occurred. The lactate itself does not have a negative impact on the muscle function but the hydrogen ions do. The anaerobic (without oxygen) generation of energy leads to a number of consequences which affect the muscle function in a negative way. Tests have clearly illustrated that the technique of a footballer is worsened when the level of lactic acid in the blood and muscles increases.

It is possible, however, to develop tolerance of anaerobic energy generation through training. To a certain extent, improved ability to withstand lactic acid depends on an increased buffer capacity — in other words, a greater capacity to neutralize the increased concentration of hydrogen ions. The greatest effect, however, is that the performance level is heightened as lactic acid starts to develop while at the same time the player can work harder without developing as much lactic acid.

### Energy renewal with access to oxygen (aerobic function)

Aerobic breakdown of fat and carbohydrates (and protein)

**4 FAT + CARBOHYDRATES + $O_2$ → $CO_2$ + $H_2O$ + ENERGY**

The most important source of energy during physical work is the aerobic renewal of energy. For hard-working muscles, exertion lasting for more than 10–20 seconds, oxygen is needed in the process. Fatty acids and sugar are broken down and release energy for the renewal of ATP. The speed of this process is relatively slow. The capacity of this energy system is high, however, since the amount of energy stored is high. The body's main energy depots are primarily fats.

*Burning fats*

The limiting factor for the burning of fat is probably the transport mechanism from the blood to the place where the energy is renewed in the muscle (the mitochondrion), possibly in combination with a disturbance in the generation of fat by various products which break it down. The access to fat is not a limiting factor and the additional fat in the diet has no value in football.

*Burning carbohydrates*

Carbohydrates (sugar) are stored in the musculature and in the liver. The muscle glycogen is stored in several places in the muscle cell. There are considerable numbers of glycogen granules at the point where the oxygen-demanding process of energy renewal occurs in the muscle which are exploited during hard physical exertion. When these stores have been used up, a lack of energy occurs and the muscles have to wait for the provision of carbohydrates from the blood or increased burning of fats. This leads to a drop in speed in the renewal of energy and lower endurance levels — the player is slower and feels tired.

Blood sugar comes partly from the liver and partly from food via the digestive tract. The longer a match has been underway, the greater the importance of this sugar supply carried in the blood. A diet rich in carbohydrates can increase the stores of muscle and liver glycogen. The better trained a player is, the better the ability to 'save' the muscle glycogen by increasing the burning of fat.

*Burning protein*

Amino acids create various proteins. Normally only a small amount of amino acids are used in generating energy since they have many other important functions to fulfil in the body. Whether or not the need for amino acids increases during exertion has been a topic of discussion for many years. As long as the energy requirement is provided for by carbohydrates and fat, the increase in the generation of amino acids during training and matches compared to while resting is probably small.

# System for transporting oxygen

In order to function optimally the working musculature requires a continuous supply of oxygen. This requires oxygen-rich (aerobic) energy production to take place.

The system for transporting oxygen is responsible for taking oxygen from the air via breathing, circulation and the blood, to the working muscles. The maximum oxygen absorption capacity is equivalent to what we normally rate as the 'fitness value' or the 'test value' and is measured in litres of oxygen per minute and kilo of body weight.

The system is no stronger than its weakest link and exactly which link represents the limitation has long been a point of discussion. These days it is widely believed that the maximum oxygen absorption capacity is mainly limited by the volume of blood the heart is able to pump per beat (the beat volume). The size of the

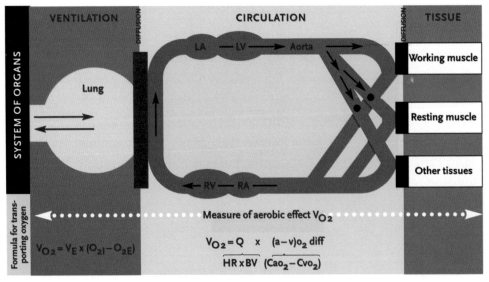

**Figure 5.3** System for transporting oxygen, LA = left atrium, LV = left ventricle, RA = right atrium, RV = right ventricle, Vo2 = oxygen intake, $V_E$ = ventilation, $O_{2I}$ and $O_{2E}$ = oxygen content in air being breathed in and out, Q = the minute volume of the heart, HR =heart rate, BV = beat volume, $CaO_2$ = oxygen content in the arterial blood, $CvO_2$= oxygen content in venous blood.

beat volume is different between individuals who have high and low maximum oxygen absorption capacity, that is, the impact of training lies in an increase in the size of the heart's beat volume. It has not been established whether hereditary factors alone are decisive for the development of the beat volume or what type of training is most important.

There are different ways of measuring the heart's capacity and function. One method is a simultaneous measurement of the oxygen intake, the heart rate and the blood pressure during physical exertion. The consumption of oxygen in the muscles rises parallel to the increase in the physical exertion. Breathing intensifies and the circulation is activated by collecting all the air exhaled and measuring the difference in the oxygen content in the air inhaled and the air exhaled.

## The heart rate

During exertion the heart rate rises relatively parallel to both the increase in exertion load and the absorption of oxygen up to maximum exertion. The maximum heart rate varies for different individuals. The average is around 200–220 beats/min (depending on age) for both fit and less fit younger men and women. The measurement of the heart rate shows how much pressure is placed on the circulation during exertion. Modifications in the heart rate during exertion can provide information about the changes in circulation functions and/or capacity. Training decreases the heart rate during exertion while nervousness, illness and tiredness increases it.

The adaptation of the circulation to exertion does not differ for men and women, nor does it differ between fit and less fit or young and adult footballers.

## Endurance

Endurance — that is, the length of time one can manage to work at a certain intensity — is the result of, among other things, how well the local circulation in the muscles functions, the capacity of the mitochondria and the access to glycogen. This can only be measured in samples from the muscle (a muscle biopsy). To get an indication of how good the adaptation to exertion is, it may also be possible to measure the lactic acid and other products from the breaking down process generating energy in the body.

**Body temperature**

When muscles work they produce heat. Only around 25 per cent of the energy renewal in the muscle is converted into mechanical energy — the rest becomes heat. The body temperature rises and the player sweats.

Surveys have shown that if a player works physically at a level equivalent to 50 per cent of the maximum oxygen absorption, the body temperature rises to around 38° C. If the exertion load is equivalent to 75 per cent of the maximum oxygen absorption capacity, the body temperature rises just as much if they exert themselves, relatively, just as hard.

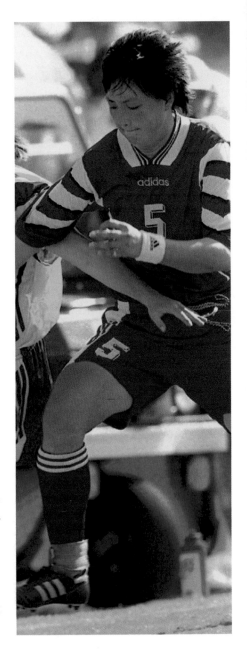

**Figure 5.4** During a match a player performs many different activities. In all, a player will 'change activity' up to 10–15 times a minute, e.g., from walking to jogging, from standing still to a rapid sprint, head the ball, receive and control the ball etc. This movement profile does not differ between divisions or between genders, nor does it differ between younger and older players.

This ratio can be used in assessing the average energy load during matches and training.

## Physiological strain during a match

In an analysis of physical strain during a match several methods can be used as discussed. The easiest method is to measure the heart rate.

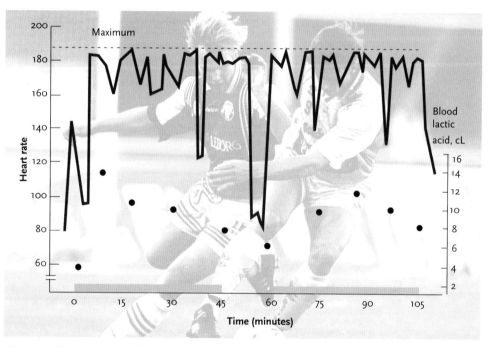

**Figure 5.5** The heart rate and lactate in the blood of a midfield player during a match in the Swedish Premier League.

Figure 5.5 shows that the heart rate is high during many parts of the match and reaches maximum rate on several occasions. The average heart rate during a top-level men's match is around 20–30 beats/min during maximum activity. There is no great difference between male and female top-level footballers or between players in the higher and lower divisions.

Measuring lactic acid concentration provides information about how much strain the player is subjected to during the match. Very high values, from 3–4 up to 10–11 mM (concentration of lactic acid in the blood) have been recorded during a regular match.

These high values show that the anaerobic generation of energy is placed under considerable pressure, mainly during the frequent bursts of speed and long stretches of running.

Measurements of the heart rate, lactic acid in the blood and body temperature show that the average strain during a top-level football match lies at around 75 per cent of maximum oxygen absorption capacity. The loss of 2–2.5 Kg through perspiration in a normal climate confirms this. In addition to this, the measurement of break down products of ATP show that very high peaks of strain occur during the game.

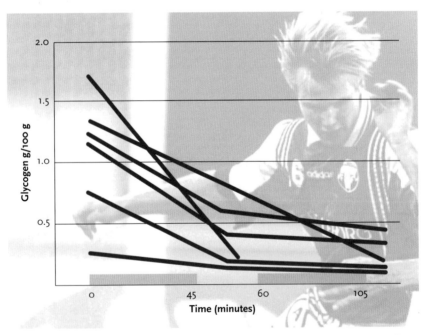

**Figure 5.6** Changes in the glycogen content of six players during a match. A muscle biopsy was taken before a match, at half-time and immediately after the match. The normal value is 1.0–1.3/100 g muscle.

An average top-level male player has a maximum oxygen absorption capacity of 4.5 l/min. If the average exertion is 75 per cent of this and the match including warming up is 100 minutes, the total energy generation for a male top-level footballer can be estimated at around 1700 calories per match. The strain for top-level female players is about 25 per cent lower (1200–1300 calories). The values for male junior players lie between these two values.

One consequence of the high energy turnover and the elements of high intensity exertion is that, for many players, the stores of muscle and liver glycogen are almost depleted by the end of the match.

Along with the considerable fluid turnover this shows that there are many physiological factors which affect the players during a match. This can lead to tiredness, impaired performance capacity, impaired technique and an increased risk of injury. The analysis of the energy strain during, primarily, a top-level match indicated the importance of good planning with regard to diet before and directly after the match including the supply of fluids and sugar during the match.

A further consequence of hard matches is that the player loses a certain amount of speed and endurance and the muscle strength becomes slightly less. The physiological factors behind these developments which impair the performance capacity are not known in detail but they should be taken into account in the planning of training after tough matches.

## A physiological profile of the football player

There is no ideal physical constitution for a footballer. Goalkeepers and central defenders should not be very short since this could lead to difficulties dominating the air space in the penalty area. It is, however, obvious that carrying excess weight is a disadvantage in a sport like football which demands fitness. Different players and different types of play should, to a certain extent, follow different training programmes. A short and relatively slim and fast forward or midfield player probably has little benefit from weight training which leads to muscle growth and an increase in the body mass. A large, heavier central defender would benefit from such training to be better able to control a heavier body.

Energy generation is an important aspect with regard to physiological demands. Anaerobic capacity is largely dependent on active muscle mass. Training practice (start and stop, five-a-side games etc.) which result in an increase in the muscle mass also lead to increased anaerobic capacity.

The maximum oxygen absorption for a top-level male footballer is around 60–65 ml/kg/min but the variations are great. Midfield players have higher values than defenders. Many junior players in the top-level junior teams have around the same values as top-level adult players of the same gender.

## Testing physical performance capacity

There are many reasons for using the various physiological and medical tests. The latter may be important to establish a medical profile when the player is healthy and in good form — for instance an ECG (registering the heart's electrical activity) during exertion, the iron status value and the values for haemoglobin in the blood, flexibility and the status of the joints (see Chapter 3).

During physiological tests it is useful to:

- Test the physical performance capacity.
- Predict performance capacity.
- Follow changes in performance capacity.
- Direct the training.
- Study the impact of different external and internal factors on the performance capacity etc.

## PHYSICAL PERFORMANCE CAPACITY IS DICTATED BY THE FOLLOWING FACTORS

1. **Energy yielding processes**
   The capacity for energy generation without the need for oxygen (anaerobic capacity)
   Maximum oxygen absorption
2. **Neuromuscular function**
   Muscle strength
   Coordination
3. **Psychological capacities**
   Determination, concentration etc.

Occasionally a coach wants to 'test' a player without having any clear idea about what the test results could be used for. It is unclear whether it is possible to direct training or predict performance capacity by using tests. It can, however, be of considerable interest to follow any changes in performance capacity over a period of time.

Generally it can be said that it is important during testing to select the method according to the questions posed. It is important to know what is to be examined or explained by means of the test and on this basis select the appropriate method. The test should be relevant for the type of sport, have a small margin of method error, the conditions around the test should be capable of being standardized and finally — the test should be accepted by the players.

Establishing physiological capacity with good precision can only be done in a laboratory. Maximum oxygen absorption, the anaerobic capacity test (the Wingate test) and measuring muscle strength are examples of what can be established in a laboratory. Few trainers or teams have such facilities. Therefore, practically adapted tests for football are better.

## The beep test

The beep test is a progressive intensity test which involves the player following instructions on a cassette and running between two lines 20 m apart. The speed of the running is controlled by signals — 'beeps' — so that the player turns at the line on each signal. As the test continues, the signals come at shorter and shorter intervals. By the end, the player doesn't manage to reach the turning line by the next signal and therefore has to stop the test. The result is presented as the level of beep speed when the player was forced to stop.

The test measures all the factors, more or less, that have been discussed concerning physical performance capacity. There are as yet no established values for the beep test which are not relevant for football. Individual values show good correlation with the maximum aerobic effect recorded on a treadmill at the same testing session. In a successful top-level football club, the average values of the A-team in January 1998 were around 13 and rose to 15–16 during the spring season. The test can be used to follow the development of training but there is a high stan-

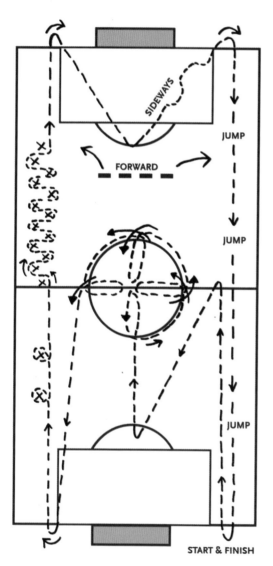

START & FINISH

**Figure 5.7** An example of a test route.

dardization requirement. Different surfaces and inappropriate weather conditions can affect the result in the same way as if the test is carried out the day after a hard training session or a match. The test is otherwise easy to use and the reproducibility is good. It takes about 10 minutes to carry out the test and is generally well accepted by players. There are other tests with movements specific to football. The test in Figure 5.7 is based on a player running a test course as quickly as possible.

The advantage of this test is that it contains different patterns of movement such as running sideways and backwards, turns and jumps. The disadvantage is that it is rather complicated and takes time to conduct.

Training has the effect of reducing the time taken by the player to run around the whole test course (in the beep test the number of levels increases). A player who had suffered a serious injury was away from training for 1 month (Figure 5.8). When he was ready to

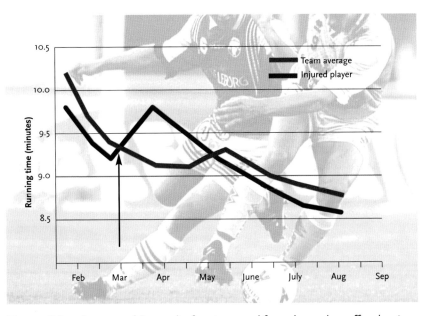

**Figure 5.8** Development of the results for a team and for a player who suffered an injury (at the arrow point).

train again, his results were the same as they were the start of the season but the rest of the team had improved. As can be seen from the red line in the figure, it took the player around 3 months to reach his previous level relative to the average for the team. This agrees with experience — it takes a well-trained player who has had to take a longer break in training around three times the 'injury time' to reach the functional level he had before the interruption caused by injury.

## Speed

The speed test from a standing position or with a flying start between 15 and 40 m can be used. The measurement of such a short time period — a few seconds — requires electronic timing equipment and well standardized test conditions.

Among the top-level players in a team, the times do not differ widely especially over such short distances — often no more than 10–15 hundredths of a second. Therefore, sprint tests of this kind cannot definitely identify the players considered fast on the pitch since speed during a game includes several different components. By speed we mean fast movements over restricted areas. These cannot be measured in sprint tests of running forward in a straight line — tests have to be used in which the players make both fast turning movements and short distances running. By speed we may also include the ability to 'be first on the ball'. This means for the most part the player is well able to predict the path of the ball, has good timing and a quick start — in brief, the player can 'read the game'.

## Elasticity

Elasticity is an important element in football. To be able to jump high in a dual in the air involves a number of qualities, in the same way that speed involves several abilities, namely timing, 'being first on the ball', elasticity etc. The latter can be tested using the jump

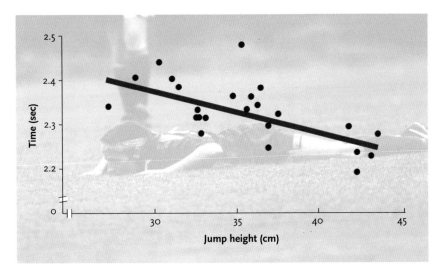

**Figure 5.9** The correlation between the height of a jump elasticity test and time in a 15 metre test.

test which measures how high a player can lift the body's central point. On average, top-level male footballers reach a jump height of around 50–55 cm and top-level women footballers reach around 30–35 cm. There is a certain correlation between the jump height test result and the result of the speed test which indicates that there is a relation between leg muscle strength and speed.

# 6. Nutrition and football

Björn Ekblom

The turnover of energy during training and matches is high. So a player's nutritional intake — for several reasons — is of great importance. It is essential that the player maintains good energy balance over long periods of time to ensure optimal development as well as to prevent various health problems. As soon as the energy balance is negative, problems arise. New studies show, for example, that a negative energy balance for long periods of time weakens the body's immune system and that the strain on the musculature and other organ systems increases.

A top-level male footballer who trains 5–6 days each week and plays a match once a week should have an average total energy intake of at least 3000 –3500 cal/day, depending on the body size and physical activity. Top-level female footballers have a daily requirement around 500–600 cal less than their male counterparts. It is difficult to ascertain with accuracy if a player has a good energy balance, but if a player with normal body weight maintains this for a long period of time, this is a clear indication that the energy balance is normal. Slight variations in body weight within the course of a few days can occur among both men and women.

Experience suggests that younger players in particular can have a negative energy balance. For various reasons they often eat irregularly and have a number of situations exerting a negative influence in their everyday life which causes them to eat too little. Keeping a record of the diet for 1 week is a simple way of checking this. Not until the correct quantities for energy requirements have been fulfilled should the qualitative aspects of diet be taken up.

# Sources of energy

Of all the energy rich substances — protein, fat and carbohydrates — carbohydrates are the most important since the glycogen stores in the liver and muscles are low after hard training and especially after a match. This means that the carbohydrate content in the diet on the days before a match should be high. Pasta, rice, potatoes and bread provide the most important sources of carbohydrates in the diet.

Previously a diet was recommended which began with 2–3 days of hard training and a low intake of carbohydrates and then switched to a diet with a high level of carbohydrates during the final 2 days. This type of carbohydrate boost is not necessary. A well-trained player has a heightened concentration of muscle glycogen if the meals after the final training session before a match include a high proportion of carbohydrates.

The process of storing glycogen in the musculature is slower after eccentric exertion. Since such exertion represents the greater

## THE ENERGY BALANCE AND NUTRITIONAL REQUIREMENTS

- The body has a good energy balance when the consumption of energy (over a long period of time) is no greater than the energy supplied to the body — *the energy requirement* is satisfactory.
- The body also places qualitative demands on the energy intake. The diet should include the essential nutritional substances — *the nutritional requirements* — to be satisfactory.

part of playing football it is possible that the player has a lower stock of glycogen than normal during periods of hard training. This can be one reason why many players are tired and worn out after tough training camps and/or several consecutive matches. Different surveys support the idea that a diet rich in carbohydrates has a positive effect on performance capacity while playing football.

### Meals in conjunction with matches

The meal eaten just hours before a match should be 'light' since the potential for increasing the glycogen content in the muscles is marginal.

After the match and training sessions, when the glycogen content in the musculature is low, the capacity for building up the muscles' store is significantly increased. After a few hours this increase in storing capacity declines. Therefore, it is recommended that players take, for example, a carbohydrate drink or eat bananas, which contain carbohydrates, as soon as possible after concluding their activities.

A snack or drink of 75–100 g of carbohydrates should be consumed within the first 30 min after a match or hard training session. This should be complemented by a well-balanced meal including

**BEFORE A MATCH**

- Main meal, such as lunch or dinner, around 3–4 hours before.
- Light snack, around 1–3 hours before.

**AFTER A MATCH**

- Carbohydrate diet or drink directly after the match (within 30 minutes) such as a banana or sports drink.
- Complete meal one or more hours later to reinforce the supply of carbohydrates.

carbohydrates, protein, fat and vitamins after an hour or so. In this way the glycogen depots in the muscles can be replenished within 24 h, which is of considerable significance during periods of hard training and matches.

# Fluids

During a match the carbohydrate stores are used up. Since the need for fluids is also great, it is appropriate for several reasons for the players to drink fluids which contain sugar as often as possible during matches. Endurance increases if a sugary drink is consumed compared with water. The players' concentration and precision are also improved. A study carried out in Britain showed that teams which received sugary drinks scored more goals and conceded fewer goals than when they drank only water.

The drinks should contain at the most 5–7 per cent sugar along with a little salt (sodium). The latter enables easier absorption of water in the small intestine. If the concentration of sugar and salt is too high along with any flavour additives in the drink, this can have a negative effect and prevent the fluid from leaving the stomach.

A player can have a sugary drink before and after warming up in connection with a match. Earlier fears that a sugary drink could have negative effects on the performance capacity if drunk before a match have not been confirmed.

# The protein requirement

Proteins are the 'building blocks' of the body and are used, among other things, to construct muscle tissue. During rest, the need for protein is around 0.7 g/kg/day — in other words 50–60 g for an adult. Since a normal diet has a relatively high content of protein the

## DRINKS DURING TRAINING AND MATCHES

- A player's basic requirement for fluid intake is 2–3 l/ day.
- Thirst signals are not a good indication of how much fluid the body needs.
- The fluid a player drinks during a match should contain up to 5–7 per cent sugar since this affects both the concentration and the precision positively.
- Drinking continually during the day, that is, not just during meals, helps the body maintain its fluid balance.

daily intake can be up to 100 g. The difference between the generation and consumption of protein and the protein intake is therefore rather extensive. The protein requirement increases somewhat during light training but does not reach especially high levels provided that the player has a good energy balance. During hard and intensive training periods the need for protein increases further but not at the same rate as the consumption of energy. This means that the difference between the protein requirement and the intake of protein increases. The more the player trains, the greater the difference. Despite this, there is no need for an extra supplement of protein in the form of tablets, powder or similar.

If the player's energy balance is negative, amino acids (protein is made up of different amino acids) are used as a source of energy. Milk, meat, many vegetables and cereal products contain most of the amino acids the body needs. The risk of the energy balance becoming negative is greatest for women and younger players. If this negative energy balance continues for a long period, the player loses the effects of training and the risk of injuries and illness increases.

Another aspect to consider is the types of amino acids in the diet. A relatively new theory states that what are known as branch chain amino acids are used by the musculature to a greater extent than other amino acids during physical exertion compared with a state of rest. As a result fewer branch chain amino acids remain in the blood. This means that the aromatic amino acids dominate the supply to the brain. These aromatic amino acids are substrate signaling substances in the brain (neuropeptides) which are related to tiredness and possibly to other reactions such as physical fatigue.

This theory may explain what is known as central fatigue during long-term exertion. On the pitch this may be expressed in not being able to maintain concentration on the game, 'hiding' and 'not wanting the ball'. The intake of branch chain amino acids may be able to counteract these signals of fatigue. Some experiments suggest that this may be the case but further studies are needed to verify this. Branch chain amino acids are found in meat etc, but are added specifically in certain sports drinks.

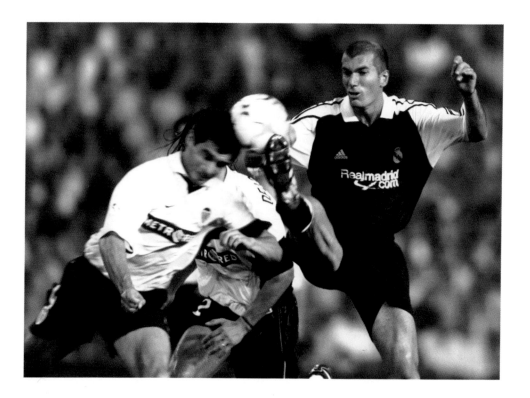

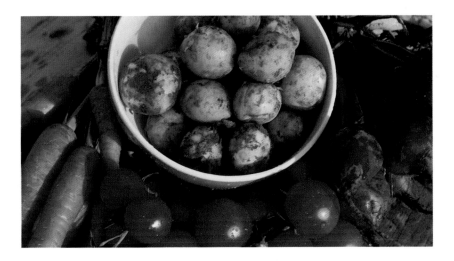

# Vitamins and minerals

The discussion of the requirement of vitamins and minerals in sport has been lively. This is partly due to the prevalence of faith in the effects of food supplements and partly due to a belief that supplements of vitamins and minerals are largely harmless but that one may as well take a supplement 'just in case'. None of these explanations can be accepted any longer.

There is much support for the view that a footballer whose energy balance is good has a higher intake of most vitamins and minerals than are utilized. The background to this is that the absorption of vitamins and minerals increases with an increase in the energy turnover if the player has a good energy balance. The exception to this is iron. The absorption of iron from food in the intestine is normally relatively low. Only 10–15 per cent of the available iron is absorbed. The absorption can be increased if, for example the food contains a lot of vitamin C. On the other hand, other components of the diet, such as wholemeal bread and tea, can inhibit absorption.

Iron is lost in small amounts in perspiration and urine as well as via bleeding in the stomach and intestinal tract. The proportion of anaemic sportsmen and women is no higher than among the population in general. This would support the view that training in itself cannot cause a lack of iron.

Women who experience heavy bleeding during menstruation may suffer from a lack of iron. It may therefore be valuable to check the ferritin (a substance which indicates how large the iron stores are in the body) and the haemoglobin values of menstruating girls and women involved in sports. If anaemia is diagnosed, supplementary iron should be taken in tablet form. To give additional supplements to a player who has not been found to suffer from lack of iron is irresponsible. An overdose of iron can have several negative effects.

There is no evidence to support the view that a sportsman or woman who has a normal diet and a good energy balance should be suffering from a lack of various minerals such as copper, zinc, magnesium etc. Selenium has been discussed for its effect as an anti-oxidant since there is a low natural occurrence of this mineral in Scandinavia. There have been no convincing studies to date which confirm that sportsmen and women might require an increased quantity of selenium.

A lack of vitamins is unusual in Europe. It is very likely that the total supply of vitamins, in common with most minerals, is greater than the utilization of these substances in the energy balance.

The theory that an extra supplement of vitamins may increase performance capacity if the basic requirement is covered has not yet been confirmed. This includes, among other things, carnitin, an excess of which is thought to increase fat depletion during exertion and therefore improve endurance. Supplements with carnitin are common in Italian football but studies have not proved the positive effects. Vitamin E has also been claimed to improve performance capacity but this has not yet been confirmed.

An excess of vitamins A, C and E are taken these days with the justification that they are able to counteract the occurrence of what are known as free oxidant radicals — which function in the same way as antioxidants. This theory is interesting but the number of studies is insufficient and the results contradictory to be able to permit us to establish any possible positive effects.

Another antioxidant is ubequinone (Q10) a substance which has many effects in the body and which is of interest during physical exertion. Q10 has a very important function in the mitochondria of the muscles and is also an important antioxidant in, for instance, different cell membranes. Considering that football places extensive demands on both anaerobic (creating lactic acid) and aerobic (requiring oxygen) energy generation, Q10 might possibly be of interest in preventing the damaging effects of oxidant radicals.

There is currently no evidence that supplements comprising antioxidants are able to prevent the occurrence of disease.

## SUMMARY

- A diet rich in carbohydrates has a tangibly positive effect on the physiological performance capacity.
- A player with a good energy balance does not require any food supplementation with the exception of iron.

# 7. The use of nutritional supplements in football

Ronald J Maughan

## Introduction

A number of physiological, biochemical, psychological and nutritional factors that may limit performance have been identified. In the pursuit of success, players and their scientific and medical advisers seek to identify ways to minimize their potential impact on the player's ability to exercise his or her skills. Nutrition cannot compensate for lack of skill, but it does have some scope to help players realize their potential. Foods and food components that can improve the capacity of an individual to perform an exercise task have been described as ergogenic aids. At one end of the spectrum of ergogenic aids are normal foods and at the other are substances that are clearly drugs: in between, however, are a number of compounds that are more difficult to classify. The term includes a number of foods, for example, those high in carbohydrate and carbohydrate-electrolyte sports drinks, whose effectiveness in improving exercise capacity is beyond doubt. It is, however, usually applied to specific nutrients or compounds rather than to whole foods.

Players who use nutritional supplements often consume these in amounts far in excess of those normally ingested. They are primarily concerned with the effectiveness of any supplement used. The amount and timing of supplementation and the specific exercise conditions under which its effects may be optimized must be considered. A second concern relates to whether there is a possibi-

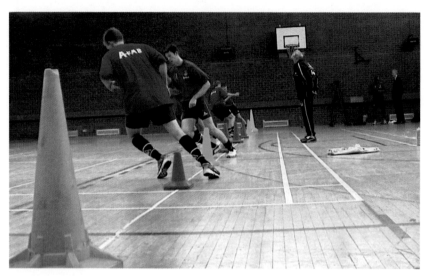

**Figure 7.1** Players train hard to improve fitness and it makes no sense to train hard without making sure that good nutrition strategy is in place.

lity of contravening the rules imposed by the governing bodies of sport, which might lead to suspension from competition. Third, and perhaps most importantly of all, the question of safety of supplementation must be considered.

As a general principle, it is safe to assume that most supplements that are effective are against the rules of the sport: this category includes drugs, pro-hormones and hormones. Any player who is liable to be called for a drugs test must recognize their responsibility for everything they eat or drink, as lack of awareness does not excuse inadvertent doping. Most substances that are not banned are not effective, and this includes most of the vitamin and mineral supplements as well as the herbal products sold in health food shops. There may, however, be some exceptions to these generalizations, and some supplements have been shown to have potentially beneficial effects. There are also grey areas, sometimes referred to as 'nutraceuticals', including compounds such as caffeine that are components of day-to-day foods but which are consumed in large doses for their pharmacological actions.

It is important to recognize that an increase in muscle mass or an improvement in stamina does not necessarily translate into an improvement in performance. It is also not possible to review all of the nutritional supplements used by players, or to consider in any detail the evidence relating to more than a few. However, consideration of some specific examples will illustrate the general principles that determine usage and the evaluation that should be applied to these supplements. This review focuses on three main categories of supplements: those that affect energy production and metabolism; those that may influence muscle hypertrophy and lean body mass; and those that can influence general health.

# Supplements that may influence energy metabolism

### Creatine

Creatine has been used by many successful athletes, and in recent years, its use has been widespread in football. Some indication of the extent of its use is gained from the fact that the estimated sales of creatine to athletes in the United States alone in 1997 amounted to over 300 000 kg. This represents a remarkable growth, as its use first became popular in sport after the 1992 Olympic Games in Barcelona. What distinguishes creatine from other ergogenic aids is that it seems to be effective in improving performance but is not banned by any of the international sports organizations, although its use has been prohibited by the French Football Federation.

*Metabolic role of creatine*

Most (95 per cent) of the body's creatine is present in skeletal muscle, and approximately two-thirds of the total is in the form of creatine phosphate. Creatine phosphate (CP) itself is present in resting muscle in a concentration approximately 3–4 times that of ATP, the immediate energy source for muscle contraction. Because muscle fatigue is associated with decreased intracellular ATP concentrations, regeneration of ATP at a rate close to that of ATP breakdown is essential to delay fatigue. The creatine kinase (CK) reaction is extremely rapid, and makes a significant contribution to the energy supply necessary for brief bursts of very high intensity exercise. The average sprint in football lasts less than 2 sec, and CP will be an important energy source, especially when the recovery between sprints is incomplete. Increasing the CP content of muscle may allow more work to be done using this energy source. In high intensity exercise, lactate (lactic acid) accumulates within the muscle. The hydrogen ions associated with lactate production cause the muscle to become more acidic, and this acidity is one of the reasons for fatigue in sprinting. An increased availability of CP for breakdown will increase the muscle buffering capacity (the CK reaction consumes a hydrogen ion), delaying the point at which the pH reaches a critically low level.

### Creatine supplementation and muscle CP concentration

Creatine occurs naturally in the diet, being present in meat: 1 kg of fresh steak contains about 5 g of creatine. The normal daily intake of meat-eaters is less than 1 g, but the estimated daily requirement for the average individual is about 2 g. The body can synthesize creatine in the liver, kidney, pancreas and in other tissues. This supplies the amount required in excess of the dietary intake, and is also the only way in which vegetarians can meet their requirement. Studies of resting human skeletal muscle have shown the CP concentration to be about 75 mmol/kg dry weight and the free creatine concentration to be about 50 mmol/kg. There is, however, quite a large range of values reported in the literature, and it seems clear that there is considerable inter-individual variability. There is some evidence that the muscle creatine content is higher in women than in men. The first study to investigate the effects of supplementation systematically of large amounts of creatine was conducted in 1992. They showed that ingestion of small amounts of creatine (1 g or less) had a negligible effect on the circulating creatine concentration, whereas intake of higher doses (5 g) resulted in a large increase. Repeated intake of creatine (5 g four times/day) over a period of 4–5 days resulted in a marked increase in the total creatine content of the quadriceps muscle. An increase in muscle creatine content was apparent within 2 days of starting this regimen, and the increase was greatest in those with a low initial level: in some cases an increase of 50 per cent was observed.

*Effects of creatine supplementation on exercise performance*
There are only a limited number of scientific studies which have reported the effects of dietary creatine supplementation on muscle function and exercise performance, and even fewer have looked at an exercise model that resembles the pattern of play in football. From these results, there appears to be no beneficial effect on the peak power output that can be achieved in a range of tests, but the balance of the available evidence suggests that performance is improved in high intensity exercise tasks, especially where repeated exercise bouts are carried out.

*Creatine and muscle strength*
There have been numerous investigations into the effects of creatine supplementation on the ability to generate high levels of muscle power, but only a few studies have looked for possible effects on muscle strength. This is surprising in view of the importance of a high force-generating capacity for the development of power. It was shown that 5 days of creatine supplementation was effective in increasing maximum voluntary isometric strength of the knee extensor muscles in individuals engaged in strength training programme. This gain was maintained in a subsequent test after a period during which a placebo was administered. In a second group

of subjects, the treatment order was reversed: no gain in strength was seen after the first period of placebo administration, but an increase was observed in the third test, after the creatine supplementation period. Isometric endurance capacity at various fractions of MVC was also increased after creatine supplementation but was not affected by the placebo treatment.

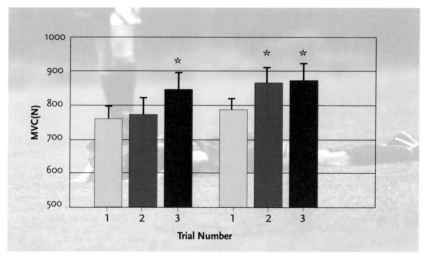

**Figure 7.2** Effects of creatine supplementation on muscle strength. Subjects received either placebo followed by creatine (Group A) or creatine followed by placebo (Group B) for 5 days. Significant increases in strength were observed after creatine supplementation. From Maganaris and Maughan (1998).

### Creatine and body mass

Many studies and anecdotal reports support the suggestion that acute supplementation with creatine is associated with a prompt gain in body mass. This typically seems to amount to about 1–2 kg over a supplementation period of 4–5 days, but may be more than this. In reviewing those studies where changes in body mass were reported, 11 studies where body mass increases were shown and three where no change in mass was reported. Because of the rapid increase in body mass, it must be assumed that this is mostly accounted for by water retention. Increasing the creatine content of muscle by 80–100 mmol/kg will increase intracellular osmolality, leading to water retention. Others found a reduction in urinary output during supplementation, tending to confirm this suggestion. The increased intramuscular osmolality due to creatine itself, however, is not likely to be sufficient to account for all of the water retention. It has been suggested that co-ingestion of creatine and carbohydrate, which results in high circulating insulin levels, may stimulate glycogen synthesis, which will further increase the water content of muscle. There is some preliminary evidence for a stimulation of protein synthesis in response to creatine supplementation.

### Health concerns of creatine supplementation

Many concerns have been raised that the effects of long-term use of large doses of creatine are unknown and that its use may pose a health risk. Studies on the response to long-term creatine use are in progress at this time, and results are not yet available. There have, however, been no reports of adverse effects in any of the studies published in the literature. One study that specifically examined renal function in individuals supplemented with creatine found no reason to believe that renal complications were likely. Anecdotal reports of an increased prevalence of muscle cramps in athletes taking creatine supplements have been circulating for some time, but there is no evidence to support this. It seems likely that any injury suffered by an athlete will be ascribed to an easily identifiable change in habit, such as the introduction of a new supplement.

It is usually recommended that athletes take 20 g/day of creatine for 4–5 days (a loading dose) followed by 1–2 g/day (maintenance dose). The muscle may be saturated with creatine when a dose as small as 10 g/day is taken for 3–4 days if this is taken together with sufficient carbohydrate to stimulate a marked elevation of the circulating insulin concentration. Many athletes, however, work on the principle that more is better and may greatly exceed these amounts. Even with very large doses, however, the possibility of adverse effects seems remote. Creatine is a small water-soluble mole-cule easily cleared by the kidney, and the additional nitrogen load resulting from supplementation is small.

## Carnitine

Depletion of the intramuscular glycogen stores is recognized as one of the primary factors involved in the fatigue that accompanies pro-longed exercise, and this is certainly true in football, which places high demands on the muscle glycogen stores. The importance of carbohydrate as a fuel for the working muscles is confirmed by the close relationship between the pre-exercise glycogen concentra-tion and the time for which exercise can be sustained. Further evidence comes from studies which show that increasing the com-bustion of fat during prolonged exercise, and thus sparing the lim-ited carbohydrate stores, can improve endurance capacity. Carnitine plays a key role in the transport of fatty acids into the mitochondria for oxidation, so it might be tempting to think that supplementation would accelerate this process, resulting in a sparing of glycogen and increased endurance.

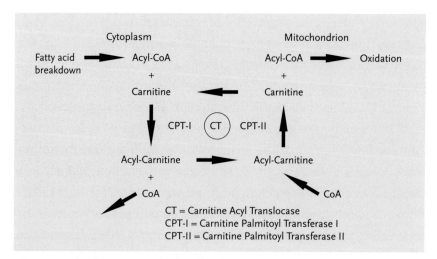

**Figure 7.3** Role of carnitine in the transfer of acyl groups across the mitochondrial membrane for oxidation.

On the basis of this logic, carnitine is widely sold in sports shops as a supplement for endurance athletes, and has also enjoyed popularity in football. There is, however, no good evidence that carnitine deficiency occurs in the general population or in athletes. Carnitine is present in the diet in red meat and dairy products, so it might be thought that individuals who follow a vegan lifestyle might be at increased risk of deficiency, but it can also be synthesized from amino acids in the liver and kidney. Measurement of the effects of exercise and diet on muscle carnitine levels in humans (muscle accounts for about 98 per cent of the total body carnitine content) has only been carried out relatively recently, and there have been few attempts to measure the effects of supplementation on the muscle carnitine level. It has been reported that short-term supplementation with carnitine (4–6 g/day for 7–14 days) had no effect on muscle carnitine levels or on the metabolic response to exercise, even when fatty acid mobilization was stimulated by high fat meals or heparin.

There are some published reports suggesting that carnitine supplementation can increase the contribution of fatty acids to oxidative metabolism and thus may have a glycogen-sparing effect. In a comprehensive review of the literature, eight studies were identified which examined the effects of supplementation on the metabolic response to endurance exercise, and found that three of those studies reported an increased rate of fat oxidation. The studies which have examined the effects of carnitine supplementation on exercise performance were also reviewed.

The findings were not generally in support of an ergogenic effect of carnitine. It must be concluded that, although there is a theoretical basis for an ergogenic effect of carnitine on performance of both high intensity and prolonged exercise, this is not supported by the experimental evidence. Supplementation of the diet with carnitine is unlikely to be beneficial for footballers or for other athletes.

## Bicarbonate

In high intensity exercise, lactate production makes a major contribution to energy metabolism, and match play is associated with increased blood lactate levels throughout the game. The metabolic acidosis that accompanies glycolysis has been implicated in the fatigue process, either by inhibition of key glycolytic enzymes, or by interfering with calcium transport and binding, or by a direct effect on the actin–myosin interaction. Because of these effects of acidosis on the muscle, an increase in the muscle buffering capacity, or an increased rate of efflux of hydrogen ions from the active muscles will all have the potential to delay fatigue and improve exercise performance.

### *Influence of induced alkalosis on exercise performance*

There is good evidence that ingestion of bicarbonate before exercise lasting about 1–10 min can enhance performance, although this was not seen in all studies. Performance of prolonged exercise seems not to be affected, and there is no good evidence of effects on intermittent exercise patterns similar to those seen in match play.

There are, of course, potential problems associated with the use of increased doses of bicarbonate. Vomiting and diarrhoea are not infrequently reported as a result of ingestion of even relatively small doses of bicarbonate, and this may limit any attempt to improve athletic performance by this method, certainly among those individuals susceptible to gastrointestinal problems. There have been reports of athletes using this intervention, which is not prohibited by the rules of sport, being unable to compete because of the severity of these symptoms. Although unpleasant and to some extent debilitating, these effects are not serious and there are no long-term adverse consequences of occasional use. Sodium citrate administration, which also results in an alkaline shift in the extracellular fluid, has also been reported to improve peak power and total work output in a 60 sec exercise test, but without any adverse gastrointestinal symptoms.

In the absence of any good evidence for a beneficial effect on performance in prolonged exercise, and with a significant risk of adverse gastrointestinal effects, there seems to be no reason for players to use bicarbonate supplements or other buffering agents before match play.

## Caffeine

Caffeine is a drug which, because of its longstanding and widespread use is considered socially acceptable. Caffeine and the related compounds theophylline and theobromine are naturally occurring food components, and for many people, these substances are part of the normal daily diet and caffeine is probably the most widely used stimulant drug in the world. The use of caffeine is not prohibited in sport, but there is a limit to the amount that may be taken by athletes in competition: any individual whose urine contains more than 12 mg/l of caffeine is guilty of a doping offence and is liable to be banned from competition.

Table 7.1 Caffeine content of varios drinks. For tea and coffee, the content varies greatly depending on the method of preparation.

| Foodstuff | Serving size | Caffeine (mg) |
|-----------|--------------|---------------|
| Coffee | 150 ml | 50–20 |
| Tea | 150 ml | 15–50 |
| Hot chocolate | 250 ml | 10 |
| Soft drinks | | |
| • Coca Cola | 330 ml | 50 |
| • Pepsi | 330 ml | 40 |
| • Jolt | 330 ml | 100 |

### Actions of caffeine

Caffeine has effects on the central nervous system and on adipose tissue and skeletal muscle that give reason to believe that it may influence exercise performance. Most interest has centred on an increased mobilization and use of fatty acids as a fuel, leading to a glycogen-sparing effect. Growing evidence of a positive effect of caffeine on performance in the absence of any glycogen sparing effect, and of effects on high intensity exercise, where glycogen availability is not a limiting factor, has stimulated the search for alternative mechanisms of action. There is speculation that caffeine directly affects the skeletal muscle and the central nervous system, either to modify the perception of effort or on the higher motor centres, but this is still to be provided.

Caffeine has a number of unwanted side effects that may limit its use by sensitive individuals: these effects include insomnia, headache, gastrointestinal irritation and bleeding, and diuresis. In the very high doses sometimes used by athletes, noticeable muscle tremor and impairment of coordination have been noted, and these are clearly unwanted effects. The diuretic action of caffeine is often stressed, particularly in situations where dehydration is a major issue. This particularly affects competitions held in hot, humid climates where the risk of dehydration is high. Players competing in these conditions are advised to increase their intake of fluid, but are usually also advised to avoid tea and coffee because of their diuretic effect. It seems likely, however, that this effect is small for those habituated to caffeine use and the negative effects caused by the symptoms of acute caffeine withdrawal may be more damaging.

*Effects of caffeine on performance*

There are several recent comprehensive reviews of the effects of caffeine on exercise performance. There are a number of studies showing beneficial effects of caffeine ingestion in a variety of laboratory tests of endurance performance. Early studies on the effects of caffeine on endurance performance focused on its role in the mobilization of free fatty acids from adipose tissue, increasing fat supply to the muscle, which in turn can increase fat oxidation, spare glycogen and thus extend exercise time. Caffeine ingestion prior to exercise to exhaustion at 80 per cent of $V_{O_2}$ max increased exercise time from 75 min on the placebo trial to 96 min on the caffeine trial. A positive effect was also observed on the total amount of work achieved in a fixed 2-hour exercise test. In this and other studies, caffeine was shown to increase circulating free fatty acid levels, increase fat oxidation and spare muscle glycogen during prolonged exercise. More recent studies have focused on exercises of shorter duration, and a number of studies have shown beneficial effects on performances lasting only a few (about 4–6) minutes. There is little information on performance in sprint tasks, and what is reported is conflicting.

It is clear from the published studies that positive effects of caffeine can be obtained in a variety of exercise situations with caffeine doses that are far below those necessary to produce a positive drug test. Doses of as little as 3 mg/kg body weight can produce ergogenic effects, but there appears to be a wide inter-individual variability in the sensitivity to caffeine. The reasons for this variability are not altogether clear, but, perhaps surprisingly, they do not appear to be related to the habitual level of caffeine consumption.

*Ethical issues in caffeine use*

Any player found to have a urine caffeine concentration of more than 12 mg/l is deemed to be guilty of a doping offence and is liable to suspension from competition. It is clear from this that caffeine is considered by the FIFA Medical Commission to be a drug, but an outright ban on its use is impractical and manifestly unfair to those who normally drink tea and coffee. It is equally clear, however, that the amount of coffee that must be drunk to exceed the permitted limit (about six cups of strong coffee consumed within a period of about 1 h) is such that it is unlikely that this would normally be achieved.

It is also clear that beneficial effects on performance can be achieved with caffeine doses that are less than those that result in a positive drug test, so players may feel justified in their view that use in these amounts is acceptable. It is difficult, but not impossible, to achieve an effective intake from drinks such as tea or coffee, but there are various products on the market that contain significant amounts of caffeine. Caffeine tablets, commonly used by over-worked students studying for examinations, are also sometimes used in sport, but these can easily lead to an intake that exceeds the per-missible limit.

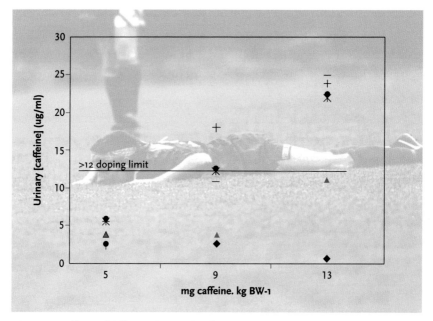

**Figure 7.4** Effects of different doses of caffeine or urine caffeine concentrations in healthy volunteers. Doses of 5 mg/kg or less are probably effective in increasing per-formance without causing a positve doping result in most people.

# Supplements that may increase muscle mass

Strength and power require a high lean body mass, and a high mus-cle mass confers a definite advantage in contact sports. Supplement use is widespread among athletes in strength sports, and a wide variety of supplements are used. The evidence for beneficial effects over those achieved by sound diet and hard training is, however, usually absent.

### Protein and amino acids

The idea that athletes need a high protein diet is intuitively attractive, and indeed there is evidence that the requirement for protein is increased by physical activity. Muscles consist largely of protein, and their involvement is fundamental to performance in all sports. It is also readily apparent that regular exercise has a number of highly specific effects on the body's protein metabolism. Strength training results in increases in muscle mass, and it is tempting to assume that this process is dependent on protein availability.

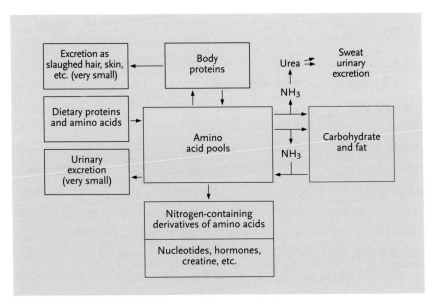

**Figure 7.5** Amino acids from the diet enter the body's amino acid pool and can be used to synthesise new proteins or can enter other metabolic pathways.

Endurance training has little effect on muscle mass, but does increase the muscle content of mitochondrial proteins, especially those involved in oxidative metabolism. Hard exercise and match play both result in muscle damage, usually at the microscopic level, and there is clearly a role for protein in the repair and recovery processes.

The contribution of protein oxidation to energy production during exercise decreases to about 5 per cent of the total energy requirement, compared with about 10–15 per cent (i.e. the normal fraction of protein in the diet) at rest, but the absolute rate of protein degradation is increased during exercise because of the high energy turnover. This leads to an increase in the minimum daily protein requirement, which will be met if a normal mixed diet adequate to meet the increased energy expenditure is consumed. The recommended protein intake for footballers has been set at about 1.4–1.7 g/kg/day, but protein may account for a lower than normal percentage of total energy intake on account of the increased total energy intake. Protein supplementation is not necessary for athletes, except perhaps in the rare situations where energy intake is restricted for example, to achieve weight loss in pre-season training.

Sales of whole protein powders account for a major part of the nutritional supplement sales to athletes, but a number of individual amino acids are also popular. Arginine and ornithine are reported to stimulate growth hormone release and to promote growth of lean tissue when taken during a period of strength training. There is some published evidence to support this, but any increase in growth hormone secretion is small compared with that which results from a bout of high intensity exercise. A number of other amino acids (including histidine, lysine, methionine and phenylalanine, are sold as 'anabolic agents', but it has been concluded after a review of the literature that 'there is little reason to believe that amino acid supplements will promote gains in muscle mass'.

In the recovery period, muscle glycogen synthesis is a priority, but synthesis of new proteins should perhaps be seen as being of equal or even greater importance. Because little attention has been paid to this area, it is not at present apparent what factors may be manipulated to influence these processes. The hormonal environment is one obvious factor that may be important, and nutritional status can influence the circulating concentration of a number of hormones that have anabolic properties, the most obvious example being insulin. It is, however, increasingly recognized that cell volume is an important regulator of metabolic processes, and there may be opportunities to manipulate this to promote tissue synthesis. During and after exercise there may be large changes in cell volume, secondary to osmotic pressure changes caused by metabolic activity, hydrostatic pressure changes, or by sweat loss. Alterations in cell volume induced by changes in osmolality are well known to alter the rate of glycogen synthesis in skeletal muscle. Amino acid transport into muscles is also affected by changes in cell volume induced by manipulation of the transmembrane osmotic gradient: skeletal muscle uptake of glutamine is stimulated by cellular swelling and inhibited by cell shrinkage.

The full significance of these findings for the post-exercise recovery process and the roles they play in adaptation to a training programme remain to be established. Manipulation of fluid and electrolyte balance and the ingestion of a variety of osmotically active substances or their precursors offers potential for optimizing the effectiveness of a training regimen.

## Chromium picolinate

Chromium is an essential trace element which has a number of functions in the body, and has been reported to potentiate the effects of insulin. Because of the anabolic effects of insulin, it might be expected that amino acid incorporation into muscle protein would be stimulated, enhancing the adaptive response to training. There is also some evidence to suggest an increased urinary chromium loss after exercise, further supporting the idea that athletes in training may have higher requirements than sedentary individuals. Chromium is widely used as a supplement by strength athletes, and is usually sold as a conjugate of picolinic acid; this form is reported to enhance chromium uptake.

Supplementation of the diet with chromium picolinate was reported to enhance the adaptive response to a strength training programme, with an increase in lean body mass. No direct measures of muscle mass were made, however, and the results of this study must be viewed with caution. A number of subsequent studies, mostly using more appropriate methodology, have failed to reproduce these results, with no effect on lean tissue accretion or on muscle performance being seen. Nonetheless, chromium supplementation remains popular.

### Beta-hydroxy beta-methyl butyrate (HMB)

ß-hydroxy ß-methylbutryrate is a metabolite of the amino acid leucine, and is also present in small amounts in some foods. There appears to be only one study published in a peer-reviewed journal in which the effects of HMB administration to humans has been investigated. This paper presented the results of two supplementation studies which showed that subjects ingesting 1.5 or 3 g/day of HMB for 3–7 weeks experienced greater gains in strength and in lean body mass compared with control groups. Although it is not easy to find any fault with these studies, it would be premature to conclude on the basis of this one report that there is an advantage to be gained from HMB supplementation. Nonetheless, it is sold in large amounts in sports nutrition stores.

## Supplements that may improve general health

Supplements such as iron, calcium and vitamin preparations are widely used by the general public and are also popular in sport. The evidence suggests that the use of these supplements is perhaps more prevalent in athletes than in the general population, but the perceived benefits are similar. Iron, of course, is important to the athlete because of the importance of haemoglobin in oxygen transport, and while anaemia is not more prevalent in athletes than in the general population the consequences may be more apparent. Nonetheless, supplementation is not warranted unless a specific deficiency is known to exist, and it must be recognized that too much iron may do more harm than good.

### Glutamine

Modest levels of regular exercise are associated with an increased sensation of physical well-being and a decreased risk of upper respiratory tract infections (URTI). The consequences of minor URTI symptoms are usually minimal, but for the athlete in hard training or preparing for a major competition, any injury or illness can have a devastating effect. There is good evidence that an active lifestyle is associated with improved health, but a number of recent epidemiological surveys have suggested that athletes in intensive training are more susceptible to minor opportunistic infections than is the sedentary individual. It has been suggested that severe exercise results in a temporary reduction in the body's ability to respond to a challenge to its immune system and that an inflammatory response similar to that occurring with sepsis and trauma is invoked. In view of the role of glutamine as a fuel for the cells of the immune system, it has been proposed that supplementation might enhance the body's ability to respond to infection. At present, the limited information on the influence of glutamine supplementation that is available provides no clear pattern of results.

In spite of the attractiveness of this hypothesis, it has not yet been established that there is a clear link between hard exercise, compromised immune function, susceptibility to infection and glutamine availability. Nonetheless, glutamine supplementation for athletes is being promoted and supplements are on widespread sale in sports nutrition outlets.

### Antioxidant nutrients

It has long been common practice for athletes to take vitamin supplements, usually without any thought as to their vitamin status. Recently there has been much interest among athletes in vitamins C and E which have been shown to have antioxidant properties, and which may be involved in protecting cells, especially muscle cells, from the harmful effects of the highly reactive free radicals that are produced when the rate of oxygen consumption is increased during exercise. It is believed that free radicals, a highly reactive chemical species, may be involved in the damage that occurs to muscle membranes. If the post-exercise damage can be reduced by an increased intake of antioxidants, then recovery after training and competition may be more rapid and more complete. The evidence for this at present suggests a possible role, but is not conclusive. Even the suggestion, however, is enough to convince many athletes to take supplements of these vitamins 'just in case'. There are, however, reports of increased, rather than decreased, levels of muscle damage in exercise after supplementation with Coenzyme Q10, so players should think carefully before using supplements. Regular training increases the effectiveness of the endogenous antioxidant mechanisms so that even extreme exercise (long distance triathlon) may not cause any indications of oxidative damage in well-trained athletes. Players in regular training may therefore not experience any benefit from antioxidant supplementation.

## Other compounds

Athletes use a wide range of nutritional supplements in their quest for improved health and performance. Even a cursory inspection of sports shops and magazines reveals the scale and diversity of supplement use. Most of the exotic supplements make extravagant claims and are sold at inflated prices. The market is, however, largely unregulated and few of the claims made for these products are based on any evidence; instead they rely on endorsement by top athletes (who are paid handsomely for doing so) and on the gullibility of the consumer.

Sales figures for exotic supplements such as ginseng, bee pollen, royal jelly and pangamic acid, together with a wide range of vitamins and minerals (including boron, vanadium, zinc, magnesium, manganese), demonstrate that many athletes remain convinced of their effectiveness. In spite of the limited and conflicting evidence, however, the balance of the available information suggests that there is no benefit of these substances for healthy individuals consuming a normal diet. Examination of the information in the bodybuilding world gives an idea of the range of products used and of the claims made for them. Some supplements are potentially harmful in large doses and their use should be actively discouraged. Many studies that purport to show beneficial effects are poorly designed, often with inadequate subject numbers and no control group, and few are published in reputable journals. The power of the placebo effect is well recognized, and athletes seem to be particularly susceptible. Where a beneficial effect is obtained, this is often due to the presence of illegal substances — for example, ephedrine and related compounds are common ingredients of many herbal remedies, and the use of these products renders the athlete liable to disqualification. Similarly, many products described as giving a feeling of 'increased energy' contain levels of caffeine that would cause the athlete to fail a drug test.

## Supplements and drug tests

Dietary supplements are not subject to the same stringent regulations that govern the manufacture and sale of medicines, and there are a number of well-documented cases of supplements being contaminated with prohibited compounds that can lead to positive drug tests. One study identified three dietary supplements that were contaminated with a number of prohibited steroids, including members of the testosterone and nandrolone families of compounds.

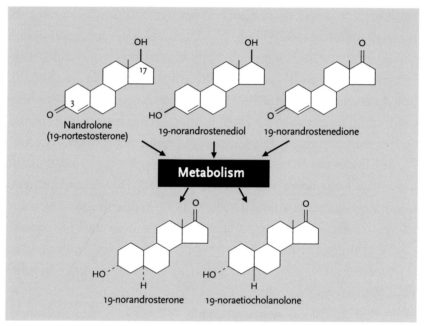

**Figure 7.6** When urine samples are tested for nandrolone, it is the metabolic 19-norandrosterone that is measured. This metabolite may also come from pro-hormones (19-norandrostenediol and 19-norandrostenedione) that have been shown to be present in many dietary supplements and which are also on sale via the internet. Players should avoid all of these products.

Subsequently another study reported results of analysis of 153 supplements: 18 different supplements contained pro-hormones that were not listed on the label. Since then there have been several other similar reports that raise concerns about the wisdom of supplement use by athletes. In some cases, it is suspected that the contamination is accidental and results from poor manufacturing practices leading to contamination of supplements with prohibited compounds but in other cases, deliberate adulteration has been sus-pected.

Although the nandrolone issue has gained most prominence, a number of other prohibited substances have been found in dietary supplements: these include ephedrine, caffeine, testosterone and methandienone. Products that have been shown to be contaminat-ed include *Tribulus terrestris*, chrysin, guarana and other herbal preparations, but also include creatine, carnitine, zinc and several others. Players and those who advise them must be aware of this risk and of the implications of a positive test. The safest option is clearly to avoid supplements altogether until such time as the con-tamination issue can be resolved. This is unrealistic, however, and many players remain committed to the use of supplements. Any player using supplements should conduct a thorough cost-benefit analysis before doing so. If a decision is made to use supplements, it seems prudent to avoid the products of companies that also man-ufacture, package or sell prohibited substances.

# 8. First aid

Åke Andrén-Sandberg and Alan Hodson

## On-field injury recognition and testing

There is a set procedure for recognizing an injury and the degree of injury i.e. minor (1st degree) or major (3rd degree) on the field of play.

The mnemonic 'VALTAPS' can be used by an 'on-field' practitioner for conducting a logical progressive injury assessment.

> **V** = Vision – see injury occur
> **A** = Ask player questions about the injury or ABC for unconscious player (emergency aid checking)
> **L** = Look at injury
> **T** = Touch — palpate the injured part
> **A** = Active movements from player
> **P** = Passive movements by therapist
> **S** = Strength — player's movements are resisted by therapist

It is easy to miss out aspects of the assessment and to fall into bad habits. Generally, if a player has suffered a major injury e.g. fracture, dislocation or severe muscle or ligament injury he or she will not be 'rolling about'. They will remain still and will probably tell you something is wrong.

Remember that there are five signs of inflammation: heat, swelling, pain, discoloration, and loss of function.

The term 'VALTAPS' explains the assessment procedure:

*V — Vision — see the injury occur*

The therapist or coach on the touchline may have seen the injury occur and will know the mechanics of the force.

*A — Ask*

The therapist asks the player what is wrong, where the injury is etc. He or she does not touch or move the injured part yet.

*L — Look*

The therapist looks at the injured site. This may mean taking the socks off to look at an ankle. One cannot see through socks, although some therapists seem to think so. Look for signs of inflammation. Do not ask for movement. There may be visible deformity which signifies a major injury. If so, the therapist should not proceed further but call for an ambulance.

*T — Touch*

If there is no visible deformity the injured part can be exposed and gently palpated. The objective is to establish quickly whether there are any signs or symptoms such as:

- Palpable pain/tenderness
- Swelling
- Loss of skin sensation
- Altered skin sensation such as pins and needles
- Any obvious deformity of the part compared to the other limb.

When palpating the part, remember to observe the player's face for response, i.e. a grimace caused by discomfort or pain. Also, remember that verbal communication is vital in order to establish whether palpation causes pain, exactly where the problem is, and also the grade or perceived level of injury (see below). No movements are asked for at this stage. The therapist may decide to go no

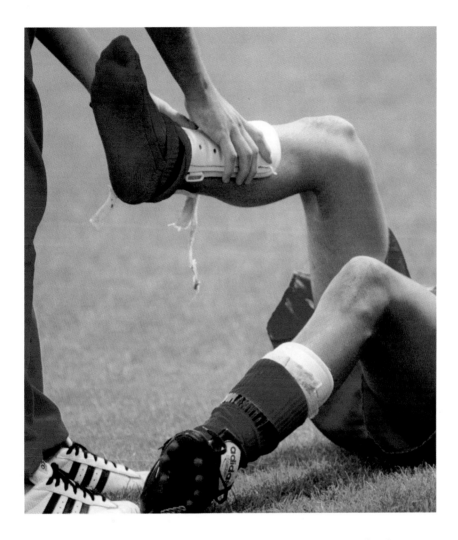

further at this stage and ensure that the player takes no further part in the training session or the game.

### A — Active movement

Up to this point, no movements of the injured part have been asked for. It may well be that the injury is of such a level that, having been through the previous testing procedures, it would be unwise to ask for active movements. However, in minor injuries, whether the player will probably be able to continue, or can at least demonstrate that there is no serious problem that would need referral to experts at a higher level and/or hospital, active movements would be the next area of the 'on-field' assessment. One may decide, following the ask, look and touch phase, to stop 'recognition' testing of the player at this point and ensure that he or she takes no further part in the session.

The player will be asked to carry out all the major movements associated with the nearest joint or joints. While he or she is carrying out these purely active movements, the therapist notes the range of movement gained in each direction and again checks the injured player's facial expression, looking out for signs of discomfort or pain.

A key sign of injury is loss of function, i.e. movement. In grade 1 (minor) injuries, a good range of active movement will be achieved by the player. However, with grade 2 (moderate) injuries, the amount of movement will be severely affected, particularly in certain directions where pain will be produced by stretching injured ligaments or muscles. Note the movement which causes discomfort, it is a good guide for what is wrong. In grade 3 injuries (severe) the player, who would be in pain, would be able to perform little or no active movement. In this case by earlier checking 'see, ask, look, touch' will probably have already found that a severe injury has been sustained, in which case further checking by movements would be pointless. In fact, it could injure the player further.

In minor injuries, particularly where the player is likely to resume playing, the range of movement will be almost full. In these cases one can progress to the next phase of the assessment.

*P — Passive movement testing*

Never move the player's injured part unless he or she demonstrated a good range of active movement. A passive movement is where the therapist performs the desired movement of a body part for the player. The player takes no active part in this at all. With knowledge of how far the player has moved his joint or body part actively, the therapist moves the part through this range and a little further, checking all the time for facial reaction. If this causes no undue problem, then the therapist will move on to strength testing. All movements available are tested.

### S — Strength testing

The decission may be taken that the player is not going to continue the game or training session and therefore there is no need for strength testing. The therapist resists the action of muscles working over the injured part. All movements available are tested.

Again, the therapist checks for pain or discomfort through facial expression and questioning.

If the player passes through the seven areas covered by the aforementioned 'on-field' assessment, the player is then assisted into the standing position for applicable weight-bearing functional tests. For an 'injury', the following progressive functional activities could be used on the touchline to confirm that the player is able to return to competitive play.

- Assisted standing
- Standing unaided
- Walking forward unaided
- Jogging on the spot
- Jogging forwards (straight line)
- Jogging backwards (straight line)
- Quarter-pace running (straight line)
- Half-pace running (straight line)
- Three-quarter pace running (straight line)
- Stopping and starting (straight line)
- Full-pace springing (straight line)
- Side to side running, i.e. 'zigzag', 'figure of eight'
- Diagonal movement changes with change of pace.

## Summary

Before leaping into action, the following guided 'on-field' recognition testing must always be followed.

**V =**   Vision – see the initial injury.

**A =**   Ask for the history.

**L =**   Look for signs of inflammation, deformity etc.

**T =**   Touch for tenderness, pain, swelling, pins and needles etc.

**A =**   Active – ask for active movements from the player.

**P =**   Passive – therapist moves the part passively.

**S =**   Strength – therapist resists movements by player of injured part.

If the player responds well to all of the above then functional weight-bearing tests can be carried out.

### *Remember*

It is very important to realize that in minor injuries where the player will carry on, all stages of the assessment will be carried out. However, in moderate to severe injuries, the full 'VALTAPS' assessment procedure will not be completed as the therapist realizes that the signs and symptoms are substantial and that to continue the assessment routine would cause further injury.

### THE THREE GRADES OF INJURY ARE

- **Grade 1** — Minor signs and symptoms of inflammation (nil to minimum).
- **Grade 2** — Moderate signs and symptoms of inflammation (noticeable and significant).
- **Grade 3** — Severe signs and symptoms of inflammation (very evident, particularly loss of movement).

As the grade of injury rises, so do the signs and symptoms of injury. At some point a decision will be made: 'Is the player fit to carry on?'. Sometimes this is a clear-cut decision, but sometimes it is not so clear. Be guided by what can be seen, touched, felt and what the player's active movement state is.

NEVER stray from the 'VALTAPS' testing routine.
NEVER continue progression through the 'VALTAPS' testing routine when a player's sign and symptoms, lack of movement or unwillingness to move the affected part indicate termination at the point reached.
NOTE: It may be that by just looking and palpation of the injury a decision is made not to ask for active movements from the player.

# SERIOUS INJURIES

## SERIOUS INJURIES AND ILLNESS WHICH CAN OCCUR IN THE CONTEXT OF FOOTBALL

- Serious concussion and haemorrhaging between the membranes of the brain.
- Blockage of the upper respiratory tract caused by the tongue blocking the throat.
- Spinal injuries to the neck.
- Sudden cardiac arrest due to blood clots or inflammation of the heart muscles.
- Puncture of the lung sack caused by broken ribs.
- Abdominal haemorrhaging after injuries to the liver or spleen.

Life-threatening injuries in the context of football are extremely unusual. There are, however, a few simple rules in connection with the immediate attention given to anyone who is seriously injured. These are rules that everyone should be aware of. In these rare cases it is essential to know what to do in the first instance until the ambulance or a doctor arrives on the scene.

## The golden hour

There is an expression in this situation — the golden hour — which means that lives can be saved if the correct attention is provided during the first hour. It is essential to be well prepared, to act systematically and to realize that cooperation between everyone present is important.

A common feature for all serious injuries is that the life-threatening complications evolve gradually. Once any bleeding is stopped and a free passage for air is secured, the injured person's life can often be saved without any serious permanent damage occuring. A significant number of deaths can be avoided if the injured person receives the correct treatment initially.

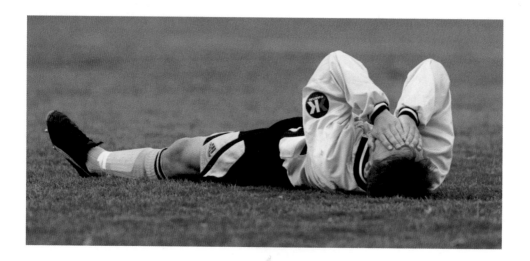

# A plan for medical treatment

When a serious injury occurs in a football situation it is not un-common that confusion arises and it is important that someone takes charge. The first task is to call for an ambulance.

The emergency treatment provided for a seriously injured person is always similar no matter how the injury has occurred and regardless of any visible external injuries. It is essential to always follow the ABC rules — the more serious the injury the more im-portant it is to follow these rules.

In many countries, the Red Cross's ABC rule has had consider-able impact. More recently, two more letters have been added to the ABC sequence — A–E is followed to ensure systematic action.

> **A.** Check the respiratory tract and spine in the neck area.
> **B.** Is breathing satisfactory?
> **C.** Is the blood circulation functioning?
> **D.** Is the brain affected?
> **E.** Make a systematic examination.

Knowledge about the symptoms and background of an illness or in-jury, which is called the past history, is the single most important factor for reaching the correct diagnosis in the shortest possible time. It is therefore important to try to describe as accurately as possible how the injury occurred. Was the body hit by a blow? Was any part of the body twisted unnaturally? What was the condition immedi-ately after the accident? How has the condition developed since the accident? A few other details are also of interest;

- Was the injured person healthy when the accident occurred?
- Are there any previous illnesses or injuries of significance?
- Is the injured person taking any medication on a regular basis?

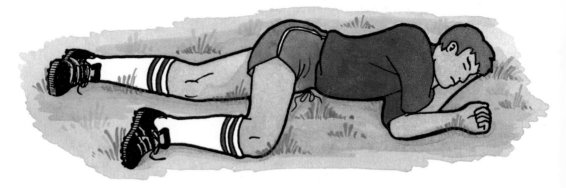

**Figure 8.1** Forward leaning side position. The injured person should be placed on their side so that one arm lies at an angle of 90° straight out from under the body and the upper arm is bent with the hand under the cheek. The upper leg should be bent at an angle of 90° at the knee and hip to prevent the injured person from rolling onto the stomach. The neck should be slightly tilted back to ensure an open air passage.

The medicines which should be particularly checked are medication for diabetes (insulin), epilepsy or psychological illness, or blood diluents.

### A — Open airway

After an accident or sudden cardiac arrest, it is important to first make sure that the air passages are not obstructed. If the person cannot breathe all other treatment is pointless. It is not always apparent whether or not the injured person can breathe. Shortage of oxygen can be suspected, however, if the injured person is pale, perspiring, anxious, confused or violent. In addition to this, rapid shallow breathing and a blue tinge to the lips can be signs of poor oxygen supply. It is important to know that this type of injury does not often worsen gradually but a serious worsening can occur suddenly and unpredictably.

First, one should always make sure that there is no alien material (dentures, dental plates, gravel etc.) in the mouth or throat. There are then several methods of opening the air passage.

## OPEN AIRWAY CAN BE ACHIEVED BY

- Forward leaning side position (rule out spinal neck injury).
- Lifting up the chin ('chin lift').
- Thrusting the jaw up and forward ('jaw thrust').

One should not put any pressure on the spinal neck area.

Note: If one is forced to choose, open airway always takes priority.

### B— Breathing

It is not enough to ensure that the injured person has open airways, they must also be able to breathe. It is best if they begin breathing spontaneously themselves but if this does not happen mouth-to-mouth respiratory assistance should be given while waiting for the ambulance.

### C — Blood circulation and bleeding

Any bleeding should be stopped as quickly as possible. If a great deal of blood is being lost, this is best done by exerting direct pressure on the area which is bleeding. Tourniquets should be avoided since they can cause more harm than good if they are fastened in the wrong way. Smaller cuts can be covered in the simplest way as cleanly as possible at the scene of the injury until more definitive treatment can be provided.

When the doctor and ambulance personnel arrive at the scene, they can provide fluids in the form of a drip to avoid shock due to loss of blood. Feeling cold and psychological anxiety can lead to poor circulation. The injured person should not, therefore, lie directly on the cold ground but should have at least one layer of material between them and the ground and if possible they should be covered with blankets. An 'internal blood transfusion' equivalent to around

(A)

(B)

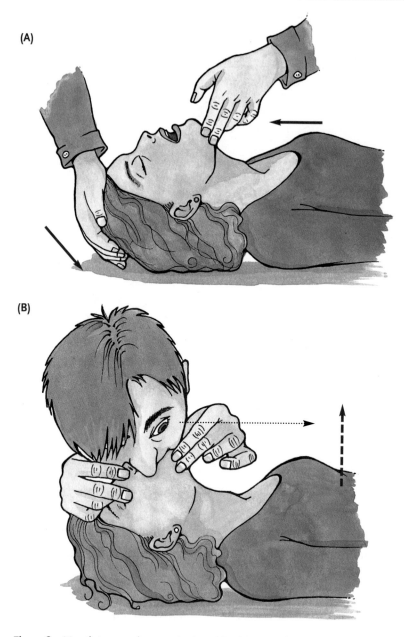

**Figure 8.2** Mouth-to-mouth resuscitation. (A) The injured person is placed on their back and the head is held tilted slightly back with the help of a hand on the forehead and two fingers under the chin. (B) The nose is pinched closed with the hand steadying the forehead. Take a deep breath and blow air forcefully through the mouth. It is important to note that the chest rises to indicate that air is really reaching the lungs. One blow every fifth second is sufficient.

one-third of the blood volume can be gained if the legs are elevated (with the feet around 30 cm above the level of the heart).

The blood pressure should be measured to evaluate the blood circulation. If it is not possible to feel any pulse in the neck, the groin or the wrist, it is often a sign that the injured person has lost a lot of blood or that the heart is not pumping efficiently. A basic rule for otherwise healthy younger people is that if the pulse can be detected at the following points, the blood pressure should be at least:

- At the neck      70 mmHg
- In the groin     80 mmHg
- At the wrist     90 mmHg.

### D — Has the brain been affected?

Haemorrhaging between the membranes of the brain is not uncommon in the event of head injuries. The correct treatment can save lives in this situation. The development of impaired brain function occurs gradually and it is therefore important to assess as early as possible whether the brain has been affected and if so, to what extent. A simple guide might be: fully conscious, slightly affected, unconscious and deeply unconscious.

The most important thing is, however, to note any changes in the degree of consciousness. The faster the degree of consciousness of the injured person falls, the more serious the injury.

### E— Examine systematically

At the scene of the injury it is not necessary to examine the injured person in detail but if the person is conscious, it is wise to ask if they are experiencing pain at any other point apart from the area obviously injured. It is important to follow the A–E routine at all times.

For those who are not medically trained, the following simple rules should be followed when serious injury occurs:

IN THE EVENT OF SERIOUS INJURY

1. Call for an ambulance.
2. Open the airways; protect the spine at the neck.
3. Prevent the injured person from getting cold.
4. Calm the injured person.

# SLIGHT INJURIES

Among the most common injuries in football are muscle injuries and joint sprains. Only a few of these are serious but many cause discomfort and can prevent the injured person from playing football for a long period if they are not treated correctly.

A plan of what can happen might look like this:

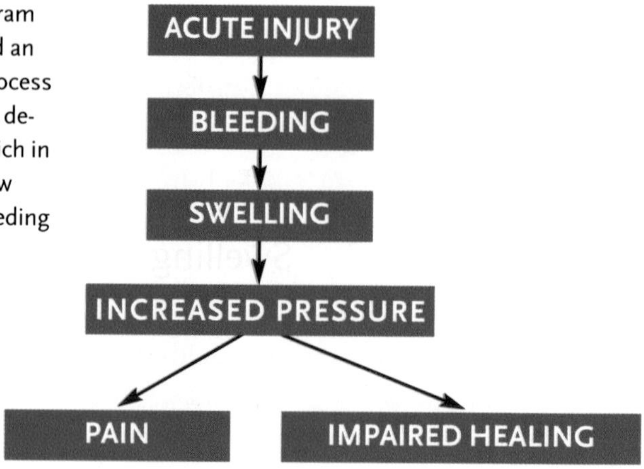

**Figure 8.3** This diagram shows how pain and an impaired healing process is dependent on the degree of swelling, which in turn depends on how pronounced the bleeding has been.

ACUTE INJURY

BLEEDING

SWELLING

INCREASED PRESSURE

PAIN     IMPAIRED HEALING

There is no direct correlation between the degree of pain and how serious, for instance, a sprain or rupture may be. It is rather the swelling which causes discomfort. The greater the swelling, the more pain experienced. Treatment in the acute situation should primarily be directed at minimizing the bleeding.

# Bleeding

With a smaller muscle rupture one can assume that the bleeding in the tissues originates from small blood vessels. The body itself generally stops the bleeding within a few minutes, partly by the platelets plugging the small blood vessels and partly by the contraction of the vessels. When an injury occurs, substances are released which cause the platelets to become stickier which allows them to stick together in small blood clots which plug the blood vessel. When the blood platelets become sticky they also affect the chemical substance in the injured walls of the blood vessels, which causes the elastic threads in the walls of the blood vessels to contract and restrict the flow of blood.

The bleeding usually stops within 6–8 min. Despite this the skin can be discoloured for several days after the injury occurred. This type of bruising, which often becomes visible after 2–4 days, is not a sign that the bleeding has continued.

# Swelling

Swelling in an injured area is not synonymous with the size of the haemorrhage but the original bleeding is an indirect cause of the swelling. The swelling is caused, to a small extent, by the increased amount of fluid in and around injured cells and, to a much greater extent, by the obstruction of blood and lymph fluid which cannot pass through the injured area. Therefore, the more extensive the bleeding, the greater the obstruction and the larger the swelling.

Swelling develops gradually during the days immediately after the injury. In cases where no treatment is given it is not uncommon for swelling to increase up to 48 h after which time the swelling slowly disappears. There are examples, however, of swelling remaining for several weeks. In such cases there is a risk that the body will adapt to the condition and reconstruct the tissues with extra connective tissue so that the swelling remains for much longer.

## Increased pressure and pain

Swelling increases the pressure in the tissues and even if the increase in pressure is moderate it can still cause damage. This is partly because the increased pressure is painful and partly because it impairs the healing process. The tissues are distended, which gives rise to pain.

An injured muscle or a damaged ligament only hurts when the tissues are stretched at the moment of injury. Afterwards the pain is due mainly to the swelling. There is a direct correlation between the degree of swelling and the degree of pain: the greater the swelling, the greater the pain.

## Impaired healing process

The increase in pressure in the tissues delays the healing process. Even if the pressure is too low to cut off the blood supply the metabolism in the area around the swelling is impaired since both the supply of nutrients and the removal of waste products becomes more difficult.

# Alternative treatments

When an injury occurs there are several methods of treatment that can be used individually or in combination:

- Rest
- Elevated position
- Cooling
- Pressure bandage
- Treatment with medication.

## Rest

An important part of the immediate treatment provided is keeping the injured part of the body still. However, this is an obsolete principle in relation to post-injury recovery.

In order to prevent bleeding out into the tissues, the injured person should keep still immediately after the injury occurs. It is particularly important to reduce the blood flow during the initial 6–8 min since this is when the blood vessels leak blood. Theoretically, it should be sufficient to keep the injured part of the body still for around 8 min but for safety's sake 10–15 min are recommended. When the bleeding has stopped, it is less important to keep still and by a day or so after the injury, this can cause more harm than good.

## Elevated position

It is not quite so urgent to move the injured part of the body into an elevated position. This can reduce the immediate bleeding but in practice the significance is negligible. On the other hand, the elevation of the injured part of the body is important to avoid swelling. Keeping the injured part of the body in an elevated position should continue for 24–28 h.

A player who has injured a foot or an ankle should walk and stand as little as possible for the first 48 h after the injury apart from when engaged in rehabilitation. When the injured person is sitting, the lower leg should be placed up on a chair, a table or an equivalent.

## Cooling

Most football players have a deep-seated faith in the value of cooling treatment for injuries. Modern research, meanwhile, has shown that the usefulness of cooling treatment can be limited. An ice pack on an injured muscle only provides a small and slow reduction in the temperature in the muscle itself since the skin insulates against cold — a reduction of 6–8° in temperature in about 45 min. This means that the reduction in the blood flow is moderate and occurs only after the bleeding has already stopped of its own accord. Cooling an injury does, however, have another useful effect, it alleviates the pain. A great part of the pain after an injury can be prevented by rendering the skin, which contains many sensory cells, insensitive.

Cooling sprays should primarily be seen as having a psychological effect, since cooling and insensitivity of the skin achieved by spraying disappears within 1–2 min. No further effect is achieved. On the other hand ice packs are effective, on condition that they are used for at least 20 min and that the pack is changed during this time to prolong the effect. Just as good, but significantly cheaper, is ordinary tap water, which is almost always at the correct temperature and can flow over exactly the part of the body that has been injured.

## Pressure bandages

Bleeding is most quickly and efficiently treated by using a pressure bandage. The greater part of the bleeding stops within a few seconds after an elastic bandage has been wound tightly around the injured area. A piece of rubber or an ice pack wrapped in cloth can be positioned on the injury to obtain the greatest pressure possible just at the point of the injury. This should be done quickly, however, for every minute that passes without a pressure bandage the bleeding will be greater! It is also important to use bandages with a high degree of elasticity.

The elastic bandage should be wound as tightly as possible. Tight pressure is not harmful if applied for a limited time. The tight bandage should be in position for around 15 min or slightly longer since it is often so painful that the pressure has to be loosened. The danger of bleeding is over by this time. The bandage can then be removed and re-applied less tightly to reduce the swelling — not to stop the bleeding. The bandage should, in principle, always be in position for the first 2 days and should be reapplied as long as the injured area is swollen.

## Treatment with medication

Footballers are used to being knocked about a bit and experience this as an unavoidable part of the game. Most of them are prepared to put up with a reasonable amount of pain and seldom seek medical assistance for this.

Paracetamol is often a sufficient painkiller for acute football injuries. Paracetamol is the medication of choice first if a player requires a painkiller. There is a very low risk of side-effects, it is widely available, cheap and reasonably effective.

Medicines for treating inflammation (known as NSAID medications = non-steroid anti-inflammatory drugs) are often used in the event of football injuries and can be bought over the counter. These drugs have a low risk of side-effects when they are given to otherwise healthy footballers for a short period of time. Distinct from the traditional painkillers, NSAIDs not only have a painkilling effect they also have an established effect in combating inflammation. This combined effect is significant when treating injuries where a painkiller is necessary to be able to start recovery training early. The anti-inflammatory element means that swelling is reduced at the same time.

## BASIC RULES FOR EMERGENCY ATTENTION

In event of slight to medium serious injuries to arms and legs

- Pressure bandage — as quickly as possible, as tight as possible for around 15 min.
- Keep still — the first minutes are most important.
- Cooling — pain treatment.
- Elevated position is effective for the first 48 h.
- Medication is seldom necessary.

# 9. Muscle injuries

Per Renström

Muscle injuries are very common in football. There are studies which show that they represent up to 30 per cent of all football injuries. Among the most common are the contusion injuries (such as internal bleeding in the thigh) which occur when the muscle is pressed against the underlying bone, for example, if a player receives a kick from another player's knee across the thigh muscle. This results in the blood vessels and muscle fibres rupturing.

Another type of muscle injury is a distension injury, in other words, a ruptured muscle due to strain. This type of injury can occur, for example, in the posterior thigh muscle during a fast burst of speed. The player suddenly experiences pain as the muscle fibres are pulled apart.

Other muscle-related problems that can arise include muscle soreness, calcification in the musculature after bleeding, and cramp.

## Distension injuries – rupturing of the muscle

Ruptures of the muscles occur when the player makes any dramatic change in the speed of running, such as during a fast burst of speed. The durability of the muscle can be exceeded during forceful eccentric muscle activation. Usually the player has to stop playing football because of an inability to contract the injured muscle. A rupture may also occur during a shot or sudden stop in mid-movement.

Studies have shown that the more energy a muscle is capable of absorbing, that is if the player is very fit, the greater the ability of the muscle to withstand injury.

Ruptures are most common in the muscles which pass over two joints such as the biceps femoris, the rectus femoris and the gastrocnemius which is part of the calf musculature. Other muscles which can be affected are, for example, the adductor longus in the groin.

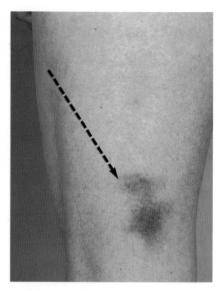

**Figure 9.1** Bleeding on the back of the thigh caused by a muscle rupture.

Ruptures usually occur at the muscle–tendon junction. A muscle/tendon junction can be assumed to be situated at the end of a muscle belly, but can extend along the length of the whole muscle on the surface or within the muscle belly. This means that a junction between a muscle and a tendon can also exist at the centre of a muscle.

The treatment of distension injuries or muscle ruptures, is the same as for contusion injuries and is described for both types of injury in the section 'The treatment of muscle injuries'.

## Contusion injuries

A contusion injury is located at the point where the impact was received. If, for example, the thigh muscle receives a kick, the injury occurs beneath the skin at the point where the kick made impact.

An injury in a contracted muscle often occurs more superficially than in a muscle which is relaxed.

A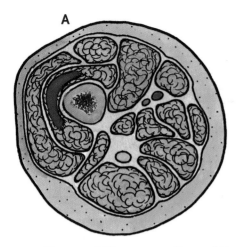  B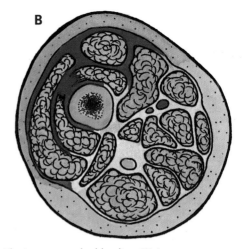

**Figure 9.2** Different types of internal bleeding. The intramuscular bleeding (A) is en-cased in the membrane of the muscle and the intermuscular bleeding (B) spreads between the muscles.

## Bleeding

When a muscle is injured, bleeding occurs. Muscles generally have a considerable flow of blood especially during activity. After 10–12 min of physical exertion, the amount of blood the heart pumps out to the muscles increases from 15 per cent, or 0.8 l/min, to 72 per cent, or 1.8 l/min. The musculature therefore has very good blood circulation when players are physically active.

Bleeding in the musculature which occurs quickly in the event of an injury, can be either intramuscular bleeding or intermuscular bleeding depending on whether the muscle membrane (fascia) which encases the musculature remains intact or not (Figure 9.2).

### Intramuscular bleeding

An intramuscular collection of blood (haematoma), often affects the more superficial musculature and has an intact muscle mem-brane which limits the extent of the bleeding. The increase in pres-sure counteracts the bleeding since the blood vessels are com-pressed. Common symptoms include pain and impaired function. This type of bleeding is more difficult to treat successfully than the

## DIFFERENT TYPES OF BLEEDING

- **Intramuscular bleeding:** The bleeding is encased in the muscle and the fascia is intact. This type of bleeding is more difficult to treat successfully since the injury is deeply embedded in the muscle.
- **Intermuscular bleeding:** If the fascia is damaged the bleeding can spread between the muscles. The potential for a quick recovery is good if the injury is correctly treated.

intermuscular type of bleeding since the musculature has little space for increasing its volume and thereby reducing pressure.

*Intermuscular bleeding*

If the fascia is damaged intermuscular bleeding occurs. The bleeding spreads between the muscle bellies and the fascia and in this way the pressure is reduced. Players affected by intermuscular bleeding experience less pain and less functional impairment. The prognosis is better for this type of bleeding and these injuries heal quickly on condition that the immediate treatment provided is correct.

# How muscle injuries heal

The way in which muscle injuries heal is influenced by two factors that work in opposite directions:

1. Regeneration of the injured muscle fibres – formation of new fibres.
2. Development of scar tissue.

A balance between these two factors is important for optimal healing. The damaged muscle fibre is pulled together while the ends are pulled apart which means that a space forms between the muscle fibres, which is filled with blood. Later this space is gradually filled by scar tissue. In the event of a serious injury, the scar tissue can be so pronounced that it creates a mechanical barrier which restricts complete regeneration of the muscle fibres across the gap. This means that it is important to restrict the extent of the bleeding and therefore the amount of scar tissue.

## The treatment of muscle injuries

Treatment consists of short rest, compression, cooling treatment and elevation of the injured area. Relieving the pressure by the use of crutches can be useful in the initial stages.

Immediate immobilization after a muscle injury is necessary to allow the new tissue to strengthen and to prevent further dam-

### EVALUATION OF THE BLEEDING – HAEMATOMA WITHIN 24–48 HOURS

- Is the injured area swollen?
- Has the bleeding spread out into the skin and caused discoloration?
- Has the muscle regained its normal contraction capacity?
- Have the joints around the muscle markedly reduced capacity for movement?

If the answers to the questions are yes, there is an intramuscular haematoma and if no, there is an intermuscular haematoma.

221

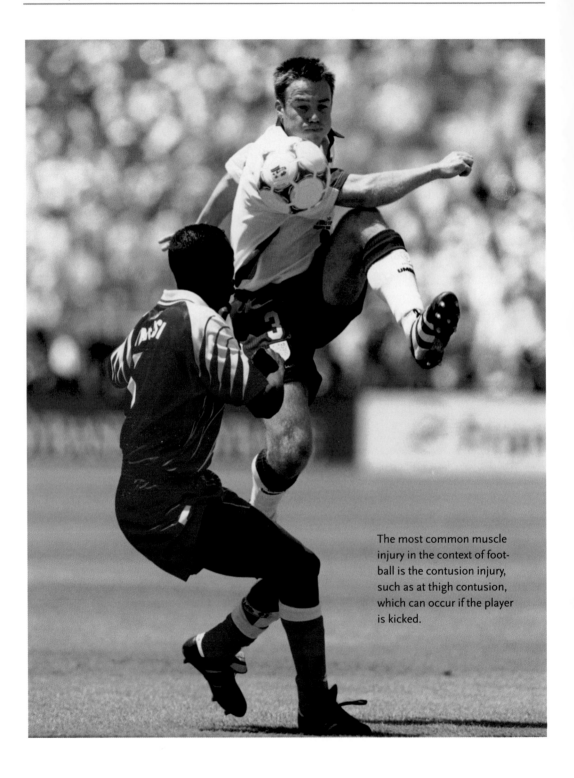

The most common muscle injury in the context of football is the contusion injury, such as at thigh contusion, which can occur if the player is kicked.

age. The length of the period of immobilization depends on the degree of the injury, in other words, the injury has to withstand certain contraction forces which takes around 2–4 days. Current studies support initial immobilization after a muscle injury for 2–4 days after which one should mobilize or activate the muscle as soon as possible. This provides optimal opportunity for healing and positive development of the new muscle fibres.

On evaluating the injury after 24–48 h, it is possible to distinguish which type of internal bleeding the player has suffered. This has important significance for recovery potential and treatment. If intermuscular bleeding is suspected quick mobilization is preferable. The recovery potential is good. If there is reason to suspect intramuscular bleeding, further examination with ultrasonography or magnetic resonance imaging (MRI) may be useful.

The recovery potential for a muscle rupture can, if the damage has occurred in the anterior thigh muscle, to a certain extent be evaluated by testing the player's ability to bend the knee. If the player can bend the knee more than 90–120° the injury is slight with good potential for recovery within the period of a week. If the player can bend the knee 45–90°, the injury is moderately serious with a recovery time of 1–4 weeks. If the player is unable to bend the knee more than 45°, the injury is serious and recovery could take 1–3 months.

## Why early mobilization?

Early mobilization provides the chance of fast and intensive muscle regeneration, or muscle reconstruction. Early mobilization also increases the growth of capillaries, the small blood vessels. The tissue grows stronger since the new muscle fibres are faster and can grow in parallel with each other at the same time as the muscle grows faster and can more easily be contracted.

The principles of a rehabilitation programme after a muscle injury should therefore initially concentrate on static exercises. After

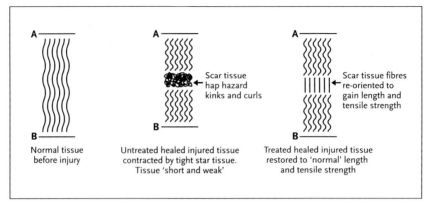

A ———
A ———
Scar tissue
hap hazard
kinks and curls
B ———

A ———
Scar tissue fibres
re-oriented to
gain length and
tensile strength
B ———

Normal tissue
before injury

Untreated healed injured tissue
contracted by tight star tissue.
Tissue 'short and weak'

Treated healed injured tissue
restored to 'normal' length
and tensile strength

**Figure 9.3** Stretching will merely straighten or re-orientate the fibres. It is a remodelling of the developing collagen as it is laid down within the limits of discomfort. Scar tissue has 'plastic' properties. Plastic stretch means that the tissue retains its new shape after the elongated stress is released.

that, rapid concentric exercises can be introduced with a low degree of resistance followed by concentric exercises with increased resistance. If the player manages to carry out the exercises without pain, eccentric exercises with gradually increased speed and resistance can be added.

If the injured player is unable to contract the musculature on his or her own, electrical stimulus may be useful.

Stretching should not be started too early. When the player manages to contract the muscle well, stretching periods of 10–15 sec can be started and subsequently increased to 1 min. Stretching of the same muscle should be done regularly every few hours.

The principles of rehabilitation of muscle injuries are described on the schedule on Page 225.

Anti-inflammatory medicine can be used for short periods. Some doctors use cortisone injections for muscle injuries. However, this results in a delay in the healing process in the area where bleeding has occurred, and the development of necrotic or dead tissue, which delays the muscle reconstruction process. Cortisone injections should therefore be avoided in connection with muscle injuries.

## REHABILITATION PROGRESS REPORT • MUSCLE RUPTURE

| | DAYS | | WEEKS | | | | |
|---|---|---|---|---|---|---|---|
| | 1–2 | 3–7 | 2 | 3 | 4 | 5 | 6 |
| **Immobilization** | | | | | | | |
| Compression bandage | ■ | | | | | | |
| Crutches | ■ | | | | | | |
| Partial load | ■ | | | | | | |
| **Mobility training** | | | | | | | |
| Passive mobility training | | ■ | | | | | |
| Light stretching | | ■ | | | | | |
| Pool | | ■ | | | | | |
| Cycling, slight load | | ■ | | | | | |
| Stretching | | | ■ | ■ | ■ | ■ | ■ |
| **Weight training** | | | | | | | |
| Static muscle tension | | ■ | | | | | |
| Endurance training | | | ■ | ■ | | | |
| Dynamic weight training | | | | ■ | ■ | | |
| Eccentric weight training | | | | | ■ | ■ | ■ |
| **Football-related training** | | | | | ■ | ■ | ■ |
| **Coordination training** | | | | | | | |
| Coordination training | | | ■ | ■ | ■ | ■ | ■ |
| Suppleness training | | | | | ■ | ■ | ■ |
| **Fitness training** | | | | | | | |
| Cycling | | | ■ | ■ | ■ | ■ | ■ |
| Pool | | | | ■ | ■ | ■ | ■ |
| Jogging, running | | | | | ■ | ■ | ■ |

225

### Prognosis for successful healing

Studies have shown that the contraction capacity and strength of the muscle are generally recovered within 1 week of a muscle injury. Around 50 per cent of the strength returns within 24 h. After 7 days, the player has regained around 90 per cent of muscle strength.

After a distension injury of medium seriousness, the muscle often takes around 3–4 weeks to recover while a contusion injury can take 4–5 weeks depending on the degree of seriousness.

### Further examination

If the injured player has suffered an intramuscular bleed or a serious injury, there is cause to examine the injury more closely. Ultrasonography has been found to be a good method for evaluating the extent of the injury as well as the degree of seriousness. Ultrasonographic examinations also allow us to follow the healing process and predict any complication which may arise.

Examination by magnetic resonance imaging can give good information during the first few weeks if a rupture is present.

### Indications for surgery

It is uncommon for muscle injuries to require surgery since rehabilitation as a rule provides sufficient support for successful recovery. If the haematoma is extensive and there is a risk of increased tissue pressure, the haematoma should be drained, which can be done relatively simply. There are also certain injuries involving muscles which do not have any agonists, such as the pectoralis major, which may require surgery. A complete detachment of the hamstring muscles usually requires surgery on the back of the thigh since rehabilitation alone does not always provide full functional recovery.

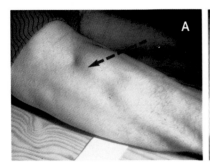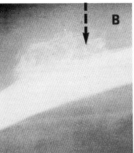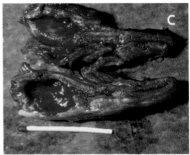

**Figure 9.4** (A) Major muscle injury, with a visible pit in the muscle. (B) X-ray showing ossification or calcification of muscle haemorrhage (myositis ossificans). (C) After surgery. The ossification has been removed.

## Complications relating to muscle injuries

Complications which can arise in relation to muscle injuries include ossification or calcification of the bleeding in a muscle, known as myositis ossificans. This complication arose earlier in about 20 per cent of cases after considerable bleeding in the anterior thigh muscles. However, the frequency has probably fallen radically, as a result of modern rehabilitation methods.

After a contusion, the haematoma in the muscles is often situated close to the bone. This collection of blood can calcify and then ossify. After 4–6 weeks extensive calcification may have occurred which means that the musculature cannot be used optimally. If the deep anterior thigh muscles have calcified, for instance, the player often finds it difficult to bend his knee.

The treatment of these injuries generally involves preventative and rehabilitation measures. Cautious training of the musculature is recommended and the player is generally free from any symptoms after a few months. If problems continue, surgery may be considered to remove the calcification. This has been shown to provide good results and the player can return to football within 4–8 weeks. It is, however, unusual that surgery is necessary.

# Other muscle-related problems

## Muscle soreness

Soreness is common especially at the start of the season. It may also arise when the playing surface is changed, such as from soft to hard or vice versa.

Soreness is often located deep inside the musculature for 1–2 days. The player affected may also experience a feeling of weakness for up to 1 week and may also experience impaired mobility. It is common that soreness can arise after repeated eccentric activities such as a great deal of jumping during training. The pain is caused by the injuries inside the muscle fibres giving rise to swelling and pain. Rest, compression and the avoidance of activities which are painful should ensure that the problems reduce within 1–2 days.

## Cramp

The exact cause of cramp in the musculature is not known and there are several explanations. One reason for cramp may be previous injuries which have left scar tissue with other mechanical properties than the rest of the musculature. This may give rise to a painful condition experienced as cramp.

Any change in the balance between the chemical substances in the tissues, such as changes in salt content, have been discussed as a further cause. Players often get cramp towards the end of a match played on a soft or wet, heavy surface. This can lead to an exhaustion phenomenon known as cramp.

Cramp is treated with rest and activation of the agonist musculature which can stop or ease the cramp condition and thereby reduce the pain. Cramp in the calf can be eased by bending the foot upwards forcefully with the knee in full extension.

# 10. Head injuries

Yelverton Tegner

Head and facial injuries constitute a problem in many sports. Between 5 and 10 per cent of all injuries reported relate to these parts of the body.

In football there are several dangerous situations which could lead to head injuries. There is, for instance, a risk of concussion when heading the ball, especially if the wrong technique is used. Considerable force is set in motion when a football is kicked with full impact and the ball can reach speeds of 100 km/h.

Injuries which can affect the head are of several different kinds: concussion, brain haemorrhaging, skeletal injuries and cuts.

## Concussion

Concussion is the most common head injury in sport. The term 'concussion' is not very accurate since it gives the impression that the injury is harmless, a mere 'shaking up' of the brain. This is not the case. Every concussion damages part of the brain tissues which is serious since damaged brain tissue does not heal in the way as, for example, muscle tissue does. Furthermore, there is also a risk that the injury is aggravated if not handled correctly. However, a single, correctly treated concussion does not generally lead to any permanent damage.

## The injury mechanism

Concussion, during football activities, can occur in a number of ways. The head can collide with an external mobile object such as a football, or can collide with an immobile object such as a goalpost, or the head can be exposed to indirect violence, for example if a player falls backwards uncontrollably resulting in whiplash injury to the neck and an uncontrolled movement of the brain within the skull. The trauma to the head that results in a concussion, always involves a combination of acceleration and deceleration. The brain has its own shock absorbers, the cerebral fluid and the neck musculature, which normally function well to protect the brain from minor trauma and from getting injured when, for example, heading a football.

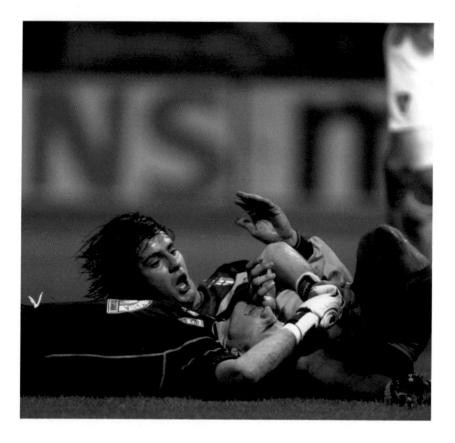

## Definition

Different definitions of concussion have been used over the years. Recently, the International Concussion in Sports Group revised the earlier definition and developed a new more accurate definition of concussion. They stated among other things that a concussion 'results in a graded set of clinical symptoms that may or may not involve loss of consciousness'. A common feature of a concussed player is confusion and loss of memory.

The most common signs of concussion are shown in Table 10.1.

**Table 10.1** Common signs of concussion

| Early signs | Common signs |
|---|---|
| • Vacant stare | **Initial** |
| • Delayed verbal response | • Headache, dizziness |
| • Confusion – can go the wrong way | • Lack of awareness |
| • Blurred speech | • Nausea and vomiting |
| • Uncoordinated | |
| • Abnormal emotional reactions | **Later (days to weeks)** |
| • Memory deficits | • Low grade of headache |
| • Loss of consciousness | • Hypersensitivity to light |
| | • Impaired attention |
| | • Memory dysfunction |
| | • Easily fatiguability |
| | • Irritated and easily frustrated |
| | • Difficulty in focusing vision |
| | • Intolerant of sound |
| | • Worry, anxiety, insomnia |
| | • Concentration difficulties |

In order to be able to treat concussion more simply and uniformly, different treatment models have been used. The most recent published models classify concussion into three different grades (Table 10.2).

**Table 10.2** Classification of concussion

**Grade 1:** Transient confusion without loss of consciousness and the symptoms resolve in less than 15 min.

**Grade 2:** Transient confusion without loss of consciousness and the symptoms last for more than 15 min. This includes instances when the player has posttraumatic amnesia after 15 min.

**Grade 3:** All concussions with unconsciousness.

Grades 1 and 2 are most common but can sometimes be difficult to identify. The player has not been unconscious and may appear completely clear in the head. The only indication can be a vacant stare, difficulty to express oneself clearly and/or reduced memory function. Headache, dizziness and nausea may occur. This is what is known as a slight temporary disturbance of the mental functions or a 'bell ringer' and it is important that even such a slight concussion receives attention so that the injury is not made worse.

Every player who suffers a suspected concussion should be carefully observed. The symptoms of concussion may first occur several minutes after the headtrauma.

The diagnosis of 'concussion' is established according to the clinical picture immediately after the injury and not after various medical tests such as radiographic examination or magnetic resonance tomography etc. These are carried out only to verify or eliminate complications in connection with the injury.

## What to do?

Concussion should always be dealt with by a doctor as soon as possible. If the player is unconscious, it is extremely important that the emergency care is correct. The first thing one should check is the breathing. If breathing is normal, the player should be moved as little as possible since there is always a risk of simultaneous injury to the neck which could be aggravated.

If the player has difficulty breathing, he or she should be placed on his or her side leaning forward (see Chapter 8) to guarantee a free passage for air. If the player cannot breathe, artificial respiration should be provided using the mouth-to-mouth technique. When the airway is guaranteed to be clear, the player should be transported to hospital as quickly as possible. During the whole procedure, the neck should be fixed, preferably with a rigid neck brace.

A player who has suffered concussion should not continue to play. The player should be taken into the changing rooms so that the level of seriousness of the injury can be assessed undisturbed.

In order to establish when a player has completely recovered one should use simple neuropsychological tests (see the test schedule on Page 240). These tests should be carried out on the whole squad before the season starts to establish the baseline performance of each player. If this has not been done, it can be difficult to evaluate the implications of what an impaired value for a test result may represent. This test and other similar tests all involve different memory components, all important when evaluating brain function. Apart from this test, a neurological screening should also be performed. Recollection of recent events should be evaluated with questions like: What team are we playing against? What is the name of the ground where the game is being played? How long has the game been in progress? Who scored the goal?

If the player manages to answer all the questions and is alert and clear within 15 min, he or she should exert him- or herself physically (for example 40 m sprint, 5 sit-ups, 5 push-ups, 5 knee bends) and then the memory test should be repeated. If everything is well, it can be concluded that the player received a grade 1 concussion. In this situation the player can return to playing football the next day.

If the player does not recover completely within 15 min this is, by definition, a grade 2 concussion. A player who has sustained a grade 2 concussion should be free from symptoms for 7 days before taking up football again. The player can begin physical training as soon as the symptoms disappear. During the rehabilitation phase the player should not expose her- or himself to any situations where there is a risk of a new concussion. This means that the player should avoid heading the ball and also avoid forceful physical contact with other players.

During rehabilitation, balance and coordination should be practised regularly as these abilites are often adversely affected following concussion.

If the player has been unconscious — even for a short time — this is defined as a grade 3 concussion. If the period of unconsciousness is shorter than 1 minute it should be treated as a grade 2 concussion. For longer periods of unconsciousness, 2 weeks absence from football is recommended.

When treating these injuries, it is important that one takes previous head injuries into consideration including those which may have occurred outside the sports arena. If the player has had a previous concussion within the last 12 months, the rest period should be longer (Table 10.3). Players who have suffered more than three concussions should undergo an extended medical examination. While awaiting the result of such an examination, the player should not be involved in football activities — to prevent any risk of chronic brain damage.

- Note that all absence from activities are counted from the first symptom-free day.

Table 10.3 Treatment schedules for the three levels of concussion

| | Definition | Treatment | Second concussion within 12 months |
|---|---|---|---|
| **Grade 1** | Stunned. No unconsciousness. Recovered within 15 minutes | Stop activities. Return to activities the next day if symptom free | Return to activities after 7 symptom free days |
| **Grade 2** | Stunned. No unconsciousness. Recovered after 15 minutes | Stop activities. Return to activities after 7 symptom free days | Return to activities after 14 symptom free days |
| **Grade 3** | A) Unconscious for less than 1 minute. B) Unconscious for more than 1 minute. | A) Same as grade 2 B) Return to activities after 14 symptom free days. | Examination. Return to activities at the earliest after 28 days with no symptoms. |

### Internet neuropsychological post-concussion test

New Web-based neuropsychological tests have been presented recently. These tests can be used in order to detect and to monitor resolution of symptoms after concussion. They can also be of use in order to provide objective information for return-to-play decision. These Web-based tests can only be used if the players have performed a baseline test before season. These tests measure memory, reaction time, and speed of information processing.

These Web-based tests are highly recommended and in the future they will be much more common than today. These Web-based tests offer the possibility of individual treatment of concussion as recommended by the Concussion in Sport Group.

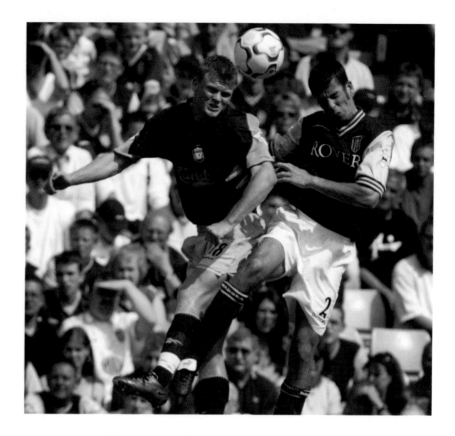

## The consequences of concussion

Each individual who suffers a concussion of a grade 2 or 3 can experience a number of subsequent symptoms. Symptoms such as headache, sensitivity to light, difficulties in concentrating etc. may persist. If the injured player's symptoms persist after 1 week, an extended examination using a computerized tomography (CAT) scan should be carried out since there may be other injuries to the head such as haemorrhaging. Furthermore, every player who has suffered a level 3 concussion with unconsciousness should always undergo such an examination immediately.

The basic principle for all concussion and brain injuries is that the player may not return to physical activities if he or she is experiencing any symptoms whatsoever. Since this type of injury leads to impaired reaction times, it is easy for new injuries to occur.

A greatly feared complication of concussion is known as the second impact syndrome. This is a special condition which is almost 100 per cent fatal. It can occur if a player is exposed to a second head injury soon after a slight concussion. All those who have been affected by this complication had returned to activities despite persistent symptoms (see Table 10.1). The second impact to the head is often very slight and would probably not have caused any injury at all if suffered by a healthy brain. Despite the mild degree of the impact the injured player quickly loses consciousness and, most frequently, dies within the space of a few hours. Fortunately this condition is rare. There have, however, been several reports of this occuring in other sports, for example, in American football, ice hockey and boxing.

Other complications of concussion include persistent impairment of psychological capacity and memory. Disturbances of memory functions can persist up to 3 months after concussion with unconsciousness. It is also possible that migraine can occur after repeated head injuries.

## Haemorrhaging in the brain

Haemorrhaging inside the head can occur as a result of external violence to the head. Three different types of haemorrhaging can be distinguished:

- Bleeding between the skull and the dura mater
  – epidural bleeding.
- Bleeding between the pia mater and the dura mater
  – subdural bleeding.
- Bleeding in the brain itself – intracerebral bleeding.

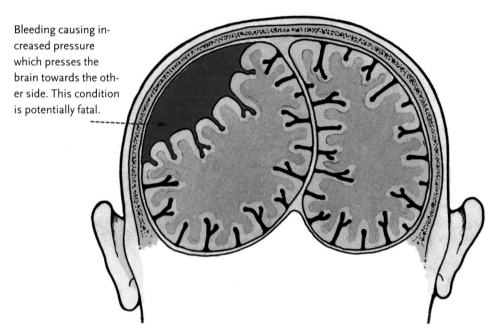

Bleeding causing increased pressure which presses the brain towards the other side. This condition is potentially fatal.

**Figure 10.1** Serious injuries to the head can lead to epidural bleeding, bleeding between the skull and the dura mater, or subdural bleeding, bleeding between the pia mater and the dura mater.

During the acute phase it is often impossible to distinguish between these types of bleeding and 'regular' concussion. All injuries which cause concussion can also give rise to bleeding inside the head. There are, however, certain clear symptoms of the different types of bleeding. It is important to know that one can never, on the basis of the medical history alone, eliminate a serious haemorrhage. All injured players should, if there is the slightest doubt, undergo a CAT scan of the brain to eliminate these types of bleeding.

Epidural bleeding is often believed, in a typical case, to have what is known as a free interval. This means that the injured player often recovers after an initial short period of unconsciousness to then — often within the hour — decline rapidly into heavy new unconsciousness. In this situation the injured player has to be operated on urgently if her or his life is to be saved. Epidural bleeding generally occurs when an artery in the temporal bone ruptures.

Subdural bleeding can also have a free interval. In the typical case this often exceeds 24 hours — sometimes several months. The progress is slower than with epidural bleeding since the bleeding is often caused by an injured vein and not by an artery. This means that anyone who experiences a persistent headache after a concussion injury should undergo an examination to eliminate bleeding.

Intracerebral bleeding is often associated with long-term unconsciousness before the injured player comes round. The patients are often very seriously ill and their need for emergency treatment is generally apparent.

# Skeletal injuries

### Skull fractures
Fractures to the skull are often an indication that the head has been exposed to extreme force. The fracture itself seldom requires attention. The treatment depends on the underlying brain injury — often concussion.

### Cheekbone fractures
The cheekbone is situated between the cheek and the ear. The bone can be fractured by a high kick or if a player collides with a goalpost. The symptoms can often include pain when chewing and the injury can sometimes require surgery. Medical personnel should check from above and the side of the face for any deformity.

### Maxillary bone fractures
This type of fracture can also be caused by a high kick and can lead to damage to the facial nerves with impaired sensitivity as a result. Double vision may also occur. The injury sometimes requires surgery and the player is then away from football for around 4 weeks.

## TEST FOR EVALUATING HEAD INJURIES

### ORIENTATION

Ask the injured player to state the: year, month, date, day of the week and time (± 1 hour). 1 point for each correct answer.
*Max points: 5*

### IMMEDIATE MEMORY

Say five 'meaningless' words for the injured player to repeat on three occasions. The words might be, for example, car, horse, house, pen and sweet. 1 point for each correct word, a total of 3 times.
*Max points: 15*

### CONCENTRATION

1. Ask the injured player to repeat the following combinations of figures backwards. Go on to the next row if the first combination is repeated correctly. Stop if both are wrong. 1 point per row.

| | |
|---|---|
| 3-8-2 | 5-1-8 |
| 2-7-9-3 | 2-1-6-8 |
| 5-1-8-6-9 | 9-4-1-7-5 |
| 6-9-7-5-3-1 | 4-2-8-9-3-7 |

2. Ask the injured player to say the months of the year in reverse order. 1 point for an entirely correct sequence.
*Max points: 5*

### DELAYED REPLY

About 5 minutes after the first immediate memory test, ask the injured player to repeat the same words. 1 point per word.
*Max points: 5*

## Total points: max 30

# 11. Injuries to the upper extremities

Jon Karlsson

## INJURIES TO THE SHOULDER

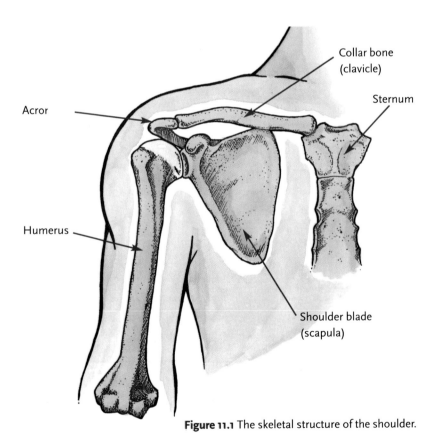

**Figure 11.1** The skeletal structure of the shoulder.

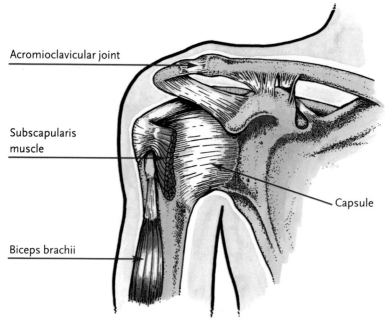

Acromioclavicular joint

Subscapularis
muscle

Capsule

Biceps brachii

**Figure 11.2** The muscles, tendons and ligaments of the shoulder.

Injuries to the upper extremities, including the shoulder, are considerably less common in football than injuries to the lower extremities. The injuries mainly encountered as acute injuries are
contusions, ligament injuries, luxation and, in rare cases, fractures.
Goalkeepers are more exposed to this type of injury than outfield
players.

The function of the shoulder is based on the delicate interplay
of movements between the upper arm, the shoulder blade, the collar
bone and the back. The interplay of muscles in a normal shoulder
is well coordinated. Any disturbance in this coordination can lead to
pain and/or instability.

The muscle groups can be divided into the larger, superficial
muscles which develop force, and the smaller, stabilizing muscles
close to the joints which have a coordinating function. The muscles
which fix and stabilize the shoulder blade are especially important
for the function of the shoulder.

In anatomical terms, the shoulder is composed of four joints —
in addition to the joint between the upper arm and the shoulder
blade, there are also joints between the collar bone and the sternum
on one side and the collar bone and the shoulder blade on the other
side. And finally, the joint between the shoulder blade and the torso
is important for the function of the shoulder. Injuries to the shoulder caused by overuse, which are common in sports involving
throwing, are caused by the supraspinatus tendon and the bursa
being trapped between the acromion and the humerus. These injuries are, however, unusual in football.

## Collar bone fractures

### Injury mechanism

Among children and younger footballers, collar bone fractures are
the most common sports injury. The injury is less common among
adults. The injury mechanism is either a direct injury, such as after
a kick to the collar bone, or — more commonly — falling with the
arm outstretched.

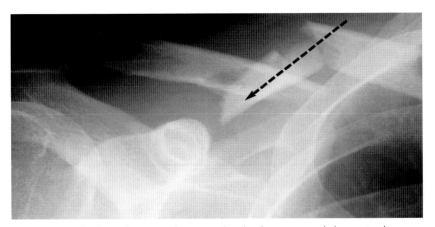

**Figure 11.3** Collar bone fractures always involve displacement and shortening between the ends of the fracture.

### Symptoms and signs

The symptoms are clear. A radiograph is seldom necessary to establish an accurate diagnosis for children. The point of the fracture is painful, swollen and it is possible to feel instability between the ends of the fracture.

### Treatment

For the youngest patients, no specific treatment is necessary. The usual treatment is immobilization to ease the pain using a figure of eight bandage for 2–3 weeks. For adults a sling is often used.

### Prognosis

Complications, such as nerve or vascular damage, are rare. The healing prospects are good. The fracture always heals, however, with some degree of shortening and a lump occurs over the injured area which can be disfiguring. The lump disappears after a while in many cases, especially in youngsters.

## Shoulder dislocation

### Injury mechanism

Shoulder dislocation is common in sport. It occurs in football both among outfield players and goalkeepers but is more common in other sports such as ice hockey. Dislocation of the shoulder is divided into anterior and posterior and 95 per cent of cases involve anterior shoulder dislocation. Posterior shoulder dislocation is unusual. During a match, the shoulder is dislocation mainly when the player rotates the arm outwards.

A Bankart injury occurs when the capsule and cartilage ring which deepen the labrum, are torn away on the anterior side of the shoulder blade. If the capsule injury fails to heal, there may be a risk of recurrent instability.

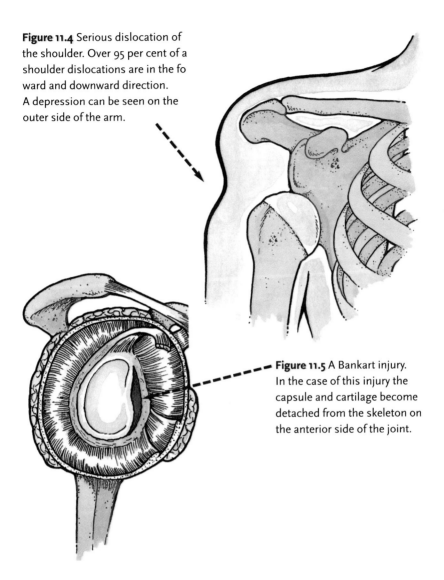

**Figure 11.4** Serious dislocation of the shoulder. Over 95 per cent of a shoulder dislocations are in the fo ward and downward direction. A depression can be seen on the outer side of the arm.

**Figure 11.5** A Bankart injury. In the case of this injury the capsule and cartilage become detached from the skeleton on the anterior side of the joint.

## Symptoms and signs

Shoulder dislocation causes immediate, severe pain and seriously impaired mobility. The contour of the shoulder is altered and a depression can be noted beneath the projection from the shoulder blade. A radiographic examination is recommended to be able to establish an accurate diagnosis, to eliminate fractures and to see the direction in which the humerus has dislocated. Thorough ex-

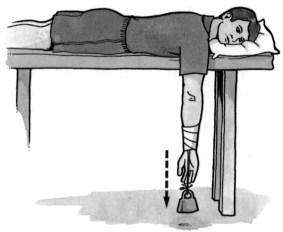

**Figure 11.6** The simplest way of setting a dislocated shoulder is by using the hanging arm technique. The player lies on his or her stomach and the arm is pulled straight downwards.

amination of sensory and muscle function and blood circulation should be made. Damage to the nerves can occur in some cases, most commonly damage to the axillary nerve, the first indication of which is reduced sensation on the outer side of the upper arm.

## Treatment

When dislocation has been established through examination, the joint should be reduced as quickly as possible. Any delay causes muscle spasm which makes setting more difficult.

There are several ways of setting the arm in the correct position. The simplest way involving least risk is the hanging arm method. The player lies on his or her stomach on an examination bench with the arm hanging over the edge. Pulling the arm downwards in the direction of the length of the arm will place the joint in the correct position. Other methods are more complicated and can require a short time in hospital especially if there has been a delay in setting the dislocation. Occasionally the player has to be anaesthetized before the arm is set.

To relieve pain a shoulder bandage can be used after the arm has been set. The bandage can be removed and rehabilitation started after 1–3 days.

### Prognosis

The most common complication is recurring instability. The risk of this is greatest among younger players between 15 and 20 years old. Some studies have calculated the risk for a recurrence of the injury at 50–70 per cent or more, but the risk of recurrences declines as the player gets older. The risk of other complications such as nerve or vascular damage is small. After adequate rehabilitation most players regain good shoulder function.

## Recurrent shoulder instability

### Injury mechanism

Recurrent shoulder instability occurs relatively often among young players after a severe dislocation. The underlying cause is often a Bankart injury.

### Symptoms and signs

Total dislocation or subluxation can occur. Instability can be noted especially during an external rotation of the arm with the arm positioned away from the body.

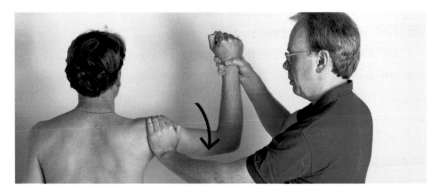

**Figure 11.7** A test to examine instability in the shoulder. The examiner stands behind the player and the arm is rotated outwards on a horizontal plain. Subluxation (or severe discomfort) occurs and the player rotates the arm inwards on reflex to avoid subluxation of the shoulder joint.

In order to assess the injury, a stability test can be done. The arm may be unstable in a forward and downward direction or rarely in a backward direction. The stability test is carried out by trying to draw or push the head in the joint back and forth. Normally, the head can only be moved around 10 mm — any more indicates instability.

A more sensitive test is known as the apprehension test. The arm is held at 90° away from the body and is rotated externally. The joint head is then pushed forward and the player either experiences discomfort or the joint head subluxates forwards. A reflex inward rotation is initiated in order to keep the arm in the correct position. This is called a positive apprehension test and is a sensitive indication of forward instability.

## Treatment

Operative treatment is generally necessary. Around 150 different methods of surgery have been described but the best method is believed to be the Bankhart operation where the injury to the capsule and cartilage (labrum) is repaired. A keyhole examination (arthroscopy) is often of great value in diagnosing the injury to examine adjacent injuries. In some cases the stabilizing operation can be done using keyhole surgery. However, the results of keyhole surgery are not yet as good as open surgery.

Rehabilitation after the operation takes 4–6 months. It is important that the shoulder has regained full strength, flexibility and coordination before football activities can be resumed.

## Prognosis

The result after surgery has been shown to be good in several studies. Over 90 per cent of players experience regained flexibility, stability and function and find it possible to return to sporting activities.

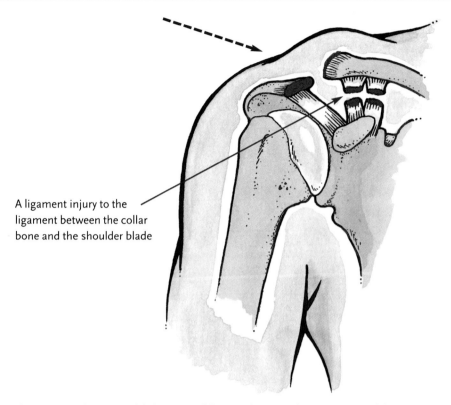

A ligament injury to the ligament between the collar bone and the shoulder blade

**Figure 11.8** In the event of dislocation of the joint between the acromion and the collar bone (dashed arrow), displacement can be seen above the joint along with instability and pain.

# Dislocation of the acromioclavicular joint

### Injury mechanism

Dislocation in the joint between the acromion and the collar bone (acromioclavicular joint) is more common in for example ice hockey, than in football. This injury occurs in contact situations such as forceful tackles or if a player falls and the impact to the shoulder is directed downwards.

Injuries to the acromioclavicular joint can be divided into six levels of seriousness depending on the severity and degree of instability. Damage to the capsule, the ligaments and the muscle attachments can occur.

## Symptoms and signs

The symptoms of an acromioclavicular joint dislocation are distinct with pain and swelling over the damaged joint. The diagnosis can often be established after a clinical examination. An instability test of the joint can also be carried out by pushing the upper arm upwards while pushing the collar bone downwards. Increased mobility can be detected between the acromion and the collar bone.

A radiograph is recommended to see the exact position of the injury and to eliminate any fracture.

## Treatment

Non-operative treatment is recommended with short-term immobilization to ease pain followed by range of motion and weight training. Only cases of a complete rupture of the deltoid muscle attachment and/or dislocation of the sternoclavicular joint call for emergency surgery. However, both these injuries are rare. The reason for surgery is, in such cases, to retain the normal function of the deltoid muscle.

If there are any persisting problems with pain or instability, it is possible to operate at a later stage. The joint is then stabilized at the same time as the outer end of the collar bone is removed.

## Prognosis

Most players can return to play around 2–4 weeks after rehabilitation. The prognosis is generally good. When surgery has been carried out the rehabilitation process takes longer, often 3–4 months.

# ELBOW INJURIES

Injuries to the elbow are unusual in football and arise almost exclusively as acute injuries.

## Elbow dislocation

### Injury mechanism

Dislocation of the elbow is considerably less common than dislocations of the shoulder. It is, however, the second most common dislocation in the body. The injury occurs when a player falls with an outstretched arm with the elbow in a half-bent position. In around 90 per cent of cases the dislocation is in a backwards direction, that is, the forearm has been forced back in relation to the upper arm. In some cases fractures of bones in the elbow can occur in combination with the dislocation.

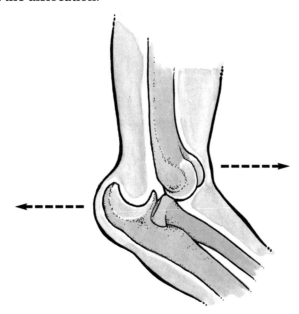

**Figure 11.9** Elbow dislocation. In cases of elbow dislocation the forearm is most often forced backwards in relation to the upper arm.

### Symptoms and signs

Immediate pain, relatively pronounced swelling and impaired mobility or an inability to move occur. The injured player keeps the elbow half bent. Examination reveals a displacement along with a depression towards the back between the upper arm and the forearm. A radiograph examination is recommended. The injured player should receive immediate attention at a casualty department. The direction of the luxation and any combined fractures can be assessed from the radiographs. The most common fracture is to the radial head.

### Treatment

An elbow dislocation should be reduced correctly as quickly as possible. The patient often has to be anaesthetized. Immobilization with plaster or a splint can be used from 1 to 3 weeks. When the immobilization has been removed, rehabilitation can begin in which emphasis should be placed on range of motion training.

### Prognosis

The prognosis for regaining function is good. A common persistent complication can involve a stretch defect. The longer the immobilization, the greater the risk of a stretch defect. Serious complications such as vascular and nerve damage along with recurring instability are, however, very rare.

# Bursitis

Bursitis above the point of the elbow occurs either as an acute or a chronic injury and is most common among goalkeepers. In an acute situation (such as a straight fall onto the elbow), bleeding can occur into the bursa. In chronic cases, the inflammation can result from repeated irritation such as may occur when a goalkeeper stretch-

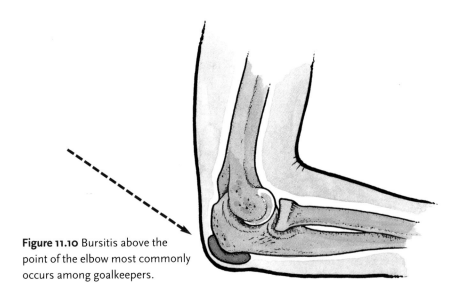

**Figure 11.10** Bursitis above the point of the elbow most commonly occurs among goalkeepers.

es for the ball and often lands on the elbow. The condition can take a long time to heal but is only seldom serious.

### Symptoms and signs

The bursa above the point of the elbow is swollen and tender when palpated or pressed. A large fluid-filled blister can often be seen.

### Treatment

If there is bleeding or an infection, it may be necessary to operate and drain the wound. However, this is rare. If infection is suspected, antibiotics should be prescribed. The discomfort from chronic bursitis usually disappears after a short period of rest and the use of elbow protection. In a few cases the bursa can be surgically removed due to recurrent problems.

### Prognosis

The prognosis is good. Many players can continue playing football despite persistent bursitis.

# Thrower's elbow

### Injury mechanism

This injury is most common among those involved in throwing sports and can occur among goalkeepers in football. The cause is degenerative changes towards the back of the elbow joint with the development of calcified osteophytes on the point of the elbow. This injury is probably the most common wear and tear injury to the elbow in the context of football.

### Symptoms and signs

The elbow joint is painful towards the back above and around the point of the elbow. The pain can radiate towards both the inside and the outside of the joint and is particularly noticeable if the elbow is stretched to its full extent. In certain cases of long-term symptoms, a stretch defect can occur, occasionally leading to fixing and/or locking of the elbow.

A radiograph to see the injury with the calcified osteophytes on the point of the elbow is recommended. A more thorough diagnosis can be established after an arthoscopic examination.

### Treatment

In the initial stages when the elbow is swollen and painful, rest is recommended combined with an anti-inflammatory medication. Since this often fails to provide satisfactory results in the long term, surgery is often necessary to remove the calcified osteophytes. This operation can be done using keyhole surgery.

### Prognosis

The prognosis is good. Many goalkeepers with thrower's arm can continue to play football despite the problem. The results of surgery are generally good.

# HAND AND WRIST INJURIES

The hand is a very complicated organ of movement. The hand and wrist consist of 27 bones altogether. These are linked in a complex system of ligaments, tendons and muscles. Injuries to the hand, for example to the fingers, are relatively frequent in football. Wrist injuries are less common.

## Injuries to the lower radius (radius fractures)

### Injury mechanism
This injury occurs when a player falls onto the hand and outstretched arm. In the case of children where the growth zones have not yet closed, the same injury mechanism results in a displacement of the growth zone, known as physiolysis. The injury mechanism and symptoms of the two conditions are therefore alike.

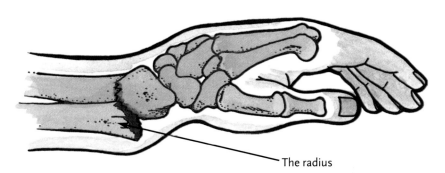

The radius

**Figure 11.11** Radius fracture. Displacement occurs since the broken fragment is wrongly positioned.

### Symptoms and signs
A typical displacement with a turn of the lower fractured fragment along with swelling and pronounced pain can be noted.

Radiographic examination is recommended if this injury is suspected. With the aid of radiographs it is possible to assess the severity of the injury and then decide on appropriate treatment.

## Treatment

If the fracture is displaced, it should be reduced as soon as possible. If there is any suspicion of a radius fracture, the player should be taken to the casualty department: the fracture can be reduced under local anaesthetic. It is important to determine the exact position for the fracture in order to achieve good results. Immobilization should be ensured using a plaster splint for around 4 weeks. A repeat radiograph should be done after 1 week to check that the position remains stable. If this is not the case, the injury should be re-reduced and sometimes surgery may be necessary.

## Prognosis

The healing process is good. Any remaining displacement can cause impaired mobility in some cases. Other complications are rare.

# Scaphoid fractures

## Injury mechanism

This injury is not that uncommon and occurs both among goalkeepers and field players. It occurs when the player falls on the hand with the arm outstretched. Unfortunately this injury can be difficult to diagnose in an initial examination.

## Symptoms and signs

Pain occurs if the area above the bone is palpated. Indirect pain occurs when the wrist is bent towards the thumb and backwards which indicates a suspected fracture. Swelling is minimal or does not occur at all.

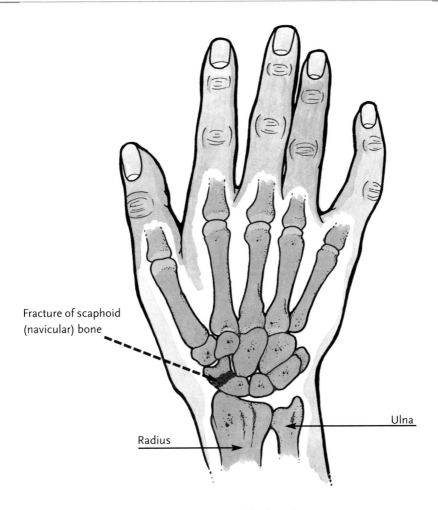

Fracture of scaphoid
(navicular) bone

Ulna

Radius

**Figure 11.12** Navicular bone fractures can be difficult to diagnose. It is sometimes
necessary to use repeated radiographs.

If the first radiographs do not show any injury, a scaphoid
bone fracture should be suspected if the pain has not disappeared
within 2–3 weeks. Radiographs should be taken once again. The injury is treated as a fracture with immobilization until a second radiographic examination has been carried out.

A diagnosis can be established with greater accuracy in the
initial phase with the aid of an isotopic scan (scintigraphy).

**Treatment**

For fractures without any displacement, immobilization with a plaster cast is recommended for around 8 weeks. Plastic protection is often used to allow the player to begin training after 1 or 2 weeks. It may even be possible to play a match with the plaster or splint padded with soft wadding.

If displacement occurs, especially if the gap between the fractured fragments is greater than 1–1.5 mm, surgery may be necessary. The healing time can be reduced and correct healing ensured. This type of treatment is sometimes preferred to speed up the return to football. From an ethical point of view this is, however, doubtful since the operation involves an element of risk.

**Prognosis**

The healing prospects are good. More than 90 per cent of all scaphoid bone fractures heal. Any impairment of mobility is rare although the rehabilitation period is long, often up to 6 months.

In some cases complications may occur when the fracture fails to heal (pseudarthrosis) or if a part of the bone dies (avascular necrosis). Surgery is always necessary in such cases. It may then be difficult for the player to continue playing football.

# Instability in the wrist

**Injury mechanism**

Instability in the wrist is probably more common than was previously believed. The cause is an injury to the ligament which attaches the lower radius with the wrist bone, or between the two rows of wrist bones. The injury is not especially common in football, however, and occurs more commonly as a wear and tear injury among gymnasts.

## Symptoms and signs

The wrist is painful if moved especially in extreme positions. The pain is diffuse, however, and a clinical diagnosis is difficult to establish. If such an injury is suspected a stability test should be carried out on the wrist. Radiographic examination does not show any fracture but can disclose displacement of the small bones in the wrist area. For a more accurate diagnosis, an MRI scan or keyhole examination may be required.

## Treatment

Strength training for the muscles in the wrist along with the use of a stabilizing support splint is recommended. Tape can also be used. In certain cases surgery is required to stabilize the wrist but this is rare.

## Prognosis

Since diagnosis is difficult many players have problems for a long period of time before the extent of their injury can be established. The prognosis is uncertain, not least if the instability is marked and surgery is necessary.

# Ligament rupture in the thumb

## Injury mechanism

A collateral ligament injury in the thumb is an acute injury which can occur both among field players and goalkeepers if the player falls onto the hand with the thumb bent outwards. The medial (ulnar) collateral ligament is torn off. The ends of the ligament lie on either side of the aponeurosis which is why this injury cannot heal without surgery.

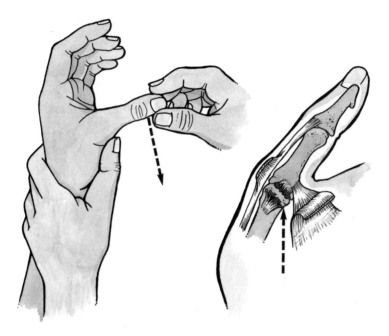

**Figure 11.13** Stability examination Instability occurs in the event of a collateral liga-ment injury in the thumb. This injury generally requires surgery.

## Symptoms and signs

Pain is elicited when the thumb joint is palpated. A diagnosis can be established by means of a stability test and comparison with the uninjured thumb. The stability test may be difficult to conduct soon after the injury has occurred due to the pain.

A simple nerve-blocking agent at wrist level should ease the pain to allow a stability test. Radiographic examination is recom-mended.

## Treatment

Surgery is usually recommended. Otherwise, there is a risk that the ligament will not heal and that the player will have persistent instability. The ends of the ligament can be re-attached to the bone or the ends can be sewn together. In some cases the ligament is torn away from the attachment along with a small fragment of bone. If the bone fragment is in the correct place this indicates that further surgery is not required. If the bone fragment has moved more than 2 mm an operation is necessary. After the operation, immobilization is necessary using a plaster splint or orthosis for 4–5 weeks.

**Prognosis**

The prognosis is good if the injury is diagnosed and treated in the correct way. The rehabilitation period after the operation is around 8–10 weeks.

If the injury is not diagnosed or if the player seeks help some time after the injury (several months) there will be chronic instability and weakness in the thumb. A goalkeeper may then find difficulty in gripping or holding the ball at which point reconstructive surgery may be necessary. The prognosis for continuing a career in sport, for example as a goalkeeper, is then doubtful, particularly after surgery.

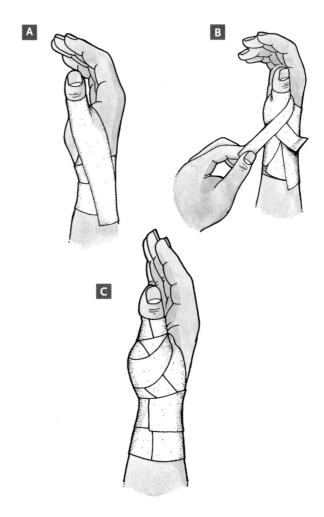

**Figure 11.14** Tape is often used – especially by goalkeepers – after a collateral ligament rupture in the thumb and in order to prevent this injury. (A) A length of tape is first placed along the length of the thumb. (B) Cross-taping then ensures stability. (C) Finally, the tape is wound around the thumb and wrist for anchorage.

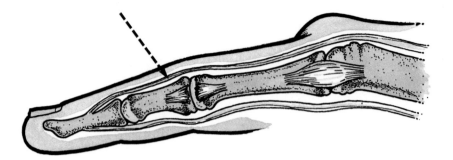

**Figure 11.15** Collateral ligament injury in the finger joint. The injury takes a long time to heal and swelling often persists around the joint.

# Ligament injuries in the finger

### Injury mechanism

This injury occurs only as an acute injury and is relatively common among goalkeepers. It is, however, more common in other ball sports than football. The injury occurs if the player falls or any other impact forces any of the fingers in a sideways direction.

### Symptoms

Ligament injuries cause acute pain and relatively pronounced swelling around the finger joint. The swelling often persists for some time. It may take 6–12 months for the injury to heal and the swelling may be permanent. During examination, instability can be noted, in addition to swelling and soreness, when the finger is moved to the side.

The injury may be associated with a more serious ligament injury and damage to the the cartilage plate on the underside of the joint. This injury should be suspected especially if the joint can be overstretched. Suspicion of this type of injury warrants an immediate referral to a hand surgeon. Radiographic examination is recommended to eliminate the suspicion of any fractures.

## Treatment

Surgery is not necessary if there is only a ligament injury. If the cartilage plates on the underside of the joint is damaged, it may be necessary to operate. The injury is treated using a two-finger dressing which involves the injured finger being taped to the finger next to it. The reason for using this type of bandage is to enable early range of motion training. The uninjured finger helps move the injured one. The player can return to football almost immediately after the injury if adequate treatment and taping with a two-finger dressing is used for 6–8 weeks. Some goalkeepers use the two-finger dressing as a preventative measure to prevent the injury from occurring.

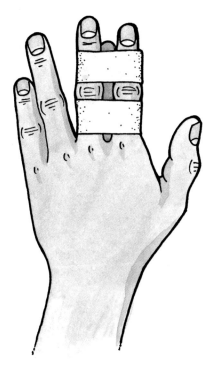

**Figure 11.16** A two-finger dressing stabilizes the injured finger by binding it to a healthy one. Rehabilitation can then be initiated to regain mobility.

# Finger joint dislocation

## Injury mechanism

This injury occurs only as an acute injury mainly among goalkeepers. It very seldom occurs in the thumb while the other fingers are more susceptible. Dislocation generally occurs when the fingers are bent back and the outer phalanx is forced backwards in relation to the closest phalanx.

263

## Symptoms and signs

A classic displacement occurs along with pronounced pain and impairment of mobility. Radiographic examination is recommended to eliminate any fractures.

## Treatment

Surgery may be necessary if the dislocation is combined with a fracture engaging the surface of the joint. If there is no fracture, the joint can be reduced as soon as possible by pulling the fingers out lengthwise after which the joint is overstretched and bent. The stability of the joint can then be tested. Further treatment consists of immobilization using a two-finger bandage. If the two-finger dressing is used range of motion training can be initiated early and the player can generally return to football within a day or a few days of the injury. Swelling and soreness over the joint often persists for 6–12 months.

## Prognosis

In some cases with slightly impaired mobility, apart from swelling and stiffness, the prognosis is good. Thorough examination to detect any possibility of more serious damage is necessary, such as tendon damage.

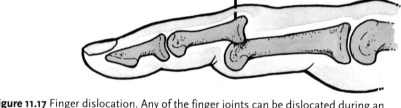

**Figure 11.17** Finger dislocation. Any of the finger joints can be dislocated during an accident. After reducing the joint, it can be supported with tape at the same time as range of motion training is initiated.

**Figure 11.18** Drop finger. The attachment of the extensor tendon is torn away, in some cases along with a bone fragment. The joint cannot be stretched actively. This injury is most common among goalkeepers.

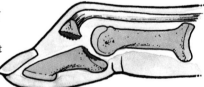

# Drop finger

### Injury mechanism

Drop finger occurs most often as an acute injury among goalkeepers. The injury occurs when the extensor tendon, which stretches the outer phalanx, is torn away taking with it a small fragment of bone from the phalanx. The player loses any ability to stretch the joint.

### Symptoms and signs

The diagnosis is clinical but a radiograph is recommended to eliminate fractures and to assess the degree of any potential fracture. Examination reveals drop finger and inability to stretch the outer phalanx of the injured finger actively.

### Treatment

If the radiographs show a fracture, the size of the bone fragment is of decisive significance for treatment. If the bone fragment engages one-third of the joint surface or more, immediate surgery is recommended. In other cases the injury can be treated using a splint to keep the joint overstretched for 5–6 weeks. During surgery the finger is held in position with a pin or suture after the bone fragment has been put back into position.

   If the injury can be treated with a splint alone, football activities can be resumed directly without risk of further problems. Even after surgery, football can be resumed after 1–3 weeks on condition that the appropriate support is used.

### Prognosis

The prognosis is good for both function and pain. A slight stretching defect may often persist, which can be cosmetically disturbing, but does not affect function.

# 12. Back injuries

Leif Swärd

Injuries which affect the spine are relatively uncommon in football. The energy generated during tackling and high challenges is, however, large enough for serious injury to occur. Young players who put too much strain on their spines while training also run the risk of developing overuse injuries in the body of the vertebrae, the discs and the vertebral arch.

## Anatomy and development

The spine consists of 24 vertebrae: seven cervical vertebrae, 12 thoracic vertebrae and five lumbar vertebrae. The top two cervical vertebrae are very distinct in appearance, while the others are very much alike and consist of the body of the vertebra and an arch. On the arch sits a bony process with facet joints — two which articulate with the vertebra above and two which articulate with the vertebra beneath.

Between each pair of vertebrae lies a disc which consists of a fibrous ring surrounding a softer core. The disk makes movement in the spine possible. The degree of movement between each pair of vertebrae is limited by the facet joints, which make the range of movement specific for each individual pair of vertebrae.

The spine's passive stability is guaranteed by a large number of ligaments which run between the body of the vertebrae and the arches. The active stability is controlled by a number of muscles, located both on the front but mainly to the rear of the spine.

The cervical spine has the largest range of movement but is also the least stable. In the thoracic spine the widest range of movement is in turning, while in the lumbar spine it is in bending.

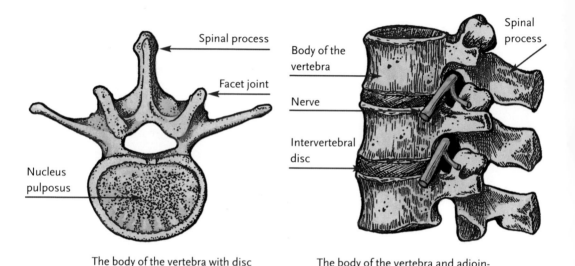

Spinal process

Facet joint

Nucleus pulposus

Body of the vertebra

Nerve

Intervertebral disc

Spinal process

The body of the vertebra with disc viewed from above. In the middle of the intervertebral disc is a gelatinous mass, the nucleus pulposus.

The body of the vertebra and adjoining nerves which run between the body of the vertebrae.

**Figure 12.1** The body of the vertebrae and adjacent nerves.

The body of the vertebrae and the discs are already well defined in the fetal stage. Each body develops from two growth plates, one upwards and one downwards. These growth plates are sensitive to injury right until the young player is fully grown, in other words until between the ages of 17 and 20. There are several studies, in which football has also been studied, which show that the strain on the back from playing high-level sport affects the growth of the body of the vertebrae, probably due to the great strain the growth plates are subjected to. The disc's attachment to the body of the vertebra, or the ring apophysis, is a weak point, which can be damaged as a result of overstraining during growth.

The spine also has a protective function for the spinal cord. In the spinal or vertebral canal, the spinal cord runs down from the brain to the first lumbar vertebra, where it devides into a tail of nerves (cauda equina). Between each pair of vertebrae run nerves which carry information to and from the brain. The spinal cord and nerves can get damaged, for example during a bad tackle in football, although this is uncommon. These injuries are serious, as it is very difficult to treat damaged nerve tissue.

## Emergency treatment of back injuries

If a footballer is subjected to a blow to the head (in a tackle or high challenge) and loses consciousness, it must always be assumed that the cervical spine may be damaged and emergency treatment must therefore be carried out accordingly (see Chapter 8). If the player is still conscious, nerve function can be tested by assessment of sensory and muscle functions. If the player suffers from pain in the cervical spine, this must be supported in a neutral position during transport to the hospital. If damage to the bone, joints or discs in the thoracic or lumbar spine is suspected, the injured player must be handled with the greatest possible care, to prevent the condition deteriorating.

Injuries to the soft parts of the spine can occur not only as the result of a direct blow, but also an indirect one due to the kinetic energy which is generated by the weight of the head and the ball, for example during tackles (especially unexpected tackles from behind). This impact can be compared to a whiplash injury in a car accident.

# INJURIES TO THE SOFT PARTS OF THE SPINE

## Muscle and ligament damage in the cervical spine

### Injury mechanism

Damage to ligaments and muscles can cause a reflex cramp in the muscula-ture. The muscles in the neck often react by going into a state of tension and a condition called wry neck or a crick in the neck (torticollis) arises.

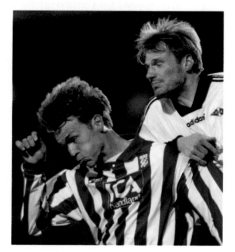

### Diagnosis

It can be difficult to diagnose muscle and ligament injuries in the cervical spine when radiographic and neuro-logical examinations are negative. It is, however, important to dif-ferentiate this condition from an injury which causes radiating pain in the arm or leg. With radiating pain, a nerve may be irritated or damaged. A player with radiating pain should therefore be exam-ined by a doctor as soon as possible.

### Symptoms and signs

Pain together with restricted movement in the neck or stiffness (wry neck).

### Treatment

Treatment of pain and stiffness in the neck where nerves are not affected involves anti-inflammatory drugs, rest, a neck brace and reha-bilitation until the patient is free from symptoms. The pain can lead to a reflex muscle cramp and consequently more limited range of move-ment compared to normal. The player should therefore not participate in match-like situations or games but instead take part in alternative training during this period to reduce the risk of new or aggravated injury.

### Prognosis

In the majority of cases, the symptoms go away after a few days' treatment and alternative training. If there is any further problem or radiating pain in the arm, examination for the possibility of a slipped disk should be considered.

# Muscle and ligament injuries in the chest and lumbar region

As the thorax is very stable, injuries to the soft parts are uncommon in this part of the back. The lumbar vertebrae have no ribs and the soft parts of the lumbar region are more susceptible to injury. Lumbago is a common painful condition which most people, including footballers, suffer from at some time in their lives.

### Injury mechanism

The direct cause of lumbago is still unclear. The structures which comprise and encompass the spine are generously supplied with nerves. Damage or irritation to any of these structures can therefore cause pain which can develop into lumbago. Studies have shown that footballers suffer from back pain more often than non-sportsmen or women, probably because the stress on the back is great in changes of pace, jerks, sudden changes in direction, tackles and headers. It is therefore important that the back's muscles are in good shape both in terms of strength and stamina.

### Symptoms

The problem often comes on suddenly following a heavy lift, a sudden twist or after standing slightly bent forward for a relatively long time. The pain is most often localized to the lumbar region and there is no radiation down into the legs. Due to muscle strain, a stiffness is felt in the lumbar region. It is also common for the muscles on one side to be more tense than on the other side, which leads to lopsidedness in the back (pain-related scoliosis), most often in the lumbar region.

### Treatment

The cycle of pain should be interrupted as quickly as possible with rest, anti-inflammatory drugs, possibly combined with heat treatment and massage. Fitness and strength training can be started after about 3–5 days if the symptoms do not worsen.

The player should refrain from playing football as long as the pain lasts. Controlled muscle training during this period can be of great value. Running should be added at an early stage and the intensity successively increased. If the symptoms increase, a more thorough examination should be carried out, which can be complemented with radiographs if required.

### Prognosis

The prognosis for lumbago is good. If the symptoms persist or return, however, follow-up examinations are important, as for example, disc damage, can develop over a long time, and although radiographic examinations are negative, in an acute stage the disc may be damaged.

# Slipped discs

### Injury mechanism

The disc is composed of a ring (annulus fibrosus) and a core (nucleus pulposus). The pressure in the core is greater than in the surrounding area as long as the ring is intact. Damage to the disc can occur, sometimes as a result of the ageing process (the disc starts to change due to ageing even during growth), sometimes following a sharp wrench, such as a severe twist or a flexion/extension wrench. The material in the nucleus is then squeezed out of the disc, due to the higher pressure and a slipped disc occurs. In the neck and thorax it is serious if the material in the nucleus is squeezed backwards towards the spinal cord. This injury, which is unusual, can in turn lead to damage to the spinal cord with paralysis as a consequence. If the slipped disc moves to one side, it can irritate a nerve which runs into the arm.

A slipped disc in the lower part of the lumbar region is much more common. As the rear of the disc ages most quickly, this is where most slipped discs occur. If the material in the nucleus presses the root of a nerve, the result is sciatica (pain radiating into one leg). In young footballers, this type of injury is uncommon (it is most common between the ages of 35–40 years).

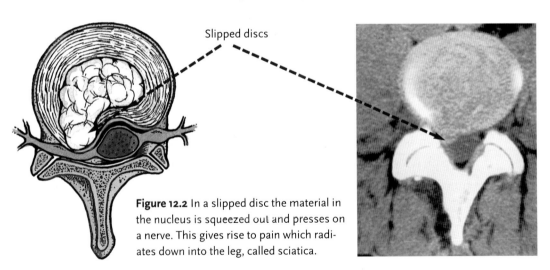

Slipped discs

**Figure 12.2** In a slipped disc the material in the nucleus is squeezed out and presses on a nerve. This gives rise to pain which radiates down into the leg, called sciatica.

If the load exceeds the strength of the disc in young players, it is relatively common for other parts of the body of the vertebra and/or disc complex to be damaged. The growth plates can be damaged and the mass of the disc can be squeezed into the body of the vertebra. This is called Schmorl's node.

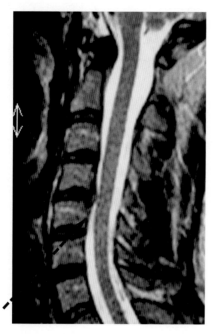

**Figure 12.3** The picture shows a slipped disc in the cervical spine between the 4th and 5th vertebrae.

## Diagnosis

Disc damage causes pain in the back and when the root of a nerve is involved, as in a slipped disc, a radiating pain in the leg or arm also arises. One problem associated with making the right diagnosis is that pressure on the nerve is located in the back, while the pain is felt far down in an arm or leg — what is known as referred pain. However, an examination including a check of reflexes, sensations and strength generally leads to the correct diagnosis. Radiographic examination should be carried out to rule out causes other than a slipped disc for the symptoms. By means of computerized tomography (CT) or magnetic resonance imaging (MRI), the appearance and size of the slipped disc can be established if necessary.

A slipped disc in the cervical spine often causes radiating pain from the neck to the shoulder and down into the arm or up to the head. In addition to pain, impaired sensations and muscle weakness can occur. A slipped disc in the lumbar region causes radiating pain in one leg with impaired sensations. It can also affect muscle functions and reflexes. The pain increases upon provocation of the irritated nerveroot, such as during the Lasègue's test.

## Treatment

The preliminary treatment is rest, quickly followed by a programme of rehabilitation with fitness and strength training. If the radiating pain is intense and does not disappear with rest and rehabilitation, surgery should be considered.

The slipped disc is removed during surgery and in this way the irritation of the nerve root subsides.

### Prognosis

Relatively soon after surgery, suitable training can begin. It takes about 6 months before the player can return to full play. Prognosis is good in most cases.

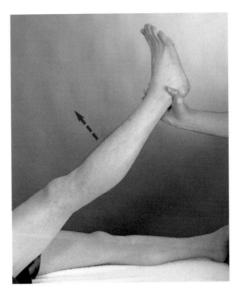

**Figure 12.4** In Lasègue's test, the leg is lifted off the couch with the knee straight. In a positive test the player feels pain radiating into the leg and foot.

# FRACTURES

Fractures of the vertebrae are very uncommon in football and are therefore dealt with only briefly in this chapter.

## Fractures of the cervical spine

### Injury mechanism

Compression injuries in the cervical spine can occur following a blow from directly above, such as during a collision in football, but are very uncommon. In this type of injury, there is a risk of fracture in the first cervical vertebra (Jefferson's fracture).

Bending injuries of the cervical spine can occur following a blow from behind, resulting in fracture or ligament injuries. If the ligament which stabilizes the second cervical vertebra in relation to the first (transverse ligament) is damaged, an instability, which in the vast majority of cases requires surgery, occurs.

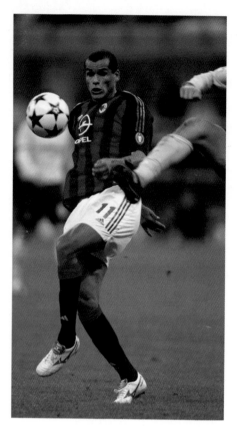

A blow from the front can lead to a extension injury in the cervical spine. As the muscles in the front are weaker than those in the back of the neck, the blow or any other force does not have to be particularly strong to result in injury. Very often ligaments and intervertebral discs are damaged, sometimes together with the breaking off of a bony fragment from the edge of the body of the vertebra.

### Diagnosis

Diagnosis can be made by means of radiographic examination. Often provocation by bending forwards and backwards is needed to detect an instability. In damage to the cervical spine, it is important to differentiate between pain localized in the cervical spine, pain which radiates out into the arms and pain or weakness in the lower extremities. Diagnosis is established by means of clinical examination and radiographic examination, and possibly computerized tomography (CT) or magnetic resonance imaging (MRT).

### Treatment

With fracture or suspected damage to the spinal cord, specialist treatment at an emergency department is required.

### Prognosis

The prognosis in cervical spine injury where there is no nerve damage is good. Where there is nerve damage, it is important that the remaining functions are exercised to minimize the spread of the nerve damage.

# Fractures of the thoracic and lumbar spine

## Injury mechanism

An acute injury as a result of a blow to the thoracic or lumbar spine is very rare in football. The spinal cord comes to an end at the level of the first lumbar vertebra and divides into a tail of nerve roots (cauda equina) beneath. There is, therefore, more space around the nerves and the risk of nerve damage in the event of a fracture of the vertebrae is less than in the event of damage above the first lumbar vertebra.

## Diagnosis

The player experiences great pain, radiating into the thorax and also, if the spinal cord is damaged, pain radiating down into the legs or a feeling of numbness and inability to activate muscles below the level of the injury.

## Treatment

In the case of suspected injury to the vertebrae, the injured individual must be moved extremely carefully. If there is any weakness in the area adjacent to the injury, damage to the spinal cord or nerves can be aggravated by careless movement.

In less serious fractures of the vertebrae, treatment with a body-brace is used in many cases. In more serious injuries, stabilizing surgery is, however, required.

## Prognosis

Prognosis is good in stable fractures of the vertebrae. If the damaged vertebra has been compressed in the front part, the end result when the fracture has healed can be a slightly greater stoop (kyphosis), which normally does not limit continued activity. In the case of damage to the spinal cord, there is, however, a risk that this will be permanent, which means that the player cannot go back to playing football.

# Scheuermann's disease

### Injury mechanism

Scheuermann's disease, which affects young players between the ages of 10 and 16 years, is very likely caused by excessive strain on the sensitive growth plates of the most exposed bodies of the vertebrae. The end result is wedge-shaped vertebrae in addition to narrowed discs, which are visible in a normal radiographic examination. Scheuermann's disease is common in sportsmen or -women who place great strain on their back, but it also occurs relatively often among football players.

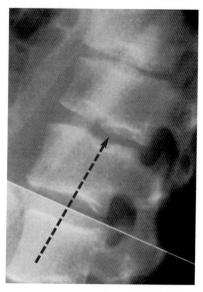

**Figure 12.5** In Scheuermann's disease, changes occur in the vertebrae as well as in the intervertebral discs.

### Diagnosis

In the course of the development of Scheuermann's disease, the young player experiences back pain on moving but not while at rest. The damage develops very slowly and can take up to 3–4 months and, in certain cases, as much as a year, before any changes are visible in a radiographic examination.

### Treatment

The player should take a break from heavy training during the healing period. This is especially important during spurts in growth, which normally occur between the ages of 12 and 16 years (slightly earlier in girls), as the growth plates are most sensitive then. Never train with more than one's own bodyweight. Place greater emphasis on technique training — less on strength and fitness.

### Prognosis

People who have had Scheuermann's disease can have slightly increased frequency of back trouble.

## Spondylolysis – spondylolisthesis

### Injury mechanism

Spondylolysis is a defect in a vertebral arch, most commonly located on the fifth lumbar vertebra. No one is born with spondylolysis but at the age of 5 years about 5 per cent of the population has spondylolysis. There is some evidence to show a hereditary component.

Spondylolysis is more common among sportsmen and women who place strain on their back, but it also occurs relatively often in football (twice as often as among non-sportsmen or women). In these cases, spondylolysis is caused by a stress fracture, which is produced by repeated overloading. If there is a defect in the vertebral arch, the risk of slipping vertebrae, i.e., spondylolisthesis, increases.

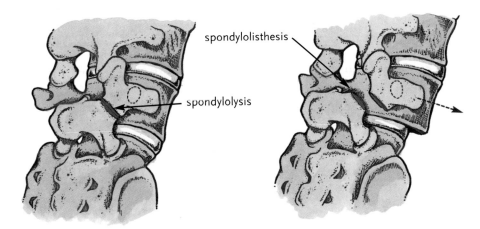

spondylolisthesis

spondylolysis

**Figure 12.6** In spondylolysis, a defect appears in a vertebral arch. In spondylolisthesis the vertebral bodies slip forward a few millimetres.

### Diagnosis

The symptom is pain where the spondylolysis develops. Radiographic examination does not reveal the fracture until the healing phase. Many stress fractures in the vertebral arch do not heal, but rather a false joint develops. Footballers with spondylolisthesis can be troubled by lower back pain which increases progressively with activity. It is primarily a backward bend in the lumbar spine which produces pain.

### Treatment

If a player complains of back pain in the lower lumbar spine, a stress fracture in the vertebral arch may be developing. Training should be individually tailored with great importance given to posture correction (to reduce curvature in the lumbar spine). Immobilization by means of a corset or plaster has no effect. The stress fracture probably has a greater chance of healing if the patient refrains from exercise which places heavy strain on the spine during a period of 2–3 months from the beginning of the symptoms.

The player should not take part in training games or matches during this period but can take part in other team training which does not involve placing strain on the spine in stretched or bent positions, such as in heading and jumping exercises.

### Prognosis

Spondylolysis probably does not lead to an increased risk of back trouble after the end of a sporting career. During the active career alternative training combined with muscle training if trouble arises, is helpful.

# 13. Chest, abdominal and skin injuries

Anders Falk

## Chest Injuries

Injuries to the thorax or thoracic cavity arise from what might be called blunt-instrument blows in football, for example following a collision or a kick.

### Injury mechanism

The mildest form of blow to the thorax simply causes bleeding in the subcutaneous tissue and rib muscles. If the blow is greater, it can result in more serious muscular haemorrhages and in the worst case fractured ribs. Following a very powerful blow, the ribs can fracture and the pleura can be damaged.

### Symptoms

An injury to the wall of the thorax causes pain, which worsens on movement, deep breathing, coughing, etc. The symptoms are fundamentally the same in milder injuries to the soft tissues as in injuries to the ribs. If the blow has caused fractured ribs and damage to the pleura, breathing difficulties and shortness of breath arise and perhaps bloody expectoration.

### Diagnosis

Following a blow to the thorax, the degree of injury can be assessed from the player's symptoms — judging from the local soreness upon touch and pressure. Even an experienced doctor can find it difficult to determine if there is only damage to the soft tissues, for example bleeding, or if a rib is fractured. In the case of a fractured rib, when pressure is applied to the area of the pain, a clicking noise can often be heard when the ends of the fracture rub against one another. If, what is known as an indirect pain reaction, can be elicited in the area of the injury by pressing on the sternum and movement can be produced in the ribs, this indicates a rib injury/fracture. Play should then be stopped. If the player's breathing is affected, the doctor should examine and above all assess the sound of breathing. If the blow has resulted in a rupture or bleeding in the pleura and the sound of breathing is reduced, prompt hospital attention is required.

The usual kind of blow in the context of football is moderate in nature. Available medical personnel can determine whether the local and indirect soreness in the area of the injury is significant. Under such circumstances the pain prevents the player from finishing the match.

## Treatment

A blow to the thorax, even fractured ribs, does not normally require any treatment other than analgesics and avoiding painful movements. Playing football involves movements in the rib muscles, which means that even minor injuries such as rib muscle bleeding prevent continued play. There is a risk that in an intense match situation the extent of the injury will be underestimated. Bandaging with elastic tape has, for example, been suggested for milder injuries, but this will probably be ineffective and is not recommended.

## Prognosis

In the case of fractured ribs, healing is estimated to take at least 4 weeks and full football activity can most often not be resumed until after this period. Simple injury to soft tissues with bleeding gives freedom from pain and permits return to full footballing activity after a shorter time. Individual variations occur. Playing with pain in the thorax from a muscular bleeding following a blow is not dangerous in itself, but negatively affects performance.

# Abdominal injuries

Abdominal injuries are uncommon in football and occur only after a blow or a kick from elbow or knee in the area of the abdomen or side or following collision with the goalposts.

### Injury mechanism

Just as with chest injuries, in less serious cases haemorrhaging can occur in the cutis and muscles. If the blow is heavy and badly placed, the abdomen's internal organs, most often the liver, spleen and kidneys can be damaged in rare instances. A player with abdominal injuries complains of local soreness when pressure is applied to the area of the injury and the symptoms intensify on movement. In abdominal wall muscle haemorrhage, the symptoms become aggravated with an increase in bleeding. If the pain is pronounced, it is difficult to differentiate between an abdominal wall muscle bleeding and damage to the internal organs.

Rupture of muscles and local bleeding are otherwise handled as other abdominal wall muscle injuries.

### Diagnosis

When a player is subjected to a blow to the area of the abdomen and is in pain, he should be taken off the pitch and examined quickly. If the pain is slight when pressure is applied to the injury, it is probably not serious. In abdominal muscle injury, the pain felt often increases when pressure is applied, as the abdominal muscles are simultaneously stretched.

The extent of movement-related pain determines whether play can be continued in this situation. If the pain felt is strong and linked to nausea and perhaps vomiting, damage to some abdominal organ should be suspected. Prompt medical examination is recommended, preferably by the match doctor, otherwise at a casualty department.

A blow to the side/flank can damage the underlying kidney. One symptom of kidney damage is blood in the player's urine. If kidney damage is suspected, the player should be taken to a casualty department without further delay for assessment of the damage.

### Treatment

As a rule, treatment of a muscle bleeding which is a result of a blow to the abdominal wall requires a few days' rest from painful movements. Thereafter the player can begin training again. No other treatment is necessary. If the liver or spleen have been damaged, the damage must be assessed by a doctor, who will give instructions as regards a return to training and play.

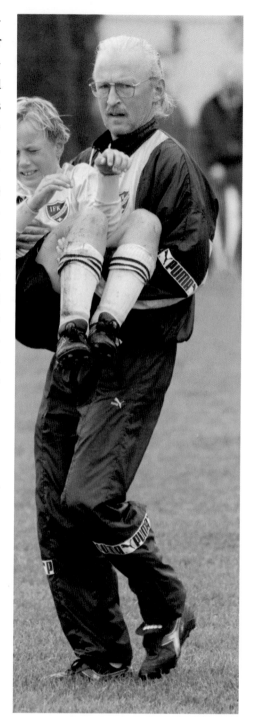

### Prognosis

The healing of injuries to the abdominal wall muscles which are more moderate in extent has a more favourable course, with a greater chance of a quick return to training and play. The extent of an injury is of significance to the healing time. If the blow has led to damage to the internal organs, a return to training can take place in consultation with a doctor.

# Skin injuries

Skin injuries in football can be divided into two fundamentally different types, on the one hand those arising from crushing and on the other, scratches and grazes. The most common injury is a crush injury, such as may occur during heading challenges between two players, with (as a rule) quite short cuts to the forehead, the eyebrows, the bridge of the nose or the scalp as a result. Grazes are most often seen during play on a gravel pitch, for example in sliding tackles. Most frequently, the knee and the outside of the thigh are affected. Grazing entails the outer layer of the skin being scraped off, while the lower part of the skin is intact. So no actual wound is there.

### Diagnosis

Skin injuries in football are insignificant on the whole and are seldom connected with concussion or any injury affecting a joint. If the injury is judged to be of uncertain depth and is near the knee joint, the doctor should assess the injury. If the match doctor is not available, serious consideration should be given to taking the player to casualty, where assessment of the depth of the injury can take place in controlled, sterile conditions.

If a player suffers a crush injury for example, during a heading challenge and at the same time loses consciousness for a short

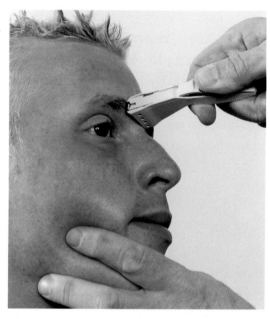

**Figure 13.1** A wound can be closed with normal stitches or the sides of the cut can also be approximated with surgical staples. The advantage of staples is that any cuts during a match can be closed quickly and simply.

time, this means that he has concussion. The player should then be assessed by a doctor as quickly as possible (see Chapter 10).

## Treatment

Skin injuries should be attended to as soon as is practically possible. If a number of hours go by before the wound is cleaned and closed, there is risk of infection. As regards crush injuries to the head area, if the wound is slight and is not bleeding, and if the player has no headache or dizziness, he can continue playing. If the wound is larger and especially if it is bleeding and causes trouble, it should be taken care of immediately. Simply applying a plaster or tape is not advisable as this does not stay in place. A pressure dressing using an elastic bandage can be applied around the whole of the head, but this slips off easily. Furthermore, it is forbidden to continue playing with a bleeding wound. The best thing to do is to clean and close the wound. Cleaning can be performed just as well using everyday materials, i.e. no sterile equipment is required — running room-temperature water is enough. The wound can then be stitched or the sides of the cut can be approximated using surgical staples. If there is no match doctor, the wound should be cleaned and a clean bandage applied. The wound should then be treated as soon as possible, which should be within 5–6 hours.

In the case of scratches and grazes it is not uncommon to get particles of gravel in the skin. It is important that the wound is cleaned thoroughly, for example with a nailbrush. Following washing, a severe graze should be covered with an ointment before putting a dressing so that the dressing does not stick to the wound. The dressing should be changed daily for a few days. If the wound is 'aired' without the bandage, it dries more quickly and the healing time is reduced.

**Prognosis**

Skin injuries of the types described heal in 1–2 weeks. Stitches in the scalp should be kept in for 10-12 days. Stitches in the face should be removed after 5–6 days and can be replaced using cross-taping to ensure healing. Risk of problems during healing such as infection is, however, small. If the skin injury is not associated with concussion or joint, training and play can, in principle, continue uninterrupted.

## Specific injury problems

One not uncommon problem is for a player to suffer from an accumulation of blood under the big toenail, due to shoes being too tight or stamping on the toes. Bleeding under the nails is very painful. Treatment is simple. The end of a paperclip is made red-hot in a flame and can then be

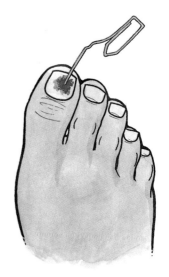

Figure 13.2 Bleeding under the toe nails can be very painful. If the blood can escape, the pain is lessened. This can be done by making a hole in the nail with a red-hot paper-clip.

used to make a hole through the nail to the nail-bed. This produces momentary discomfort, but subsequently relief as the blood drains away. The nail is then covered with a dressing and surgical tape.

After about 1 week the nail will separate from the nail-bed. The process occurs gradually and without any problem. If the nail is more or less loose from the beginning, consideration can be given to removing it completely. This can be painful and it may be necessary for it to be done under local anaesthetic. The nail-bed should then be covered with a bandage for a few days.

Sores can also cause foot trouble. If a sore is in the form of a painful blister, most commonly on the heel, it is best to keep the blister intact and to cover it with some form of sore dressing such as Duoderm (the whole blister should be well covered). The sore dressing should remain in place for a few days and should be covered with tape, so that it does not stick to the sock. After a few days the dressing can be changed and after a further few days the sore has usually healed. With a sore which is treated like this, the player can usually continue playing without any problem.

# 14. Groin injuries

Jan Ekstrand

The term groin injuries is used generically for a number of different conditions, all of which cause pain in the groin area. Groin injuries make up between 5 and 13 per cent of all football injuries in men and 4 per cent in women. If groin injuries are defined as absence from training or matches due to pain in the groin area, the risk of injury is estimated at 0.8/1000 h of footballing activity. The problem is, however, probably greater than this. A player with groin trouble can often take part in training and match play even though the pain prevents a 100 per cent performance.

## Symptoms and diagnosis

Groin injuries can be acute, but are most common after chronic (prolonged) overuse. Pain is the primary symptom of both acute and chronic groin injuries. The key to success in diagnosis and treatment consists of analysing which structure or structures cause the player pain.

In chronic groin injuries, the underlying causes can be difficult to find. The symptoms are generally diffuse. In addition, the picture often changes during the course of the problem. The pain changes in character and location, as the player unevenly loads other parts of the pelvis in an attempt to compensate for the original pain. It is therefore common for secondary symptoms such as pain in the muscular attachment to be treated, while the underlying condition remains untreated.

# Tendon and muscle injuries

Muscle injuries in the groin area can occur in many different muscles. The most common is damage to the leg adductors, especially the long adductor muscle (adductor longus). In football, these muscles are subjected to great stress during side-foot shots and lay-offs. Other muscles which can be damaged or overstrained are the upper part of the thigh muscle (rectus femoris muscle), which is severely strained during shooting, the hip joint muscle (iliopsoas muscle) and the abdominal muscle (rectus abdominis muscle).

Thigh muscle
(rectus femoris)

Abdominal muscle
(rectus abdominis)

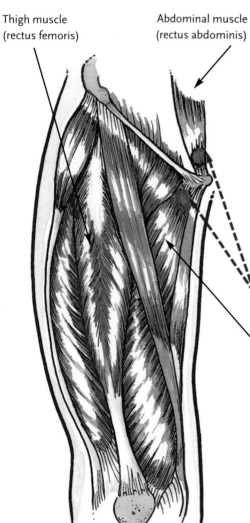

Rupture in the tendons of the muscle and the leg adductor muscle.

Leg adductor muscle
(adductor longus)

**Figure 14.1** The groin muscles viewed from the front. Example of localization of muscle ruptures in the abdominal muscle (rectus abdominis) and the leg adductor muscle (adductor longus).

## Acute injuries (muscle ruptures)

### Diagnosis

In acute muscle or tendon rupture, sudden stabbing pain appears in association with strain, very often when the muscle is stretched. On clinical examination, local soreness is noted and when pressure is applied there is pain if the player tries to contract the muscle against resistance. If the rupture is large, a defect can sometimes be felt in the muscle or tendon. Sometimes a bluish discoloration (haematoma) can appear about a day after the injury. In this case the diagnosis of muscle rupture can be considered confirmed.

The diagnosis can be verified by means of ultrasonographic examination and/or magnetic resonance imaging if required.

### Treatment

Treatment follows the principles for treatment of acute injury to the soft tissues (see Chapter 8). These injuries rarely require surgery.

### Prognosis

Prognosis is good. The problem with these injuries, just as with other muscle injuries, is assessing the extent of the injury and recovery time. The reason for a muscle injury 'flaring up' is very often that the extent of the injury was underestimated from the beginning.

## Chronic injuries (overuse)

### Injury mechanism

A footballer can easily overstrain the muscular attachment in the groin and pelvic areas. As with all overuse injuries, the strain, for however short or long a time, has been greater than the limit the body can stand. The surrounding tissues then react with inflammation, i.e. soreness, swelling, pain and reduced function.

It has not been investigated if groin injuries are due to increased stress or reduced stress tolerance in the tissues. It is important to analyse whether the type or amount of stress has changed or whether the conditions are different. The mechanism which triggers the injury can be an external or internal factor or a combination of several factors (see Chapter 3). Excessive strain leads to tissue damage and local inflammation in strained muscular/tendinous attachments.

There are symptoms typical of inflammation, e.g. insidious first appearance, reduced pain after warming up and increased pain and stiffness at the end of activity. There is a risk that the player will end up in a vicious circle of pain, with continuous aches and pains.

## Diagnosis

On examination, soreness is noted on the affected muscular attachment and pain when the muscle is tensed in response to resistance.

## Treatment

Treatment is the same as for chronic tendon inflammations. The player should refrain from activities which cause pain. Alternative exercise such as cycling, pool-exercise and exercise on a balance board are recommended. If there is soreness in the muscular or tendinous attachments, cortisone injections can be given. All activities which produce pain should then be avoided for 2 weeks. It is important to develop flexibility, muscle strength and coordination before a return to training.

Surgery can be considered if other treatments have been ineffective. With chronic pain, division of the adductor muscle at its attachment (adductor tenotomy) has proved successful. Rehabilitation takes around 2–3 months. Analysis of the underlying causes is essential to prevent new injuries.

## Prognosis

Chronic groin injuries are often difficult to treat. In players who have had trouble for more than 3–4 months and who have not improved despite treatment, surgery is often required. The result is generally good.

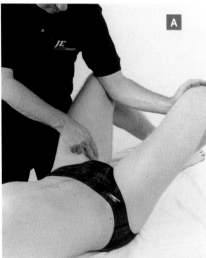

**Figure 14.2** Provocation tests of the groin muscles. (A) The hip adductor. The examiner places his forearm between the player's knees. The player pushes his knees together. (B) The thigh muscle. The player tries to raise his leg while the examiner offers resistance. (C) The abdominal muscle. The player tries to do a sit-up while the examiner offers resistance.

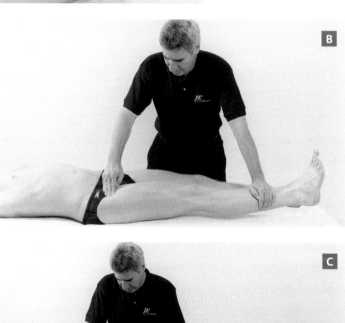

## SURGERY TO DIVIDE THE HIP ADDUCTOR MUSCLE (ADDUCTOR TENOTOMY)

This aims to eliminate painful stress on the muscular attachment to the symphysis. The following criteria must be met.

- Persistent trouble for more than 3 months.
- Clinical findings indicate tendon/muscle damage.
- Changes indicating tendon/muscle damage revealed by sonographic examination or magnetic resonance imaging.
- Other treatment has had no effect.
- Other diagnoses have been ruled out.

# Trapped nerves ('entrapment')

### Injury mechanism

Nerves in the groin area can be subjected to strain or pressure. The nerves which are most often trapped are the ilioinguinal and iliohypogastric. Abdominal nerves can become trapped on contraction of the abdominal muscle or in connection with abdominal strain.

The ilioinguinal and iliohypogastric nerves originate from the nerve roots at the twelfth thoracic vertebra (Th 12) and the first lumbar vertebra (L1), respectively. The nerves run on the inside of the abdomen, and subsequently zig-zag through the three layers of the abdominal musculature to then supply the lower abdomen and the inside of the thigh. The greatest risk of entrapment is either in the zig-zagging path through the layers of the abdominal muscle or when the nerves run through the outermost layer of the oblique abdominal musculatur (outer aponeurosis). When trapped, the nerve is irritated and pain arises in the groin area. The nerve is rarely affected to the extent that the player notices altered sense.

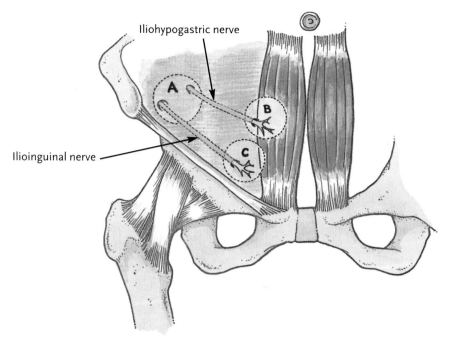

**Figure 14.3** The course of the ilioinguinal and the iliohypogastric nerves. The nerves run between the oblique abdominal muscles in the lower abdomen. The circles indicate the most common locations for entrapment. At A, the branches of both nerves zig-zag through both deep muscle layers to then run under the outermost layer of the oblique abdominal muscles (the outer aponeurosis), indicated by lilac colour in the figure.

## Diagnosis

Diagnosis is suspected with local soreness and is confirmed by a desensitization test. In the desensitization test, the player must first perform a straight-leg lift or another exercise which produces pain. The nerve is subsequently anaesthetized. If the straight-leg lift can be performed without pain, the injection test indicates that there may be a trapped nerve.

## Treatment

Sometimes a cortisone injection together with the injection test gives lasting improvement, but often surgery is required. During the operation, a part of the affected nerve is removed (neurotomy). Rehabilitation time following a neurotomy is 3–4 weeks.

**Prognosis**

Prognosis is good. Around 75–80 per cent are completely trouble-free if the diagnosis has been correct. Sometimes the pain can remain or return directly after surgery but normally disappears within a 6-month period. Following surgery, there is very often a reduction in sensations around the surgery scar, which does not generally, however, cause the player any bother.

Surgery is often performed on football players after the end of the season, as a player with trapped nerve trouble can play normally despite the pain. It is not considered that play, even with pain, prolongs or aggravates the problem and does not do any lasting harm.

# Inguinal hernia

An inguinal hernia is a protuberance of peritoneum due to a weakening of the abdominal wall muscles and the connective tissue layer.

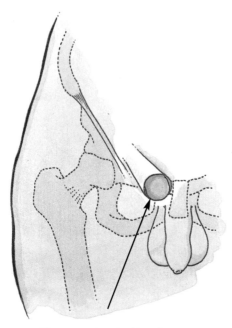

**Figure 14.4** Inguinal hernia

**Injury mechanism**

A hernia can cause pain in the groin area when the abdomen is under pressure, for example when jumping, shooting and jerking. The pain is similar to that experienced with other groin problems such as muscle injury and trapped nerves. The problem is making the right diagnosis. An inguinal hernia/ abdominal wall weakness may be suspected if it can be produced by coughing, sneezing or contraction of the abdominal muscles.

## Diagnosis

Clinical examination is carried out when the player stands upright and coughs or contracts the abdominal muscles. An inguinal hernia appears as a protuberance in the lower abdomen. The examiner can palpate the external hernial orifice with a finger (annulus externus), which should normally be a finger-tip in size. In players with an inguinal hernia or an abdominal wall weakness, an enlarged hernial orifice is often noted and the contents of the hernia push against the finger on coughing. Less than 10 per cent of players with chronic groin pain have inguinal hernias that appear clearly on clinical examination.

With a clear inguinal hernia, no further examinations need be performed. In the event of doubt, a herniography examination may be warranted.

## Treatment

An inguinal hernia is treated by surgery. The surgery can be open or by using laparoscopy.

## Prognosis

Prognosis is good. Play can be returned to after 4–6 weeks.

# Abdominal wall weakness ('Sportsman's hernia')

## Injury mechanism

Weakness in the abdominal wall is common in footballers. By means of herniography, it has been shown that 80 per cent of players with chronic groin pains have a weakness in the abdominal wall. There are a number of theories regarding the reasons for this. One theory states that it is an innate weakness. According to another (scientifically unproven) theory, footballers have an imbalance in muscle strength with weak abdominal muscles in relation to strong leg muscles. It has been maintained that weakness in the abdominal wall arises as a result of earlier muscle rupture in the area. On contraction of the sagging abdominal wall, the abdominal nerves are stretched over the abdominal muscles, and are subjected to mechanical irritation, which may explain why abdominal wall weakness and nerve irritation often occur simultaneously.

### Diagnosis

Diagnosis of a suspected inguinal hernia can be made if the player has a relative muscle weakness in the abdominal wall and at the same time soreness on palpation of the outer hernia opening. The diagnosis can be confirmed by means of herniography examination.

### Treatment

Abdominal muscle exercise can sometimes have an effect, but chronic groin pain which is caused by abdominal wall weakness is normally best treated with surgical reinforcement of the abdominal wall.

### Prognosis

Following surgery, cycling and pool exercise are started when the wound has healed (after about 2 weeks), jogging can be recommended after 4 weeks and football training after about 5–6 weeks.

# Inflammation of the pubic bone (symphysitis, osteitis pubis)

### Injury mechanism

Symphysitis is a chronic inflammation around the pubic bone (symphysis), which causes pain when placed under stress. The pelvis and the area around the symphysis are strained a great deal in football.

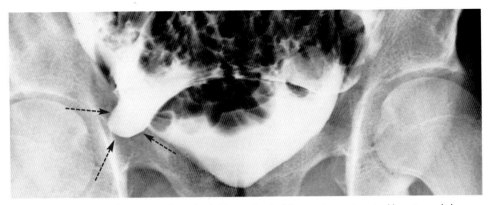

**Figure 14.5** Herniography is a simple and reliable method of diagnosing an inguinal hernia or abdominal wall weakness. Contrast medium is injected into the abdomen (white in the picture) via a fine needle. Weakness in the abdominal wall is then seen as a contrast-medium filled protuberance (red arrows). The herniography shows the anatomy, not the symptoms. The herniography findings must be correlated with the clinical symptoms before a decision is made regarding treatment.

## Diagnosis

On clinical examination, there is severe soreness when pressure is applied to the symphysis. Normally the surrounding muscular attachment is also tender. On radiographic examination, skeletal changes are also found. Many consider that these changes are a sign of excessive strain on the pelvic ring which is usual in footballers and that this has led to a local reaction in the symphysis with permanent changes visible on radiographs. However, similar changes have also been found on radiographs of healthy footballers who do not have groin trouble.

If radiographs of the pelvis shows changes in the symphysis, it can be a sign of excessive strain but it is not certain that there is any connection with the player's current problem. In magnetic resonance imaging scans, a swelling has been found in many players in the bone around the symphysis, which indicates excessive strain or overuse injury. In these players, however, no signs of tendon or muscle damage have been found, which suggests that the biggest problem is excessive loading of the bone and not irritation in the tendinous or muscular attachments.

### Treatment

Treatment consists of rest from painful activities and correction of the internal and external factors. Alternative exercises such as cycling and pool exercise are recommended.

### Prognosis

Prognosis in the majority of cases is good.

# Stress fractures

Prolonged excessive overuse can lead to stress fractures, for example, in the neck of the femur or in the pelvic ring. The line between excessive stress (oedema or swelling of the bone) and stress fractures (cracks in the bone) is vague. The symptoms are pain in the groin area when placed under stress. The player can normally walk without any difficulty, but feels pain in the groin while running. Initially there is no pain when the player is at rest but with continued training pain arises even while at rest.

### Diagnosis

Stress fractures in the pelvic ring should be suspected where there is severe local soreness when pressure is applied to the symphysis or other parts of the pelvis. Stress fractures in the neck of the femur may be suspected where there is severe pain in the groin when pressure is applied longitudinally or under rotation.

Radiographic examination at an early stage often reveals no damage. If a stress fracture is still suspected, another radiographic examination should be performed after about 2 weeks. The diagnosis can also be confirmed by means of scintigraphy or magnetic resonance imaging.

## Treatment

Treatment of stress-related symphysitis and stress fractures is rest from pain-inducing activities (running, jumping, kicking etc). Alternative forms of exercise such as cycling with low resistance are permitted if they can be done without causing pain.

If a stress fracture is suspected in the neck of the femur the player should avoid putting pressure on the leg by using crutches until the diagnosis has been confirmed or excluded. Continued stress can lead to displacement of the fracture fragments. If the diagnosis is confirmed, emergency surgery is recommended.

## Prognosis

Prognosis for a stress fracture in the pelvis is good. Return to football training should, however, not take place before the local soreness (when pressure is applied to the symphysis) has gone.

For stress fractures in the neck of the femur, prognosis is worse and setbacks in recovery occur in certain cases.

# Hip joint pain

Groin pain can be caused by hip joint disease. In growing adolescents with pain in the groin (and/or knee), the cause can be growth disturbance in the head of the femur (Perthe's disease, coxa plana) or physeolysis (slippage in the growth plates of the neck of the femur).

In fully grown players, groin pain can be caused by incipient wear in a hip joint. Hip joint disease can be confirmed or excluded by means of radiographic examination.

# Bursitis ('snapping hip')

Inflammation of the bursa (bursitis) in the upper exterior process of the femur (greater trochanter) and 'snapping hip', irritation between the tendon on the outside of the thigh (iliotibial tract) and the upper exterior process of the femur (greater trochanter) can also cause pain in the groin area.

# Back problems

Groin pain can be caused by a variety of different back problems. A slipped disc which affects the L4 root produces radiating pain in the groin and thigh (see Chapter 12).

Defects in the vertebral arches (spondylolysis) or slippage between the lumbar vertebrae (spondylolisthesis) can, in addition to pain in the lumbar spine itself, also produce pain in the groin, especially while heading, throwing in or during other activities where the player bends the lumbar spine backwards.

# Other causes of groin pain

There can be many possible causes of chronic groin pain. Women with groin pain should be referred to a gynaecologist to exclude possible gynaecological reasons.

In men, inflammation of the prostate gland (prostatitis) can cause pain in the groin. A player who experiences pain on passing water and groin pain should be examined further by a doctor. If prostatitis is suspected a urine test and palpation of the prostate should be performed.

Groin pain can, in exceptional cases, be caused by a cancerous tumour. A radiographic examination of the pelvis should always be done when there is chronic pain.

# Distribution of different diagnoses

Table 14.1 shows the criteria used in a study of footballers for clinical and objective diagnosis of groin pain. The most common clinical diagnosis was tendon/muscle damage (56 per cent) while clinical suspicion of hernia or abdominal wall weakness occurred in only 8 per cent.

By using ultrasonography or magnetic resonance imaging, tendon/muscle damage could only be established in 8 per cent, while 60 per cent with either hernia or abdominal wall weakness revealed changes in herniographic examination. Findings indicated that a diagnosis of tendon/muscle damage may perhaps be overestimated in clinical examination and that alternative diagnoses such as hernia, abdominal wall weakness and trapped nerve should also be considered.

Herniography as well as ultrasonography and magnetic resonance imaging examinations are very reliable and even small changes can be detected. If tendon/muscle damage cannot be confirmed by ultrasonography or magnetic resonance imaging, other diagnoses should be considered. The findings from a radiographic examination do not necessarily have any connection with the player's problem. Therefore, the radiographic results should be carefully compared with the player's clinical problem.

# Examination and treatment

Examination of a player with groin pain may well take place in primary care. In the case of acute groin pain, diagnosis may be made easier if secondary symptoms have not yet had time to develop. Diagnosis is made by taking the patient's medical history and clinical examination. Treatment is non-surgical with the emphasis on advice, pain-free exercise and anti-inflammatory drugs. Physiotherapy treatment is often of value.

If the problem persists, the patient's medical history, examination findings and analysis of the effects of previous treatment may have to be supplemented by further investigation. A radiographic examination of the pelvis, hip joints and pubic bone may be required. If it is suspected that the groin pain is triggered by the lumbar spine, radiographic examination of the lumbar spine is advised. Herniography is suggested if there is any suspicion of hernia or abdominal wall weakness. Nerve desensitization (blockade) may be used if it is suspected that the abdominal nerves are trapped. Treatment is still non-surgical and is focused on weighing up the findings from the medical history, clinical and radiographic examination .

A player with chronic pain (symptoms which have lasted for more than 3 months) is difficult to assess. In general there is no reason to continue using anti-inflammatory drugs. The cause of the pain must be identified and eliminated for the treatment to have effect. Referral to an orthopaedic surgeon with a good knowledge of sports medicine may be justified.

Surgery may be considered at this stage. In one study, it was found that only one-third of players who had had groin pain for more than 3 months recovered with non-surgical treatment. In another study of footballers with chronic groin pain, surgical and non-surgical treatments were compared. The study shows that surgery gave excellent results while non-surgical treatment such as physiotherapy or independent exercise by the patient, was generally ineffective.

Table 14.1 Criteria for the diagnosis of groin pain

| Diagnosis | Clinical examination | Objective findings |
|---|---|---|
| Tendon/muscle damage | Soreness when pressure is applied to the muscular attachment and pain when there is muscle tension in response to resistance. | Changes revealed by examination using ultrasonography or magnetic resonance imaging. |
| Entrapment of ilioinguinalis or iliohypogastric nerves | Palpation soreness on the ilioinguinalis or iliohypogastricus nerves. | Relief from pain following desensitization of the nerve by means of local anaesthetic nerve blockade. |
| Inguinal hernia or abdominal wall weakness, 'sportsman's hernia' | Visible inguinal hernia or pain when pressure is applied to the external hernia orifice in the lower part of the abdomen. | Hernia or abdominal wall weakness established by means of herniography. |
| Symphysitis | Soreness in response to pressure on the symphysis, pain on compression of the leg in response to resistance. | Changes revealed on radiographs in or around the symphysis. |
| Stress fracture | Distinct local soreness in response to pressure. | Increased isotope absorption revealed by scintigraphy. |
| Hip joint wear | Restricted hip joint rotation. | Wear revealed by radiographic examination or magnetic resonance imaging. |

# 15. Knee injuries

Jon Karlsson

Knee injuries, in particular ligament injuries, are very common in football. The knee joint is stabilized by ligaments on both the outside and the inside of the knee. In addition, the lower leg is stabilized in relationship to the femur by the anterior and posterior cruciate ligaments. Damage to any of these ligaments, especially the medial collateral ligament and the anterior cruciate ligament, are common football injuries. In addition, cartilage to cartilage and meniscus and the surfaces of the joint can occur.

It is well known that knee injuries can often produce permanent symptoms and that in many cases changes due to wear occur, e.g. following cartilage damage. Women football players are affected to a greater extent than men.

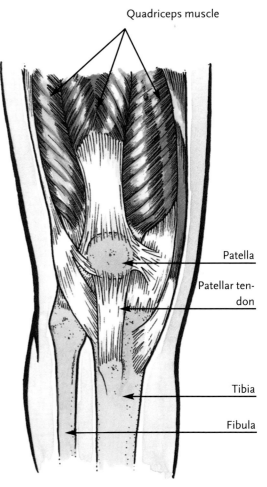

**Figure 15.1** Anatomy of the knee joint viewed from the front.

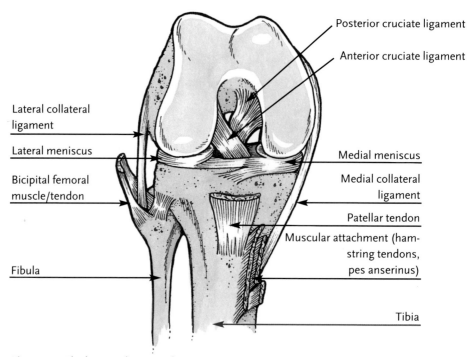

Figure 15.2 The knee and cruciate ligaments.

Approximately 75 per cent of all disability benefits in sport are a result of different knee injuries. The most common reason is damage to the anterior cruciate ligament. Football is one of those sports which are most affected by this injury and in many cases there is a risk that a player's career will come to a premature end.

## Ligament injuries

### Injury mechanism

Damage to the medial or lateral collateral ligaments occurs mainly during collisions or tackles where the lower leg bends inwards or outwards in relation to the femur. Often the damage is combined with other knee injuries, such as anterior or posterior cruciate ligament damage and meniscus and/or articular cartilage damage.

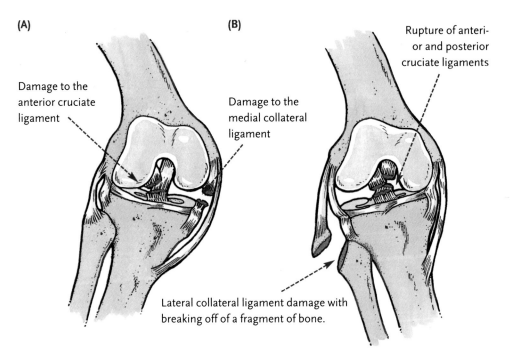

**(A)**

Damage to the anterior cruciate ligament

**(B)**

Damage to the medial collateral ligament

Rupture of anterior and posterior cruciate ligaments

Lateral collateral ligament damage with breaking off of a fragment of bone.

**Figure 15.3** (A) Rupture of the medial collateral ligament and the anterior cruciate ligament. (B) Rupture of both cruciate ligaments and of the lateral collateral ligament with a fragment of bone from the attachment on the fibula.

Damage to the medial collateral ligament is approximately 5–10 times more common than to the lateral ligament. Injuries can be divided into three degrees, depending on the extent of the instability. With a degree I injury, instability is slight (up to 5 mm), with degree II moderate (5–10 mm) and with degree III, the instability is pronounced (over 10 mm). Comparison is made with the healthy side.

### Diagnosis

The player experiences immediate pain, instability on loading and often difficulty in walking. Swelling is moderate. If, however, the swelling is severe, this generally indicates serious injury, often cruciate ligament damage.

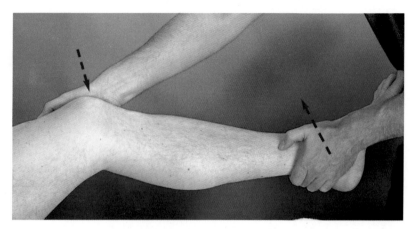

**Figure 15.4** Checking stability by performing a displacement test. When there is damage to the medial collateral ligament, the lower leg can be displaced outwards in relation to the femur.

Diagnosis is based on clinical examination. There is pain over the ligament or its point of attachment on the femur and/or the tibia. If the pain is principally in the joint space, the injury can be difficult to distinguish from meniscus damage. It can be confirmed by checking stability by performing an instability test. With increased instability, known as varus or valgus instability, where the lower leg moves outwards and inwards in relation to the femur respectively, the medial and lateral collateral ligaments are damaged. The instability examination can be hard to perform in an acute case because of pain. The examination can then be postponed for a few days. In exceptional cases, arthroscopic examination is necessary to confirm diagnosis. Very often, neither a stability examination under anaesthetic nor arthroscopy is required.

Radiographs should be taken to exclude fracture. Magnetic resonance imaging is not necessary.

### Treatment

The best treatment for collateral ligament damage, regardless of the degree of instability, is rehabilitation based on range of motion, strength and coordination exercises. Neither rapid surgical intervention nor immobilization in plaster is necessary following this injury. Stabilizing bandages, such as a knee brace which allows full movement, are recommended for 1–3 weeks. Muscle training can begin at the same time.

## Prognosis

With isolated ligament, damage prognosis is good. Most footballers recover completely without surgical intervention. Chronic problems are rare. Most players can return to normal activity after 10–12 weeks, without risk of future pain or recurrent instability.

# Anterior cruciate ligament damage

### Injury mechanism

Anterior cruciate ligament damage is very common in football. The injury occurs on rotation and/or overstretching of the knee joint. Twisting, even when not as a result of a tackle or body contact is also a common cause of injury. The injury can arise in isolation or in combination with other knee injuries such as damage to the collateral ligament and/or meniscus. On exceptional occasions, the injury occurs during extreme overstretching or overbending of the knee joint.

### Diagnosis

When there is suspicion of anterior cruciate ligament injury, acute examination is recommended. Because of swelling and pain, stability testing can, however, be difficult to perform in an acute case. The best time to make the right diagnosis is directly after the injury has occurred, before swelling and pain make examination impossible.

Approximately 75 per cent of all players with acute blood extravasation in the knee joint have anterior cruciate ligament damage. The joint can be extremely tense and tender. Where there is acute blood extravasation, there should be strong suspicions of anterior cruciate ligament damage.

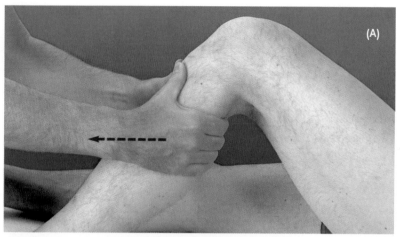

(A)

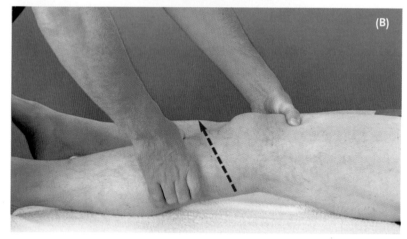

(B)

**Figure 15.5** (A) Anterior drawer test. This is carried out with the knee bent at 90°. Increased forward movement of the lower leg in relation to the femur indicates anterior cruciate ligament damage. (B) Lachman drawer test. This test is more precise in diagnosing anterior cruciate ligament damage than the anterior drawer test. The test is performed with the knee bent to around 20–30°.

Diagnosis is based on a stability test, such as the drawer test. An examination of this nature can be performed in a number of ways.

Immediately after the injury acute pain occurs in the knee. It is also difficult to put weight on the knee. Movement is limited and the knee swells up within a few hours. The swelling, which is due to bleeding in the knee, is very often pronounced. *Players who have injured their knees and where there is bloody extravasation (haemarthrosis), should always be suspected of having anterior cruciate ligament damage.* Puncture of the knee joint under sterile conditions is recommended.

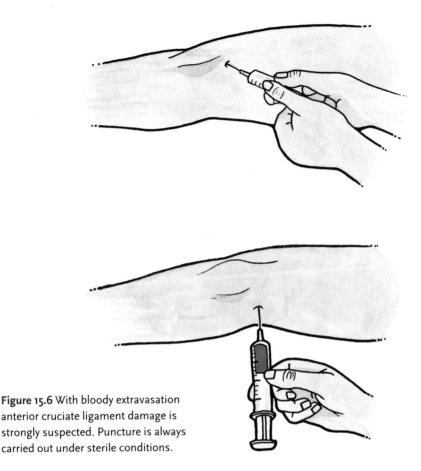

**Figure 15.6** With bloody extravasation anterior cruciate ligament damage is strongly suspected. Puncture is always carried out under sterile conditions.

Radiographic examination is carried out in order to exclude fracture. This is especially important in growing players where anterior cruciate ligament damage occurs as an avulsion fracture, i.e. the cruciate ligament's attachment to the tibia becomes detached. This damage is visible on a plain radiograph.

More advanced investigations such as magnetic resonance imaging are rarely necessary. This examination can, however, show cartilage damage, which often occurs and is of great significance for prognosis, but is not visible on radiographs.

Although arthroscopy can be of diagnostic value in acute cases, it is seldom necessary. One of the reasons for carrying out arthroscopic inspection is to examine possible meniscus or cartilage damage.

**Figure 15.7** This picture was taken during arthroscopy of the knee and shows a damaged interior meniscus in the knee, a flap rupture, which gives rise to catching/locking and pain.

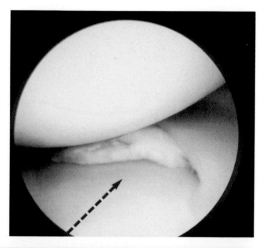

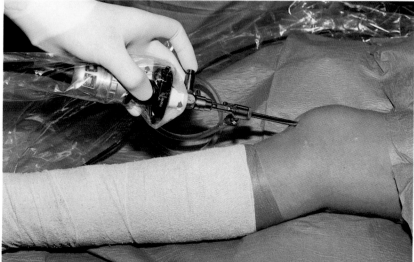

**Figure 15.8** By means of arthroscopy a thorough and reliable diagnosis can be made in the majority of knee injuries.

Approximately 50 per cent of footballers with cruciate ligament damage also have damage to the meniscus. Around 30 per cent have some other injury to the knee such as cartilage or joint capsule damage, in addition to the cruciate ligament damage.

Suspected cruciate ligament damage should be attended to by an orthopaedic surgeon with good knowledge of knee injuries.

## Treatment

The treatment for this injury depends on the player's level of activity and age. It is, however, hard or even impossible to continue playing football without a well-functioning anterior cruciate ligament. Surgery, therefore, often becomes necessary. Surgery is often carried out when the knee has regained full mobility and the swelling and inflammation have disappeared, usually around 3–6 weeks after the injury.

If surgery is performed earlier, there is a risk of cicatrization in the joint capsule (arthrofibrosis), which gives rise to stiffness, reduced motion and pain. The best time for surgery varies from individual to individual. The only exception to this rule is cruciate ligament damage in children, who should be operated on as quickly as possible. In these cases the damage involves the cruciate ligament's lower attachment, which gets detached from the tibia together with a fragment of bone.

The techniques of modern surgery are gentle and are performed using arthroscopy. Either a piece of the patellar tendon or one of the tendons in the back of the knee (hamstring tendons, semitendinosus gracilis) or a tendon on the outside of the knee (ileotibial tract) is used. Following surgery, immediate range of motion training and full weighting are allowed. Often the new cruciate ligament is protected with a knee brace after surgery, although recent studies have not proved the value of this and nowadays many players do not use any knee braces after surgery. With modern surgical techniques, the scar on the front of the knee is minimal.

Most players attain full range of motion and regain muscle strength. Rehabilitation can begin directly after the surgery.

## Prognosis

Rehabilitation time is generally about 6 months. Although surgery can restore stability and the player regains full function, there is a significant risk of changes due to wear associated with continued play.

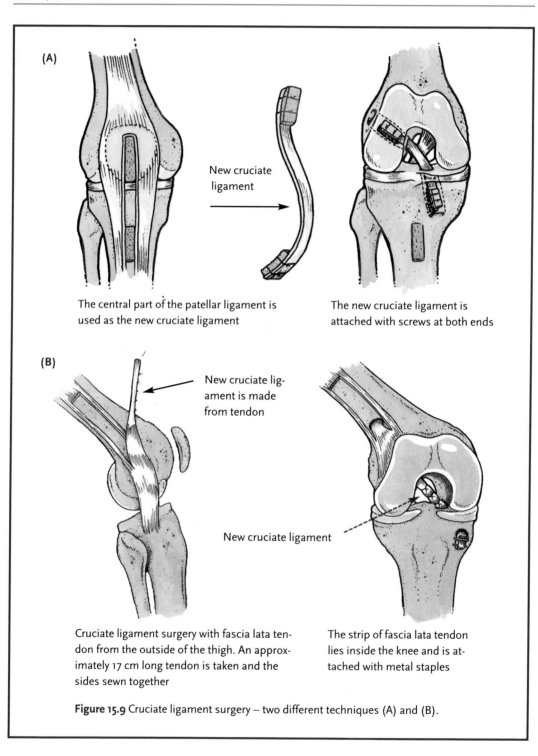

**(A)**

New cruciate ligament

The central part of the patellar ligament is used as the new cruciate ligament

The new cruciate ligament is attached with screws at both ends

**(B)**

New cruciate ligament is made from tendon

New cruciate ligament

Cruciate ligament surgery with fascia lata tendon from the outside of the thigh. An approximately 17 cm long tendon is taken and the sides sewn together

The strip of fascia lata tendon lies inside the knee and is attached with metal staples

**Figure 15.9** Cruciate ligament surgery – two different techniques (A) and (B).

## REHABILITATION PROGRESS REPORT • CRUCIATE LIGAMENT DAMAGE

| | WEEK | | | | MONTH | | |
|---|---|---|---|---|---|---|---|
| | 1–2 | 3–4 | 5–6 | 7–12 | 4 | 5 | 6 |
| **Immobilization** | | | | | | | |
| Brace | Rigid | Flexible | | | | | |
| Crutches | ■ | ■ | ■ | | | | |
| Partial load | ■ | ■ | ■ | | | | |
| **Agility exercises** | | | | | | | |
| Passive stretching | ■ | | | | | | |
| Motion exercises | 0–90° | 120° | 140° | ■ | | | |
| Retained patella movement | ■ | | | | | | |
| Light stretching of hamstrings and calf muscles | ■ | ■ | | | | | |
| Pool exercise | | | ■ | | | | |
| Cycling with low resistance | | ■ | | | | | |
| **Strength training** | | | | | | | |
| Straight leg lifts | ■ | ■ | | | | | |
| Closed chain, feet in contact with the floor | | | ■ | ■ | ■ | ■ | |
| **Sports-related exercise** | | | | | | | |
| **Coordination training** | | | | | | | |
| Walking in pool | | ■ | | | | | |
| Balance and coordination | | | ■ | ■ | ■ | ■ | |
| Range of motion training | | | | ■ | ■ | ■ | ■ |
| **Fitness training** | | | | | | | |
| Cycling | | | ■ | ■ | ■ | | |
| Pool (running in deep water) | | | ■ | ■ | | | |
| Jogging, running | | | | | | ■ | ■ |

# Posterior cruciate ligament injury

### Injury mechanism

Posterior cruciate ligament damage is relatively uncommon in football. Anterior cruciate ligament damage is considered to be about 20 times more common. The injury mechanism is a direct blow to the lower leg, which is driven straight back in relation to the femur. In exceptional cases, the injury occurs on overbending of the knee joint. Goalkeepers are especially subject to this kind of injury.

### Diagnosis

Symptoms are generally milder than with anterior cruciate ligament damage. There is less swelling. Upon palpation, the player feels an unusual soreness deep inside the back of the knee.

Diagnosis is based on a stability test. While checking stability, a posterior drawer movement is observed. The lower leg has slipped back in relation to the femur or can be displaced backwards when the knee joint is bent to 90°.

Backward stability can, as with other ligament damage to the knee, be divided into degrees I, II and III, depending on the amount of displacement. Other clinical signs of cruciate ligament damage are a pronounced ability to overstretch the leg and increased outward rotation of the lower leg. Comparison should always be made with the healthy leg.

Radiographic examination is carried out to exclude fracture. In certain cases, a fragment of bone has broken off the attachment to the tibia. Magnetic resonance imaging is a very precise method of evaluating the posterior cruciate ligament and can, in certain cases, be necessary to confirm the diagnosis.

In other cases, stability testing under anaesthetic is necessary. Arthroscopy may be carried out.

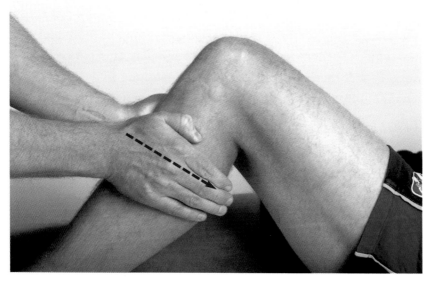

**Figure 15.10** Posterior cruciate ligament injury. The lower leg slips backward in relation to the femur and to the unaffected side. This is called posterior drawer test.

### Treatment

The recommended treatment for posterior cruciate ligament damage in footballers is rehabilitation. Only in exceptional cases is surgery necessary – especially when there is combined damage to the posterior cruciate ligament, collateral ligament and meniscus.

Another exception to the rehabilitation rule is made if the cruciate ligament attachment to the rear of the tibia has broken off with a fragment of bone. In this case it is easy to reattach the fragment of bone with a screw.

### Prognosis

In general the results of rehabilitation after posterior cruciate ligament damage are good. In spite of this, in certain cases chronic posterior cruciate ligament insufficiency, or reduced function, occurs. Most footballers, however, cope well with playing despite the injury and a certain lasting instability.

Because posterior cruciate ligament damage is relatively rare, there are few studies which describe the results following surgery. There is, however, a consensus of opinion that most footballers do not require surgery to be able to return to play. It is not certain, if surgery will increase their chance of resuming playing football. The rehabilitation period with or without surgery is long.

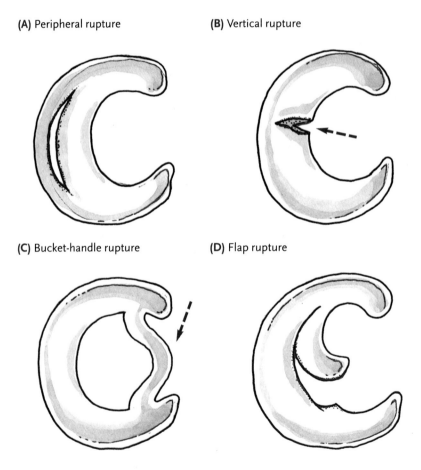

**(A)** Peripheral rupture

**(B)** Vertical rupture

**(C)** Bucket-handle rupture

**(D)** Flap rupture

**Figure 15.11** Different types of meniscus damage. (A) Peripheral rupture, near the attachment to the joint capsule, can often be repaired. (B) Vertical rupture generally occurs in the lateral meniscus. It more often causes pain than locking. (C) Bucket-handle rupture generally gives rise to locking of the knee. (D) Flap rupture occurs more often in connection with wear than with acute injury. Gives rise to catching in the knee, and pain.

# Meniscus damage

The menisci work like shock absorbers in the knee joint. If the whole meniscus is removed, the stress on the surfaces of the cartilage increases sharply. Weight is also concentrated on a smaller area of the joint cartilage, which leads to an increased risk of wear. Damage to the medial meniscus is approximately five times more common than to the lateral. Damage to the meniscus can occur in isolation, or in combination with collateral ligament and/or cruciate ligament damage.

### Injury mechanism

The most common injury mechanism is twisting, for example during a tackle. Medial meniscus damage occurs on outward rotation of the lower leg, while lateral meniscus damage occurs on inward rotation of the lower leg in relation to the femur.

There are different types of meniscus damage. In young players, a bucket-handle rupture of the meniscus is the most common, where a large part of the meniscus is driven in between the surfaces of the joint formed by the tibia and the femur.

## SYMPTOMS OF MENISCUS DAMAGE

• Pain   • Catching   • Locking   • Swelling

### Symptoms and signs

Symptoms are generally typical. In addition to reduced stretching and pain, locking, catching and swelling also occur. Swelling, however, unlike the case of anterior cruciate ligament damage, does not occur until the day after. With a bucket-handle meniscus, the knee joint locks up acutely and the player cannot stretch the knee completely. The reduction in stretching can be of the order of 20–30°

and the knee becomes painful if an attempt is made to perform passive stretching.

With lateral meniscus damage, symptoms are less typical. The most common symptoms are pain in the outside of the knee joint, over the joint space. Locking and swelling are less common. During examination, there is generally distinct pain on palpation over the joint space. Pain on movement, especially on overstretching or overbending, also occurs in many cases.

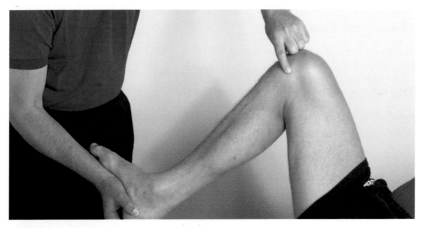

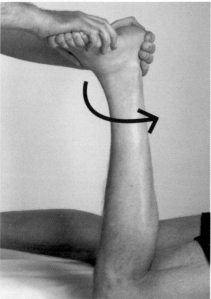

**Figure 15.12** McMurray's test. Test for meniscus damage. The player lies on his back. When stretching the knee from a completely bent position and simultaneously rotating the foot (outwards to test for medial meniscus damage and inwards to test for lateral meniscus damage) there is pain and in certain cases clicking in the joint space where the meniscus is damaged.

**Figure 15.13** Apley's test. In Apley's test, the player lies on his stomach and the knee is bent to 90°. The lower leg is rotated inward and outward. If there is meniscus damage, pain occurs in the knee, in the joint space.

## EXAMINATION FINDINGS IN MENISCUS DAMAGE

- Palpation pain over the joint space.
- Pain upon hyperextension/hyperflexion (overstretching/overbending).
- Pain and possible clicking during McMurray's test.
- Pain during Apley's test.

Specific rotation tests, called McMurray's test and Apley's test, increase the certainty when making clinical diagnosis. With medial meniscus damage, there is pain over the medial joint space on outward rotation of the lower leg, while pain with lateral meniscus damage is located over the lateral joint space on inward rotation of the lower leg.

In exceptional cases, there is a meniscal ganglion. This is a fluid-filled sac, which forms from an underlying meniscus rupture.

Radiographs reveal no bone damage. Other examinations using contrast media and/or magnetic resonance imaging are unnecessary, especially because arthroscopic examination confirms the diagnosis and is generally required for treatment.

### Treatment

In general, meniscus damage requires surgery. In most cases, the damaged part of the meniscus is removed. In exceptional cases, however, it can be repaired. This has been somewhat debated as the rehabilitation time after suturing of the meniscus is long (several months) and there are no studies at present, which with any certainty, show better long-term results with reduced risk of wear of the joint.

Meniscus surgery is performed by arthroscopy, which allows the damage to be surveyed clearly and the operation can be done in the outpatient department, and the patient can go home the same day. In certain cases, the operation can be performed under local anaesthetic. With acute locking of the knee joint, i.e. extension deficit of the order of 20–30°, surgery is recommended within a few days. With acute locking, the player should take the weight off the knee by using crutches until the operation has been performed, to reduce the risk of cartilage damage and prolonged inflammation. In isolated cases, for example if the meniscus rupture is small and the symptoms mild, surgery can wait until after the end of the football season.

### Prognosis

Prognosis after surgery on the meniscus is considered good. Following satisfactorily performed rehabilitation, most footballers can return to playing after 2–4 weeks. It is, however, important not to begin sporting exercise before the knee joint has regained full movement and is no longer swollen. In the case of suturing of the meniscus, rehabilitation time is considerably longer, as the repaired meniscus must be protected. Total rehabilitation time can then often be up to 6 months long.

# Osteochondritis dissecans

### Injury mechanism

Osteochondritis dissecans can occur in many joints but is most common in the knee joint. The underlying cause is unknown. A pice of cartilage, either with or without bone, becomes partially detached from the bone underneath. The condition is more common in young people and in most cases the damage is located on the medial surface of the joint on the femur but can also be found on the lateral side. Sometimes cartilage/bone fragments become detached and lie as a loose body in the knee. In the majority of cases, however, the focus of the osteochondritis is covered by an intact cartilage surface.

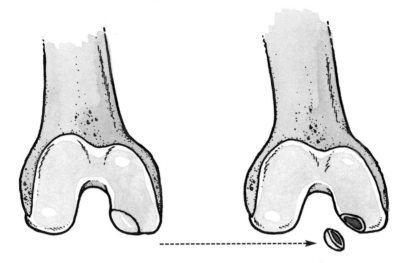

**Figure 15.14** Osteochondritis dissecans. A cartilage-covered fragment of bone can become detached from its attachment and give rise to pain or locking.

### Symptoms and signs

Unlike for example, meniscus damage, symptoms are more diffuse with pain and — especially when there is a loose body — catching and regular locking. Swelling is also common. Pain on movement and, in isolated cases, restricted range of motion also occur.

Radiographic examination is required to confirm diagnosis. In certain cases, indepth arthroscopic examination and/or computerized tomography or magnetic resonance imaging are necessary to assess the extent of the damage and to decide on treatment.

### Treatment

Symptoms, together with the radiographs, are decisive for treatment. If there is a loose body and the player is bothered by locking and catching, it can be removed by arthroscopy. If a fragment has become detached, there is an open bone surface which is not covered with cartilage inside the joint. This problem can often be difficult to solve. Possible attempts at treatment include covering the surface with periosteum or with cultured cartilage cells. One further possibility with this and other cartilage injuries is mosaic plasty.

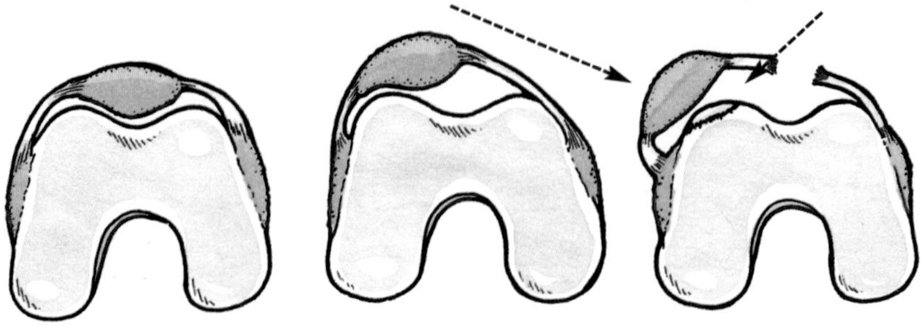

The patella always dislocates towards the outside of the knee

Bone fragment which can become detached from the lateral part of the femur

**Figure 15.15** Dislocation of the patella. The patella always dislocates outwards. Sometimes a bony fragment becomes detached and can float around in the knee-joint.

In this procedure cylinders of cartilage and bone are taken from another part of the knee and implanted to cover the damaged surface. Similar operations can be used to repair joint surface damage which has occurred following a blow to the knee, most often in combination with meniscus or cruciate ligament damage.

If the cartilage surface is intact in osteochondritis healing can be stimulated by means of surgical treatment where the fragment is fixed in place or with a number of small drill holes.

### Prognosis

Prognosis is better if the bone fragment is in place and the cartilage surface is intact. Prognosis is also better in children and adolescents than in older people. If the bony fragment has become detached and is floating as a loose body in the joint, prognosis is worse. The load-bearing surface loses its ability to take stress and wear can occur. Nowadays surgeons attempt to replace the lost cartilage surface in a variety of ways. Short-term results after these operations have shown themselves to be good but the long-term results are not known. It is also not known how these operations affect the chances of resuming an active footballing career. Whether these operations have any effect on the course of events in the long term or reduce the risk of wear is unknown at this time.

# Dislocation of the patella

Luxation of the patella is not common in football. Women footballers are affected more often than men.

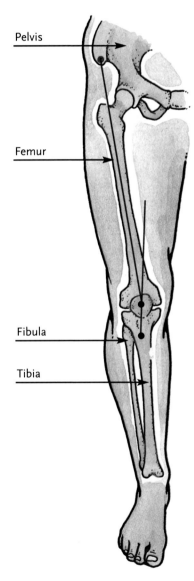

**Injury mechanism**

Injury occurs especially as the result of a blow to the knee joint on body contact, tackling or a collision and is most common in the 15–20-year-old age group. Injury occurs following a blow to the inside of the patella, with simultaneous outward rotation of the lower leg and contraction of the thigh muscle. Underlying factors are often anatomical defects such as knock-knees,

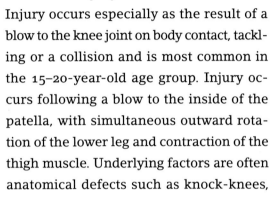

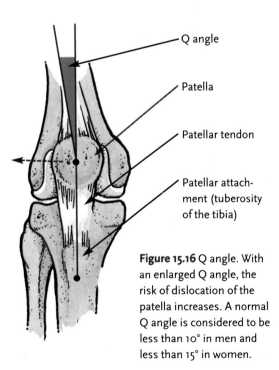

**Figure 15.16** Q angle. With an enlarged Q angle, the risk of dislocation of the patella increases. A normal Q angle is considered to be less than 10° in men and less than 15° in women.

the knee joint with underdevelopment or dysplasia of the joint surface of the femur and outward rotation of the lower leg.

The Q angle (quadriceps angle) is formed between the iliac crest, the central point of the patella and the patellar attachment to the tibia (tuberositas tibiae). If this angle is greatly increased, the risk of dislocation of the patella is also increased.

When the patella dislocates, there is always a rupture of the joint capsule and joint capsule reinforcement on the inside of the joint.

## Diagnosis

In addition to joint capsule damage on the inside of the knee, a fracture can occur on the medial edge of the patella and/or the lateral edge of the joint surface on the femur. The patella either lies out of place on the outside of the knee joint or may jump back into place of its own accord (spontaneously reduce).

Upon examination, there is relatively severe pain on the medial edge of the patella where the ligament has been damaged. Swelling and haemorrhaging also occur. In certain cases recurrent instability develops. Lateral movement of the patella, especially outwards, is increased.

Radiographic examination is recommended. This can either be completely negative or reveal bony fragments, which may be floating in the joint at the edge of the patella or at the outside of the femoral joint surface. In isolated cases arthroscopic inspection is carried out, which can confirm diagnosis. Examination can be valuable in revealing other damage such as to ligaments, cruciate ligaments, cartilage or menisci. Additional damage to cartilage is, however, relatively uncommon.

With recurrent instability, computerized tomography or magnetic resonance imaging can be of value, primarily in making decisions about possible surgery. In these examinations, the condition of the patella and any cartilage damage can be assessed.

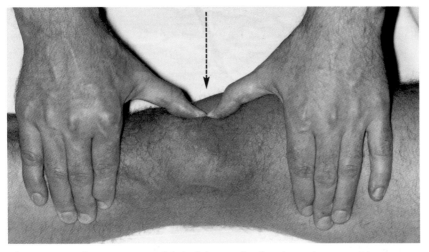

**Figure 15.17** With recurrent instability of the patella, the player gives a positive reaction to the apprehension test when the examiner presses the patella laterally. This movement is counteracted by reflex muscle action in the thigh muscle.

## Treatment

Treatment of first-time luxation of the patella consists of short-term immobilization, for example with a support brace. If radiographs reveal a bony fragment, this can probably be reattached in the right position or removed by arthroscopic surgery. Large bone fragments are not common. Generally, there is a small bony fragment which confirms diagnosis but which does not require treatment. Following immobilization, treatment consists of rehabilitation, starting with range of motion training and followed by strength and coordination training. Exercise can be increased successively. Functional exercises, such as pool exercise, is recommended. Rehabilitation training takes approximately 6–12 weeks.

With recurrent instability, stabilizing surgery may be necessary. The ligament and joint capsule on the medial side of the patella are shortened and the ligament on the lateral side is lengthened. The patellar attachment on the tibia generally needs to be moved approximately 10 mm inwards and reattached with a screw, to normalize the Q angle.

### Prognosis

Prognosis is variable. If only dislocation has occurred, prognosis after properly performed rehabilitation is often good. The player can
then return to play after approximately 2–3 months. It is, however,
very important to complete the rehabilitation and not to start any
activity before the knee is free from pain and normal range of motion and muscle strength have been achieved.

With recurrent instability where surgery has been necessary,
treatment is often long and a sporting career may be endangered.
Rehabilitation time may be up to 12 months. It is often difficult to
develop full muscle strength in the knee joint. The final outcome
after surgery in many cases is, however, relatively good.

# Patello-femoral pain

The most common pain in the knee joint in sportsmen and women
is patello-femoral pain (PFP), a condition which occurs as an
overuse injury. This condition is more common in many sports
other than football.

Patello-femoral pain can be troublesome and protracted and
leads to a long absence from footballing activity. Formerly this condition was known as 'chondromalacia patellae' (uneven cartilage
on the rear of the patella). However, because changes in the cartilage do not always appear in the surface of the patellar joint of a
player with PFP, this is a better term for the condition. Many
patients with PFP have completely normal joint cartilage. Although
PFP is more common among girls, it also occurs in boys. It is most
common in those aged between 14 and 18 years.

### Injury mechanism

Scientific evidence for the suggested underlying causes, such as
weakened thigh muscles, a large Q angle and incorrect position of

the patella in the joint between the patella and the femur, is weak. Overloading of the joint is probably the most common and most significant cause of pain.

### Symptoms and signs

It is typical for symptoms of PFP to be diffuse and to vary in intensity. The pain is mainly in the front of the patella, quite widespread and more pronounced on weight bearing. It is also typical for pain to occur during rest as well as while walking on steps and inclines, especially going down. Many players with PFP report that they find it difficult to squat, sit for a long time with their knees bent or to stand up after sitting for a long time. The latter is called 'movie sign'. In exceptional cases there is sign of locking and clicking as well as a tendency towards swelling. A tendency towards instability is atypical and real locking does not occur.

On examination there is pain when the patella is pressed against the femoral surface of the joint, especially when the thigh muscle is activated at the same time. When both sides of the patella are sore it is known as lateral pain. This is probably due to a slight inflammation in the joint capsule. On movement there is crunching (crepitation). This symptom is, however, atypical and can also occur without pain and even in completely normal joints. In certain cases malposition can be noted, especially in connection with an increased Q angle. In these cases reduced strength in the quadriceps muscle is often noted.

Radiographic examination reveals no specific changes in most cases. In exceptional cases computerized tomography and/or magnetic resonance imaging are performed. These are, however, not necessary, either to confirm the diagnosis or to start treatment. The same is true for arthroscopic inspection, which can be performed to survey changes to the cartilage on the joint surface of the patella. Diagnosis is made by a thorough clinical examination and by looking through the player's medical history.

## Treatment

Patients should adhere closely to a rehabilitation programme. Surgery very seldom needs to be performed and never before rehabilitation, which should last for at least 3–6 months.

In those cases where surgery is considered necessary, arthroscopic inspection can be performed to survey the cartilage damage. If there has been cartilage damage, 'shaving' may be performed, where the cartilage is shaved down until a smooth surface is created. The results are uncertain. In other cases 'lateral release', i.e. lengthening of the ligament which keeps the patella on the lateral side of the knee joint, can be appropriate. However, the value of this operation is also uncertain and the results variable.

## Prognosis

Prognosis in youths, especially girls with PFP, is good. Even if there is pain, there is no reason for patients to give up playing football. Training and match play at the right level are even an important part of treatment. The younger the player is when the problem arises, the better the prognosis.

# Bursitis

## Injury mechanism

The most common form of bursitis occurs in the front of the patella, i.e. pre-patellar bursitis. The cause is direct external pressure, such as when a goalkeeper dives onto a hard surface. Bursitis can also come about as the result of excessive loading.

## Symptoms

There is swelling and pain. Diagnosis is clinical. Occasionally, there is infection in the bursa. In these cases there is pronounced redness, a rise in temperature and severe pain.

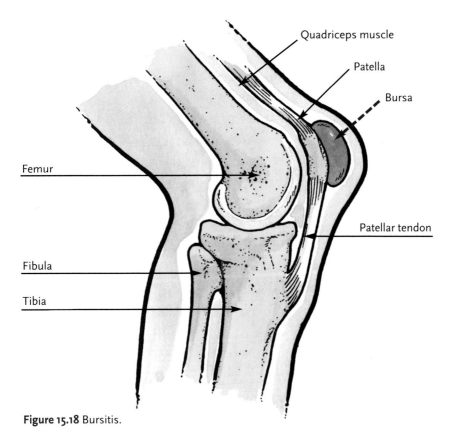

Quadriceps muscle

Patella

Bursa

Femur

Patellar tendon

Fibula

Tibia

**Figure 15.18** Bursitis.

## Treatment

If the bursa is inflamed, acute treatment including draining and the use of antibiotics is recommended.

If the problem is protracted, brief rest and cold-treatment are recommended. Anti-inflammatory drugs and possibly even cortisone injections into the bursa are appropriate. In exceptional cases, the bursa is removed surgically.

## Prognosis

This is generally good.

# Inflammation of the popliteal tendon

## Injury mechanism

Inflammation of the popliteal tendon is relatively uncommon in football, and can be difficult to differentiate from lateral meniscus damage. The popliteal tendon's attachment to the outside and rear of the femur is inflamed. The injury is, however, more common among runners.

## Symptoms

There is pain, which is very localized over the tendinous attachment behind the lateral collateral ligament on the outside or back of the femur. There is an increase in pain upon weight bearing of the bent knee.

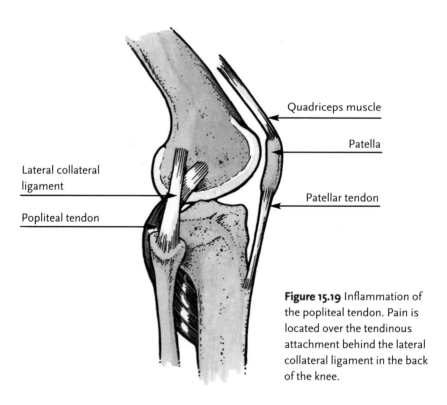

Quadriceps muscle

Patella

Lateral collateral ligament

Patellar tendon

Popliteal tendon

**Figure 15.19** Inflammation of the popliteal tendon. Pain is located over the tendinous attachment behind the lateral collateral ligament in the back of the knee.

### Diagnosis

The tendinous attachment is most easily palpated directly behind the lateral collateral ligament when the knee is bent to 90° and there is a small area where the pain occurs.

### Treatment

Recommended treatment is brief rest and rehabilitation combined with alternative training such as cycling and pool exercise, together with anti-inflammatory drugs. If ligament or meniscus damage are not suspected, one to three cortisone injections can be given. These are given at the most painful points, just behind the lateral ligament attachment.

### Prognosis

With the right diagnosis, prognosis is good and most players can return to play after around 4–6 weeks.

## Damage to the bicipital femoral tendon

### Injury mechanism

Damage to the bicipital femoral tendon, which attaches to the fibula at exactly the same point as the lateral collateral ligament's attachment, is probably more common in football than was previously considered. The injury occurs during shooting or tackling, where there is powerful muscle activation in response to resistance.

### Symptoms

Either the muscle or tendon is painful during muscle contraction. Swelling and haemorrhaging also occur. The injury can either be partial or total. With total rupture, muscle strength in knee flexion is reduced. Radiographic examination is recommended, as a small bone fragment can become detached from the attachment on the

fibula. For a precise diagnosis, ultrasonography or magnetic resonance imaging may be necessary.

## Treatment

On partial rupture of the bicipital femoral muscle or tendon, rehabilitation is recommended. After a short rest, range of motion,
coordination and strength training are started. If there is swelling,
anti-inflammatory drugs can be used, either in the form of tablets
or locally applied gel. If a bone fragment has broken off the tendinous attachment, surgery is recommended whereby the bone fragment is reattached.

## Prognosis

Unfortunately, diagnosis is hard to make, which often causes delay
and renders treatment more difficult. Emergency surgery probably
gives better results than surgery at a later stage. With prompt,
proper treatment, results are generally good. Rehabilitation time in
the case of partial rupture is around 6–8 weeks and for complete
rupture 3–4 months.

# Rupture of the patellar tendon (jumper's knee)

Damage to the patellar tendon occurs in many sports and is sometimes called 'jumper's knee' as it is considered especially common
among high jumpers. It has also been shown, however, that the
injury is just as common among football players. It is an overuse injury where there is partial rupture of the patellar tendon at the
tendinous attachment to the lower patella (tendinosis). Initially, the
symptoms are mild and the player can continue sporting activity in
spite of the pain. The problem can then often become protracted
and slow to heal.

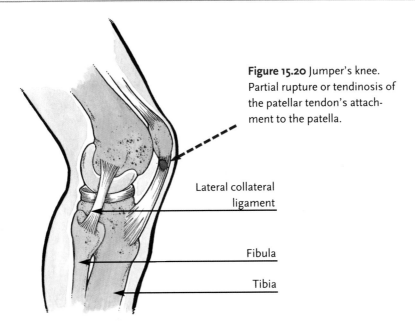

**Figure 15.20** Jumper's knee. Partial rupture or tendinosis of the patellar tendon's attachment to the patella.

Lateral collateral ligament

Fibula

Tibia

### Injury mechanism

The injury occurs in connection with excessive strain during varying muscle activity and recurrent high stress. Despite the partial rupture/tendinosis and pain, the player can often be active for varying lengths of time.

### Diagnosis

If there is only inflammation, the footballer generally has no trouble when playing but feels stiffness in the mornings and pain following strain. In the case of rupture, on the other hand, stress-related pain is the most common symptom. The pain becomes gradually more pronounced and makes play impossible. Strength in the quadriceps muscle is often reduced.

During clinical examination, pain is noted directly under the patella. There is pain when the knee joint is stretched against resistance and there is a slight swelling in the upper patellar tendon. There are no changes to be seen on radiographs. For a precise diagnosis, either sonography or magnetic resonance imaging is recommended. Both of these give good, certain diagnosis. Rupture of the patellar tendon can be divided into a variety of degrees, depending on the extent of this — the greater the rupture, the more likely it is that surgery will be necessary.

### Treatment

When the rupture is small or of medium size, it can generally be successfully treated with rehabilitation. The first step is brief rest combined with alternative forms of exercise until the player is free from pain. Taping and/or a small knee brace can be of help. Cortisone injections into the tendon are not recommended due to the risk of complete rupture of the tendon.

The injury often requires exercise beyond the pain threshold (eccentric exercise). This exercise should be done in consultation with an experienced physiotherapist. Rehabilitation time is often several months long.

In certain cases surgery is necessary and can be performed under local anaesthetic. During surgery the tendon is divided and the damaged part removed. In some cases, the operation can be done using arthroscopy. Directly after surgery rehabilitation is begun with range of motion and strength training. Immobilization, such as by means of a plaster cast, is not necessary.

### Prognosis

Although rehabilitation time is long, often 6–12 months, prognosis is good in most cases.

## Quadriceps tendinosis (inverted jumper's knee)

A similar condition, called quadriceps tendinosis or inverted jumper's knee, can occur directly above the patella. In addition to the location, the symptoms, treatment and prognosis are the same as for jumper's knee. However, surgery is rarely necessary.

# Osgood-Schlatter's disease

### Injury mechanism

Osgood-Schlatter's disease, is an apophysitis 'overuse' injury, which occurs particularly often in football-playing boys aged 15–16 years, but also in girls.

### Diagnosis

The knee hurts when placed under stress. On examination, swelling is observed and soreness on palpation as well as a relatively pronounced protuberance on the patellar tendon's attachment to the tibia. The condition often occurs in both knees. Even though the diagnosis is clinical, radiographic examination is often carried out, which shows fragmentation or loosening of the patellar tendon's attachment in the tibia.

### Treatment

Treatment is focused on the symptoms. Relieving pressure on the area which causes pain is recommended. The player should not take part in jumping, heading and shooting practice. It is extremely important, however, to say that the condition is benign and that the symptoms disappear when the player is fully grown. Training and match play, despite the pain they cause, are not contraindicated.

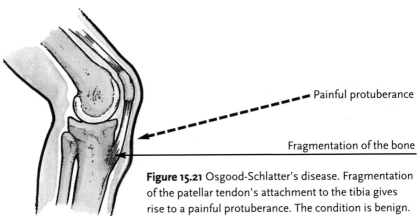

Painful protuberance

Fragmentation of the bone

**Figure 15.21** Osgood-Schlatter's disease. Fragmentation of the patellar tendon's attachment to the tibia gives rise to a painful protuberance. The condition is benign.

### Prognosis

Prognosis is good. In isolated instances, however very rare, the problem remains once growth has stopped. In these cases radiographic examination is recommended. If a large bone fragment is then found at the attachment of the patellar tendon, it can be removed.

# Runner's knee

### Injury mechanism

Runner's knee occurs most often in long-distance runners but also among footballers. The lowest part of the tendon (ileotibial tract), which slides over the outside of the femur, causes irritation of the underlying tissue. In a few cases bursitis occurs between the tendon and femur.

The underlying causes are thought to be outward rotation of the tibia and/or malalignment of the ankle as well as tightness in the ileotibial tract. People with legs of different lengths are thought to be especially at risk of developing runner's knee. The risk is greater in the longer leg. In footballers this problem generally arises during pre-season training where there is a great deal of running. Unsuitable shoes and a hard surface are also significant.

### Diagnosis

The outside of the knee joint causes considerable pain on examination. Crepitation, or a crunching sound, occurs in rare cases.

### Treatment

With acute inflammation rest, cooling and anti-inflammatory drugs are recommended. Thereafter treatment consists of rehabilitation, with special emphasis on range of motion and stamina training and stretching of the outer thigh muscle. Cortisone injections can give good results. In rare cases, surgery is appropriate.

## Prognosis

Prognosis is generally good. With treatment in the acute phase, the injured player can be back after 2–3 weeks, while recovery time following surgery is at least twice as long.

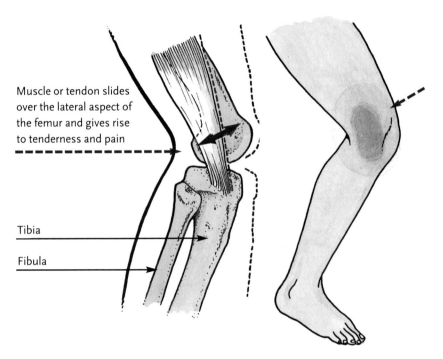

**Figure 15.22** Runner's knee. Pain in the outside of the lower femur caused by irritation of the tendon sliding over the bone.

# 16. Lower leg injuries

Jon Karlsson

The lower leg is composed of the tibia and fibula (bones), together with 12 different muscles which control movement in the ankle and foot. Some of the muscles have functions in both the knee and ankle.

The lower leg is sensitive to stress. There are four closed connective tissue compartments in the lower leg, which comprise muscles, nerves and blood vessels. If tissue pressure rises in these enclosed spaces, a condition called compartment syndrome occurs.

## Fractures

Fracture of the lower leg, while playing football, occurs either as a result of a direct blow to the tibia or indirectly by a blow which fractures the ankle. However, none of these injuries is especially common in the context of football.

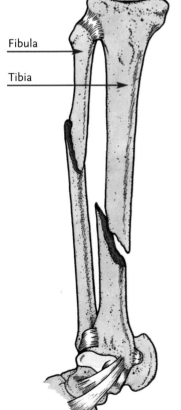

Fibula

Tibia

**Figure 16.1** Lower leg fracture. The picture shows a spiral fracture of the both tibia and fibula.

343

## Injury mechanism

A direct blow, generally the result of a kick, can give rise to a transverse fracture of the tibia and/or fibula. Following an indirect blow (twisting), a spiral fracture usually occurs. Fractures of the lower leg and ankle are classified according to appearance and malposition and whether the fracture is closed or open. The kind of blow which has given rise to the fracture, the number of bone fragments and whether the fracture is open (there is a skin wound too) or closed is of great significance to treatment, healing and prognosis. Splinter (comminuted) fractures can be associated with damage to the soft parts and healing time is much longer in this case.

## Diagnosis

With a transverse fracture, there is generally visible malposition. With fracture of the fibula and/or ankle joint, there is generally no pronounced dislocation, but there is swelling. More often than not, the player cannot put weight on the leg due to the pain. It is recommended that suspected fracture be radiographed to assess how serious the damage is, and to decide what treatment is required.

## Treatment

If there is visible and pronounced malposition, reduction is recommended on the scene of the accident itself, i.e. putting the fractured bones roughly in place and stabilizing the fracture with some form of external support. A team doctor should be able to perform a rough reduction of a lower leg fracture. Risk of further damage to the soft parts is thus diminished and the pain is also relieved.

If the fracture is open with a skin wound, the haemorrhaging should be stopped by means of compression (a pressure dressing). The wound is then covered with a clean dressing before transportation to the hospital, where the definitive treatment takes place. The extent of the injury, both in terms of bone and soft part damage, is determined for treatment. Simple fractures where there

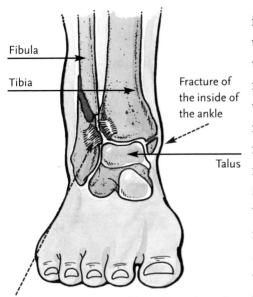

Fibula

Tibia

Fracture of the inside of the ankle

Talus

Fracture of the outside of the ankle and simultaneous rupture of the anterior syndesmosis

**Figure 16.2** Ankle fracture. As the result of twisting, a fracture has occurred in both the outside and inside of the ankle. In addition, the syndesmosis is damaged.

is no malposition can often be treated using a plaster cast, while unstable fractures where there is malposition and compound fractures often require surgical treatment. Ankle fractures generally require surgical treatment if the malposition is greater than 2 mm. Slightly greater malposition can be tolerated in fractures in the middle of the tibia or fibula. There are several surgical techniques where screws, steel plates and/or pins are used.

## Prognosis

Lower leg fractures generally heal without complications. Fracture of the fibula, which occur as a result of a direct blow, heals in approximately 3–6 weeks without any specific treatment. Healing time for a fracture of the tibia is longer, depending on how serious the injury, and not least the degree of damage to the soft tissues. The healing time varies from 8 to 16 weeks, or even longer. Rehabilitation time until a player can be back in play is, however, considerably longer, generally 6–12 months.

Fractures of the ankle generally heal without problems. In many cases, 6 weeks in plaster are recommended irrespective of whether the fracture has been operated on or not. Recent studies have shown, however, that if a stable internal fixation is performed, range of motion training can be begun earlier, as soon as 2–3 weeks after the injury. The same applies in the case of a fracture where there is little or no malposition which does not require surgery. A support brace such as an inflatable orthotic device (Aircast), is recommended in this case. Rehabilitation after an ankle fracture is similar to that after acute ligament damage in the ankle. A return to football can be made after approximately 3–4 months.

# Achilles' tendon damage

Achilles' tendon damage is either an acute injury or an overuse injury. Acute rupture of the Achilles' tendon is not especially common in active footballers, but overuse injuries, on the other hand, are.

## Complete rupture of the Achilles' tendon

### Injury mechanism

Complete rupture of the Achilles' tendon is uncommon in the context of football, but common in many other sports, such as badminton. The damage occurs acutely in a tendon which is, however, often probably degenerate, i.e. the tissue is already damaged internally. The player describes an audible snap in the tendon when the rupture occurs, simultaneously loses strength, has difficulty walking and standing normally and cannot walk on tiptoe.

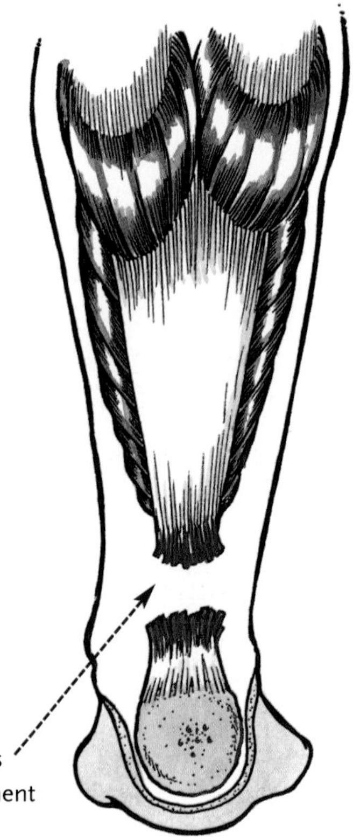

Figure 16.3 Complete rupture of the Achilles' tendon occurs approximately 3–5 cm above the Achilles' tendon's attachment to the heel bone.

## Diagnosis

A gap can be observed in the tendon in the damaged area as well as moderate haemorrhaging. Despite this relatively sure sign of acute rupture of the Achilles' tendon, several cases are not detected on the first visit to the doctor. A positive Thompson's test is a sure sign of rupture. When the calf muscle is compressed from side to side, if the Achilles' tendon is normal, there is a downward reflex movement of the foot, which is not the case if there is a rupture. This is a very sure diagnostic test.

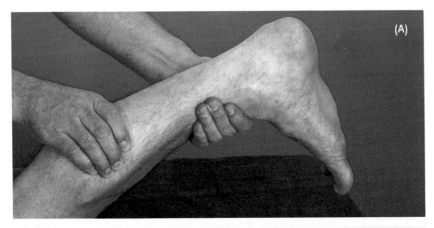

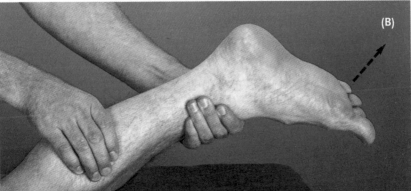

**Figure 16.4** Thompson's test. The test is performed to detect a complete rupture of the Achilles' tendon. (A) With the player lying face down, the calf is compressed from side to side. (B) If the Achilles' tendon is intact, in a reflex reaction the foot moves downwards. If the Achilles' tendon has snapped, no such movement takes place.

## Treatment

Recommended treatment for active players is surgery. Non-surgical treatment is possible, but the risk of complications in the form of renewed rupture is higher. With non-surgical treatment, the foot is put in plaster for 4 weeks with the toe pointed and thereafter subsequently in a neutral position for a further 4 weeks. When the plaster has been removed, there then follows rehabilitation with careful range of motion training as well as strength and balance training. It is recommended that flat shoes are not worn for several weeks to months once the plaster has been taken off. During surgery, the damaged ends of the tendon are sewn together. The operation can be performed under local anaesthetic and is technically simple. The advantage with surgery is that range of motion training and loading of the tendon can start early and rehabilitation time is shortened. Furthermore, the tendon retains its normal length, which gives a better chance of full function being recovered, including maximal strength.

## Prognosis

Prognosis for recovery is good, irrespective of whether the rupture of the Achilles' tendon is treated surgically or not. The risk of renewed rupture is between 20 and 30 per cent higher with non-surgical treatment. In the event of renewed rupture, surgical treatment and reconstruction are recommended. This can be done using a variety of surgical techniques. Whatever the treatment, rehabilitation time is always very long. It can be 6–12 months before the player can return to play.

# Overuse injury to the Achilles' tendon and the tendon attachment

Inflammation in the Achilles' tendon attachment or partial rupture of the Achilles' tendon are relatively common overuse injuries in footballers. The injury is more common in players who run a lot during matches. Often there is a protruding bump on the back of the heel and, because football boots are tight and relatively hard, also pronounced local pain.

In many cases a condition called tendinosis occurs. Tendinosis is a collective term for degenerative changes in the tendon. There is, unfortunately, great confusion regarding injuries surrounding the

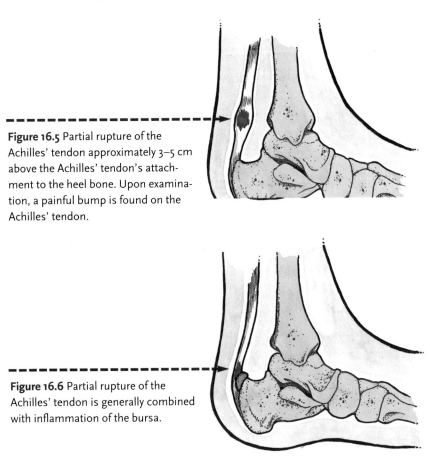

**Figure 16.5** Partial rupture of the Achilles' tendon approximately 3–5 cm above the Achilles' tendon's attachment to the heel bone. Upon examination, a painful bump is found on the Achilles' tendon.

**Figure 16.6** Partial rupture of the Achilles' tendon is generally combined with inflammation of the bursa.

Achilles' tendon, particularly regarding inflammation. Inflammation in the Achilles' tendon and its attachment occur most of all in the tendon sheath and the bursae around the Achilles' tendon. Inflammation in the Achilles' tendon itself, however, is rare and the term tendinitis should therefore be avoided.

## Injury mechanism

The cause is repeated, unilateral stress and a large amount of training, often in combination with tight footwear. Certain biomechanical factors are also considered significant, for example pronation of the back foot. In rare cases, inflammation of the tendon sheath is acute with crepitations, which feel like gravel or air bubbles under the skin when the player moves the foot up and down.

Generally, however, the symptoms are prolonged with repeated minor injuries. Thus, the problem increases gradually with pain and swelling at the attachment of the tendon and the surrounding bursae. External pressure on a protruding bump on the back of the heel bone also adds to the pain.

With inflammation of the tendon sheath, there is pressure pain at the base of the Achilles' tendon. With partial rupture or tendinosis, on the other hand, the soreness is distinctly within a smaller area. In addition, a clear swelling with a painful protuberance is observed on the Achilles' tendon itself approximately 3–5 cm above the Achilles' tendon's attachment to the heel bone. With bursitis, either to the front or the rear of the tendon attachment, the bursae are filled with fluid and swollen.

In order to be able to make a precise diagnosis, especially where rupture and/or tendinosis are concerned, sonography and/or magnetic resonance imaging can be necessary. These investigations do not have to be performed in the acute stage, however.

## Treatment

It is extremely important to review the contributing factors such as the amount of training, exercise strain as well as footwear and insoles if symptoms are noted from the Achilles' tendon. In certain cases an insole, which raises the heel around 5 mm is used to reduce strain.

With acute inflammation, anti-inflammatory drugs are prescribed. With crepitation around the tendon, heparin injections (15 000 units intravenously, for 3 consecutive days) give good results. The footballer can return to play directly after treatment finishes. The most important part of treatment, besides prevention, is rehabilitation, which should involve developing flexibility, coordination and strength. Rehabilitation should also be combined with adjusting footwear and insoles.

It is of great significance for both prognosis and treatment whether the damage lies in the Achilles' tendon itself (generally 3–5 cm above the where it attaches to the heel bone) or in the Achilles' tendon attachment. The latter quite often gives rise to protracted problems and can be difficult to treat.

In certain prolonged cases surgery can be necessary. Before a decision is made regarding surgery, the Achilles' tendon and its attachment should be examined by means of ultrasonography or

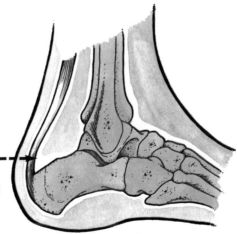

**Figure 16.7** After excision of the protruding bump on the back of the heel bone. The deep bursa has also been removed.

magnetic resonance imaging. With partial rupture or tendinosis, the damaged tissue is removed. If the player has a large protruding bump on the heel bone, this is excised. At the same time, the deep bursa can be removed.

### Prognosis

Recovery time in many cases is long, often many months, especially after surgery. It can be vitally important not to resume footballing activity before the rehabilitation is complete. The player should have complete range of motion, coordination, strength and elasticity in the calf muscles before he or she is allowed to play again. Correction of a variety of external injury factors, such as the training surface, stress, amount of training and footwear, is also very important.

## Rupture of the calf muscle

### Injury mechanism

Muscle damage in the calf is relatively common in football. Damage can either occur as a contusion injury following a direct blow to the muscle, e.g. a kick, or a distortion injury from stretching, e.g. following a jump. In addition to haemorrhaging, rupture also occurs in the crossover between muscle fibre and tendon fibre. The injury occurs following rapid muscle activation.

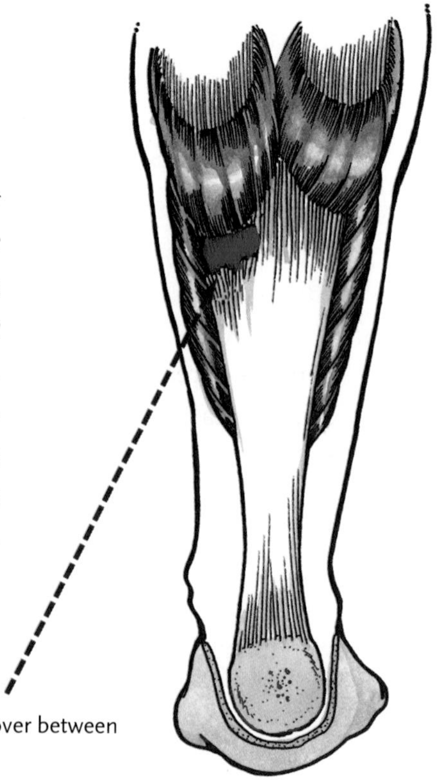

**Figure 16.8** Muscle rupture in the calf in the crossover between muscle and tendon (aponeurosis).

## Diagnosis

Upon rupture, there is acute pain on the inside of the calf, in the middle of the lower leg. Occasionally rupture of the Achilles' tendon is suspected. The player may have difficulty walking or feel that it is better to walk on tiptoe.

On examination there is swelling and haemorrhaging as well as pain in a small area in the inside of the calf muscle, with a gap in the muscle and a reduction in strength.

## Treatment

The injury never needs to be treated surgically. In acute cases, a pressure dressing and possibly ice-packs are recommended, especially with the aim of easing pain. In a few days, range of motion training is begun, followed by coordination and strength training.

It is extremely important to develop full flexibility and to stretch the muscle to its full length, in order to reduce the risk of renewed injury. Immobilization or surgery are never appropriate. In order to reduce the risk of relapse, gradually more intensive rehabilitation is recommended, with successively increased loading.

## Prognosis

Prognosis is good and rehabilitation takes approximately 4–8 weeks. Adequate rehabilitation is very important. If treatment only consists of rest, the injury heals with shortening of the muscles and scar formation. This increases the risk of relapse, with persistent pain and reduced function for a relatively long period.

# Periostitis (medial tibia syndrome)

### Injury mechanism

There is a certain confusion regarding pain in the lower leg. What is known as medial tibia syndrome is often called periostitis. Although the condition is more common among long-distance runners, it also occurs relatively often in footballers. It is especially common during the pre-season when the training surface is often changed. Thus method, the amount of training, surface, footwear and running technique are of great importance. It is also thought that training on hard pitches for example, especially training indoors and on artificial grass, are often associated with periostitis.

The condition is sometimes thought to be a preliminary stage of a stress fracture.

### Diagnosis

There is pain around the rear of the inside edge of the tibia. The pain is most intense approximately 10 cm above the inside of the ankle. The problem occurs and increases gradually, initially only after physical activity but then as time goes on in connection with and during training, too, until playing is impossible.

With pronounced symptoms, it can be difficult to distinguish medial tibia syndrome from a stress fracture. Radiographs generally show no damage. In certain cases there is, however, a thickening of the bone. Isotope scans (scintigraphy) can reveal increased absorption of radioactive isotopes, which points to increased stress on the bone. If the prob-

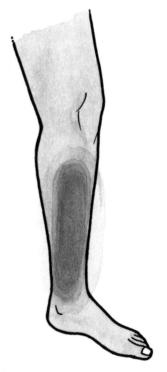

**Figure 16.9** With periostitis the player feels pain on the inside of the lower leg.

lem is protracted, there is increased absorption in large sections of the bone.

## Treatment

The most important aspect of treatment is correcting the factors which contribute to the pain, such as reducing the amount of training and possibly changing the surface. Rest from play for 2–4 weeks in acute cases is often necessary. Alternative exercise is recommended.

Anti-inflammatory drugs are often used, even if it is not certain that there is any actual inflammation. These drugs can be taken in the form of tablets or applied as a cream or gel on the area in question. If the gel or cream are used, they are applied morning and evening and are rubbed gently into the skin for about 30 seconds. These anti-inflammatory drugs are then absorbed only in the tissue where they have been rubbed in, but not in the blood circulation. In rare cases, surgery can be necessary when the pain is chronic. Then, a slit is made in the muscle membrane into the posterior muscle compartments (fasciotomy).

## Prognosis

Prognosis in most cases is good. Pain with periostitis is generally transitory. Correction of contributing factors such as the amount of training and surface are of vital importance.

The results of surgery are considered good in approximately 75 per cent of cases. It is always necessary, however, to correct contributing factors such as biomechanical malalignment.

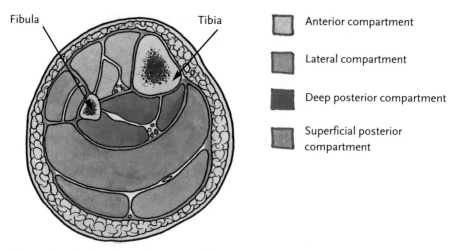

Fibula

Tibia

Anterior compartment

Lateral compartment

Deep posterior compartment

Superficial posterior compartment

**Figure 16.10** The lower leg is divided into four enclosed or closed tissue areas (compartments). The figure shows a cross-section of the lower leg.

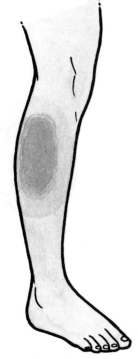

**Figure 16.11** With compartment syndrome there is pain on the front/outside of the lower leg.

# Chronic compartment syndrome (chronically high tissue pressure)

### Injury mechanism

Increased pressure in any of the enclosed or closed compartments in the muscles of the lower leg can occur during intensive muscle exertion. This is especially common in the lateral and anterior compartments. The condition occurs particularly in runners, especially those who run long distances, but also in footballers who run a great deal, such as midfielders. It is particularly common during the basic training period when players often do a great deal of training on hard and/or variable surfaces.

### Symptoms

The dominant symptom is pain which occurs after a certain amount of exertion, such as after running a certain distance or a certain time. In some cases, there can be a feeling of numbness in the foot or an altered sense of feeling. The player is often forced to interrupt the activity or slow down. The swelling subsides after approximately 30 minutes and the pain disappears, but returns when activity is resumed.

Upon clinical examination, there is soreness and swelling in the affected area. Diagnosis can be established by measuring muscle pressure under exertion.

In order to differentiate between compartment syndrome, medial tibial syndrome and stress fracture, the following description of symptoms is used.

| | Compartment syndrome | Medial tibia syndrome | Stress fracture syndrome |
|---|---|---|---|
| Pain after ... | 3 km | 300 m | Directly with every step |
| Need to stop | Yes | No | Yes |
| Pain after activity | No | Yes | No |

Another problem in the lower leg is what is called muscular hypertension syndrome. This is a kind of prolonged cramp which is caused by an inability to relax the muscles and is often misinterpreted as compartment syndrome.

## Treatment

Rest is recommended to begin with and possibly even anti-inflammatory drugs. It is important to analyse and adjust both external and internal factors such as the amount of training, surface and footwear. Training factors which can be adjusted include reducing the impact from running and jumping and adding alternative forms of exercise such as cycling and pool exercise instead. A rehabilitation programme can have a positive effect, which is also the case with custom made insoles. Sometimes surgery (fasciotomy) where a slit is made in the taut muscle membrane of the compartment in question to increase the volume for the existing muscle to work in, is necessary. In the course of fasciotomy, an incision is made approximately 4 cm from the rear edge of the tibia. The incision is made large, as it is important to be able to see the nerves and vessels, so that there is no haemorrhaging after the operation. Following surgery, crutches are used for 3 days and full weight bearing is not recommended for the first 12 hours. Running is not recommended for around 3 weeks.

With muscular hypertension syndrome, fasciotomy does not help, but it is treated with stretching exercises.

### Prognosis

Prognosis following surgery is satisfactory in approximately 70 per cent of cases. Women have slightly worse prognosis than men. It is important not to operate if there is any sign of varicose veins.

# Stress fracture

In certain cases it is thought that medial tibia syndrome, or periostitis, is a preliminary stage to a stress fracture. A stress fracture occurs due to repeated stress, which gradually exceeds the bone's ability to withstand the physiological stress of normal movement. Stress fractures are more common in runners, but they also occur in footballers, usually in the lower leg, tibia or fibula.

### Injury mechanism

A number of different causes can contribute to a stress fracture. The underlying causes may be internal factors, such as malalignment of the foot or a difference in the length of the legs or external factors such as training surface, too much training and/or the wrong equipment such as footwear. The triggering factor, however, is always stress (overuse), which gives rise to weakness in the bone and which thus eventually, when left untreated, leads to a fracture.

Where the injury is located is of great significance. A stress fracture of the tibia is a much more serious problem than a stress fracture of the fibula, which has a better prognosis. The most common location for a stress fracture of the tibia is the upper third of the bone. A stress fracture of the fibula is generally located approximately 10 cm above the outside of the ankle. Symptoms develop gradually. Often continued training and playing are feasible for a certain period, but eventually it is no longer possible because of the pain.

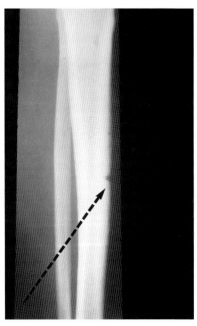

**Figure 16.12** Stress fracture of the tibia.

### Diagnosis

There is pain within a small area on palpation or provocation of the bone. On rare occasions, there is localized swelling. The pain always increases when placed under strain, but disappears when at rest, at least in the beginning.

It can often be difficult to detect the fracture on radiographs. Careful examination and comparison with the healthy side can, however, reveal bone deposits and thickening of the bone. In the event of uncertainty, isotope scans, in the majority of cases show up a stress fracture which is already in the acute phase. Radiographs are always necessary in diagnostic evaluation of lower leg pain, especially if a stress fracture is suspected.

Scans such as magnetic resonance imaging and computerized tomography can also reveal a possible stress fracture with a high degree of certainty. These scans are not recommended, however, until radiographs and isotope scans have not revealed a stress fracture, or are unequivocal.

## Treatment

Rest and alleviation of stress are an essential part of treatment. In certain cases, immobilization by means of a splint or plaster is required. The length of the immobilization ranges from 4 to 8 weeks. During the healing period, the player can do alternative forms of exercise such as in the pool. Modern treatment with shock waves has been shown to give good results in slow-healing stress fractures. This alternative form of treatment is, however, new and further studies are needed before the value of the treatment can be confirmed. Various surgical techniques for example, with intramedullary nails/pins or steel plates, are of dubious value.

## Prognosis

Healing time varies according to the location and extent of the injury. It is of great significance for treatment and prognosis whether the damage is on the front (anterior) or back (posterior) of the tibia. A stress fracture on the front of the tibia always heals much more slowly than a stress fracture on the back. Most stress fractures of the fibula and the rear of the tibia heal without complications. Stress fractures on the front of the tibia are very slow to heal with setbacks to the healing process and lingering pain.

It is very important that rehabilitation is completed before the player can return to sporting activity. Correction of the underlying factors is necessary to prevent the injury re-occurring.

Stress fractures occur to a greater extent in women and a connection has been found here between eating disorders and stress fractures.

# 17. Ankle injuries

Jon Karlsson

The outside of the ankle is stabilized by three ligaments — the anterior ligament between the fibula and the talus (anterior talofibular ligament), the ligament between the fibula and the calcaneus (calcaneofibular ligament) and the posterior ligament between the fibula and the talus (posterior talofibular ligament).

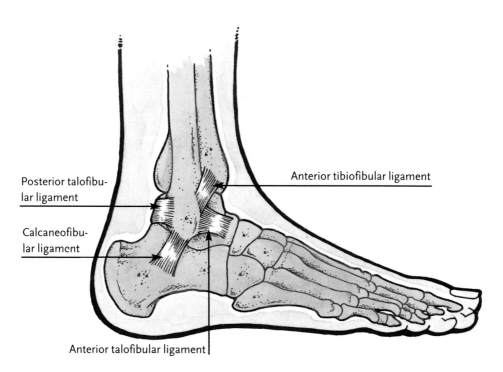

Posterior talofibular ligament

Calcaneofibular ligament

Anterior tibiofibular ligament

Anterior talofibular ligament

**Figure 17.1** The outside of the ankle.

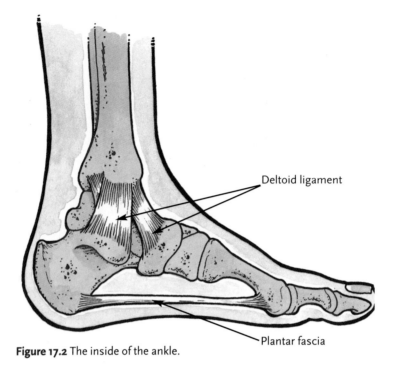

**Figure 17.2** The inside of the ankle.

# Acute ligament damage

Ligament damage in the ankle is very common in sport. Approximately one in four sports injuries is an acute ligament injury in the ankle. It is especially common in football, both as an acute and a recurrent injury.

### Injury mechanism

The injury occurs when the ankle is twisted inward with the foot pointing away. Around two-thirds of all ligament injuries in the ankle involve damage to the anterior talofibular ligament. In around 20 per cent of cases, there is combined damage to the anterior talofibular ligament and the underlying calcaneofibular ligament. Isolated ligament damage to the posterior talofibular ligament and calcaneofibular ligament is rare. Joint capsule damage can occur at the same time as ligament damage.

## Diagnosis

When this damage occurs, there is rapid, pronounced swelling. The player experiences pain and finds it difficult to bear weight on his foot.

Bleeding from the damaged ligament can be marked. The bleeding spreads around the tissues in 1–2 days, and is often seen as a bruise on the outside of the foot.

Pain occurs on palpation over the damaged ligament and joint capsule. On examination there is instability, both drawer and increased inversion. The stability test can, however, be difficult to perform in the acute phase because of pain. As the degree of instability with acute damage does not affect treatment and if the stability test is painful, it is not necessary to do it in the acute phase.

Diagnosis is clinical. Radiographs are only necessary if there is suspected bony damage. Bony damage should be suspected especially when there is 'indirect pain' i.e. pain in the ankle area which occurs when the fibula and tibia are pressed together slightly above the ankle.

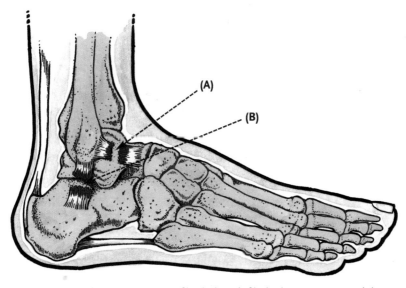

**Figure 17.3** Ligament damage. Rupture of both the talofibular ligament (A), and the calcaneofibular ligament (B).

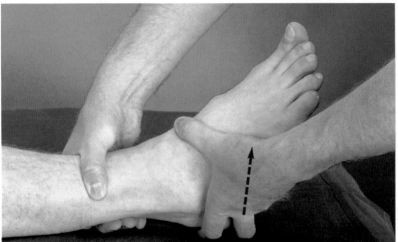

**Figure 17.4** Anterior drawer test. The test measures forward movement of the talus in relation to the tibia. When there is damage to the anterior talofibular ligament there is increased anterior drawer movement.

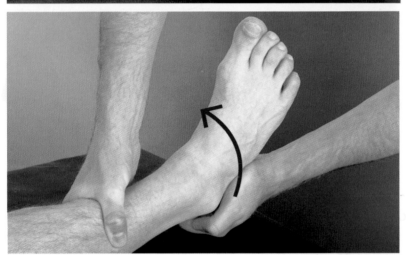

**Figure 17.5** Inversion test. The test measures inward twisting of the talus in relation to the lower leg. With increased inward twisting there is damage to both the anterior talofibular ligament and to the posterior calcaneofibular ligament. In both these tests comparison should be made with the other, healthy side.

## Treatment

Preliminary treatment follows the principles for the treatment of injury to the soft tissues. Even if the ligament is completely torn, emergency surgery is not necessary. Following treatment with a compression bandage and keeping the foot raised, the injury is best treated with early range of motion training and weight bearing. As soon as possible a pressure dressing should be applied. The pressure dressing can be combined with cooling. Within 1–2 days, the foot should be weighted until the pain threshold is reached and the

| | DAY | | | WEEK | | |
|---|---|---|---|---|---|---|
| | 1–2 | 3–4 | 5–7 | 2–4 | 5–6 | 7–12 |
| **Immobilization** | | | | | | |
| Compression dressing | ■ | | | | | |
| Crutches | ■ | | | | | |
| Partial weight bearing | ■ | | | | | |
| Taping | | ■ | ■ | | ■ | ■ |
| **Agility training** | | | | | | |
| Aerobic exercise | | ■ | | | | |
| Stretching calf muscles | | ■ | ■ | ■ | | |
| Cycling exercise | | ■ | ■ | | | |
| Pool | | ■ | | | | |
| **Weight training** | | | | | | |
| Heel raising | | | | ■ | | |
| Rubber tube (outside of the foot) | | | | ■ | | |
| **Football-related training** | | | | | ■ | |
| **Coordination training** | | | | | | |
| Standing on one leg | | ■ | ■ | | | |
| Balance board | | | | ■ | ■ | |
| Sideways jump | | | | | ■ | |
| **Fitness training** | | | | | | |
| Cycling | | | | ■ | | |
| Pool | | | | ■ | | |
| Jogging, running | | | | | ■ | ■ |

player encouraged to walk normally, without crutches if possible. Agility training can be begun after 1–2 days and balance training using a balance board a day or so later. Thereafter strength training can start.

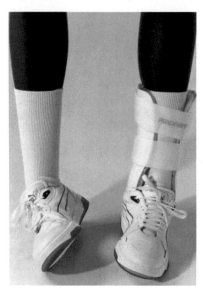

**Figure 17.6** Inflatable brace (Aircast) can be used following ligament damage to the ankle.

To prevent the injury recurring, rehabilitation is recommended for at least 12 weeks, with continued strength and coordination training. Playing football can be resumed much earlier, however, generally after around 7–10 days. For this to be possible external support is required e.g. tape (see Chapter 20) or a stabilizing ankle brace. Inflatable supports have been shown to be effective in the early stage of rehabilitation and has been shown to reduce time spent on sick level.

## Prognosis

Approximately 80–90 per cent of sportsmen and women who have suffered acute ligament injury to the ankle make a good recovery. In certain cases there is some instability and/or pain left. The total healing time is 6–12 months and continued rehabilitation is therefore important. Footballing activities can begin while the player is still under treatment, as the risk of serious residual damage is small.

With early, active treatment, absence from football and even time spent on sick leave can be shortened, without the risk of recurrent instability or pain increasing in the future.

# Chronic ligament instability

The most common consequence of ligament injury in the ankle is a feeling of unsteadiness — or functional instability — which can be described as a recurring tendency for the joint to give way. The reasons for functional instability are not entirely clear. A combination or several factors such as lengthening or rupture of the ligament, disturbance of nerve or muscle functions and impaired coordination and/or muscle weakness are contributing factors.

### Injury mechanism

Chronic ligament instability occurs as a result of recurrent ligament damage. Poor treatment or even a complete lack of treatment probably play an important role following acute injury, although there is no conclusive scientific evidence for this.

### Diagnosis

The player is troubled by a tendency for the joint to give way when placed under strain and a feeling of unsteadiness, for example when walking or running on uneven ground. Periodically (between sprains) the ankle is completely pain free. Pain and swelling occur with each new sprain, when the ligament is stretched further. Pain, generally combined with a certain degree of swelling, is observed on the outside of the ankle over the ligament.

Clinical examination consists mostly of stability tests. An examination of stability is easier to perform with chronic ligament instability than with acute injury, which is due to the fact that pain is relatively uncommon with chronic ligament damage.

In order to make a better diagnosis, gauging the degree of instability by means of stress radiographs can be of value. Scans such as computerized tomography or magnetic resonance imaging, on the other hand, do not increase the degree of certainty in diagnosis.

## Treatment

The initial treatment of a player with chronic ligament instability in the ankle is rehabilitation. After a well-executed rehabilitation programme, which is based on range of motion training, strength training and balance training for a minimum of 3 months, the symptoms abate in approximately 50 per cent of those affected. In those with persisting symptoms, even despite well-executed rehabili-

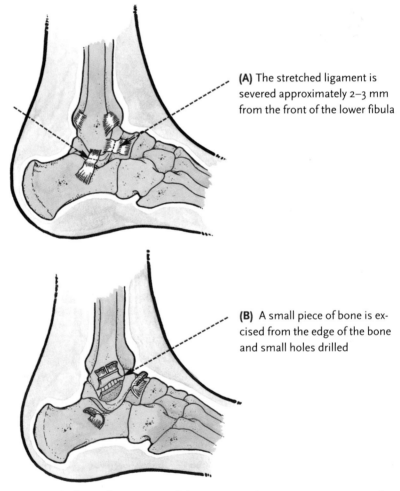

**(A)** The stretched ligament is severed approximately 2–3 mm from the front of the lower fibula

**(B)** A small piece of bone is excised from the edge of the bone and small holes drilled

**Figure 17.7** With chronic ligament instability, anatomical reconstruction is most often used. Surgery is performed by means of shortening (A–C) and new attachment (D) of the damaged ligament to the bone.

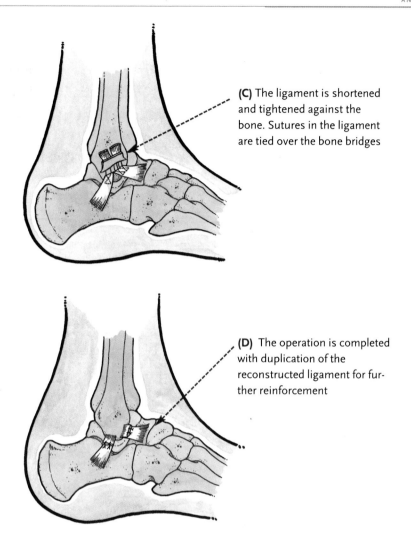

(C) The ligament is shortened and tightened against the bone. Sutures in the ligament are tied over the bone bridges

(D) The operation is completed with duplication of the reconstructed ligament for further reinforcement

tation, surgery can be necessary. Several surgical methods are used. These are based on either anatomical reconstruction or moving a tendon on the outside of the ankle. Anatomical reconstruction makes use of the remaining stretched ligaments. Following severing and shortening, a new attachment to the bone is made.

Early range of motion training following surgery has been shown to result in a player being able to return to football training and play earlier and is therefore recommended.

**Prognosis**

Approximately half of all footballers with chronic ligament instability can expect satisfactory results with normal functional stability after a programme of rehabilitation lasting around 12 weeks. In other cases, surgery is necessary.

Approximately 80–85 per cent of those who undergo surgery achieve satisfactory results, both in the short and long term. Rehabilitation time after surgery is 8–12 weeks, and the majority of footballers can return to the same level of activity as before injury.

## Ligament damage on the inside of the ankle

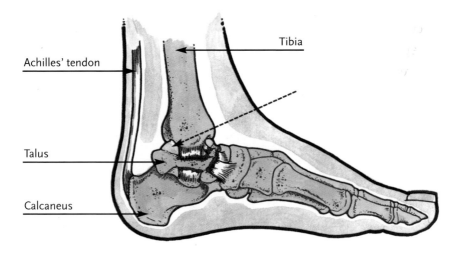

**Figure 17.8** Rupture of the deltoid ligament.

The deltoid ligament is located on the inside of the ankle. This ligament is substantial and strong and in addition, is on two different planes, both superficial and deep. Damage to this ligament is therefore much more uncommon than to those ligaments on the outside of the ankle.

## Injury mechanism

The injury occurs following outward twisting of the foot. There can be partial or total rupture of the ligament depending on the amount of force and the direction. Ligament injury can occur in isolation, but is, however, more common in association with a fracture of the ankle.

## Diagnosis

There is pain and swelling in the inside of the ankle. The pain is most pronounced in the front of the ligament. A test of stability is difficult to perform, even for an experienced examiner. Definite instability can therefore often not be established. Radiographic examination is often necessary, in order to rule out fracture.

## Treatment

Acute treatment is a pressure dressing, possibly ice packs and keeping the foot raised. After the pressure dressing has been removed, a compression bandage is applied. As soon as the pain allows rehabilitation with range of motion, balance and strength training can be begun.

There are no studies which show that immobilization or emergency surgery improve results, either in the short or long term.

## Prognosis

Healing time is significantly longer and the discomfort greater than with acute ligament damage to the outside of the ankle. Swelling and pain often persist for several weeks or months. It is important to give the injury a chance to heal without forcing treatment, to reduce the risk of prolonged inflammation together with pain and a reduction in function. Inverted taping is used for the first few weeks when the player returns to footballing activity. First of all, a stirrup is made, which stabilizes the outside of the ankle and then it is pulled tight on the inside of the ankle.

There is very little need for surgery.

# Syndesmosis rupture

Rupture of syndesmosis ligaments is uncommon. The injury generally occurs in association with a fracture, but can in rare cases also occur as an isolated injury.

## Injury mechanism

Damage to syndesmosis ligaments occurs upon forced outward rotation of the ankle. In most cases it is the anterior syndesmosis ligament (anterior tibiofibular ligament) which is damaged. Emergency surgery is generally necessary to prevent future reduction of function.

## Diagnosis

Rupture of syndesmosis ligaments can be difficult to detect. Careful clinical examination is therefore important. There is swelling and pain over the ligament. The pain is further forward and higher up the lower leg than with a usual acute ligament injury. Severe pain occurs on provocation of the syndesmosis ligaments during forced outward rotation of the foot in relation to the lower leg. This test can, however, be difficult to carry out in acute cases. It should therefore be complemented with radiographs to rule out a fracture and examination for instability by means of fluoroscopy. The provocation test reveals instability between the tibia and fibula on maximum outward rotation of the foot if the syndesmosis ligaments are damaged.

There can be a fracture of the fibula directly below the knee joint. Careful examination with palpation of the whole fibula is therefore necessary if there is suspected rupture of syndesmosis ligaments.

## Treatment

Emergency surgery to stabilize syndesmosis and suturing of the ligament are recommended. Early range of motion training is possible

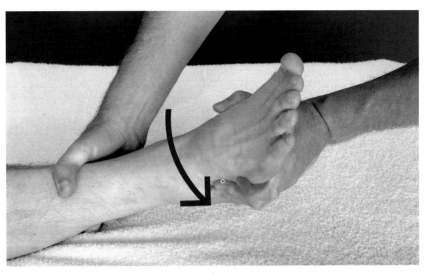

**Figure 17.9** Provocation of syndesmosis is carried out by means of outward rotation of the foot in relation to the lower leg. In the event of equivocal result, the test can be performed under local anaesthetic.

if surgery achieves good stability. In rare cases, there is chronic pain following syndesmosis damage, which has not been detected in the acute phase. The damage is very difficult to diagnose with certainty.

### Prognosis

Healing time is approximately 10–12 weeks. With early range of motion training, a return to play can be brought forward by a few days. There are a number of other diagnoses for lingering ankle pain after ligament injury. The most common differential diagnosis are given on page 374.

To make an accurate diagnosis and thereby determine which treatment is necessary, various in-depth examinations can be necessary in rare cases. Of these, ultrasonography and magnetic resonance imaging can be mentioned. Arthroscopy of the ankle is a relatively new addition to investigation and treatment, but can be of great value, for example to detect cartilage damage, bony outgrowths (anterior tibial bone spurs) and loose bodies.

**CHRONIC ANKLE PROBLEMS – DIFFERENTIAL DIAGNOSIS**

- Cartilage damage (especially on the joint surface of the talus).
- Synovitis/impingement (inflammation and entrapment).
- Entrapment of a nerve behind the inner ankle bone (medial malleolus).
  (Tarsal tunnel syndrome, see Chapter 18).
- Partial rupture of the short peroneal tendon behind the outer ankle bone (lateral malleolus).
- Bony outgrowths (osteophytes) in the joint.
- Loose bodies in the joint.

## Dislocation of the peroneal tendon

Dislocation of the peroneal tendon is a relatively rare injury in footballers.

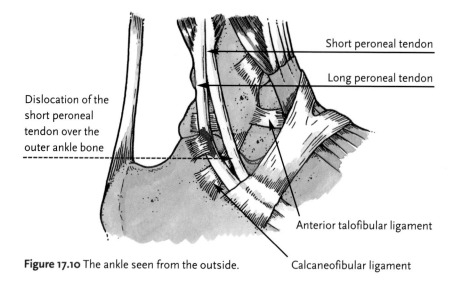

**Figure 17.10** The ankle seen from the outside.

Short peroneal tendon

Long peroneal tendon

Dislocation of the short peroneal tendon over the outer ankle bone

Anterior talofibular ligament

Calcaneofibular ligament

## Injury mechanism

Dislocation of one of the peroneal tendons, in most cases the short peroneal tendon, occurs when the tendon moves or dislocates out of the shallow groove located behind the outer ankle bone. The ligament reinforcement, which holds the tendon in place, ruptures. The injury occur on inward rotation and simultaneous inward twisting of the foot in relation to the lower leg.

## Diagnosis

The acute symptoms are almost identical to those of acute ligament damage, i.e. pain and swelling around the outer ankle bone. Clinical diagnosis is generally difficult and the injury is therefore not always detected. With suspected dislocation of the peroneal tendon, the foot is rotated inward at the same time as the peroneal muscles in the outside of the lower leg are actively contracted. Movement of the peroneal tendon over the ankle bone can then be seen and felt.

If there is recurrent instability, the tendon can move (dislocate) over the ankle bone with a perceptible clicking and be seen to do so. The condition is often painful.

## Treatment

Initial treatment of acute dislocation of the peroneal tendon is a compression dressing and ice packs. Immobilization using a plaster cast or an orthotic device is recommended for 4–6 weeks and is then followed with range of motion, strength and balance training.

With recurrent instability surgical stabilization of the tendon is necessary. Several different methods can be used. Recent studies have shown that simple reconstruction of the ligament and ligament reinforcement in the rear of the ankle give good results.

## Prognosis

Prognosis is good in most cases. If acute damage heals spontaneously, the player can return to activity after 8–10 weeks. Results following surgery are generally good. The majority of players regain normal mobility and strength in the ankle and can return to the same level of activity as before the injury.

# Os trigonum

### Injury mechanism

One of the accessory bones in the foot which can give rise to problems is the os trigonum, which is located behind the ankle joint, between the talus and the Achilles' tendon. On violent downward bending of the foot (plantar flexion), the bone can become trapped and produce pain. This bone is usually found in approximately 10 per cent of the population, but only causes problems if the area is subjected to high stress or pinching.

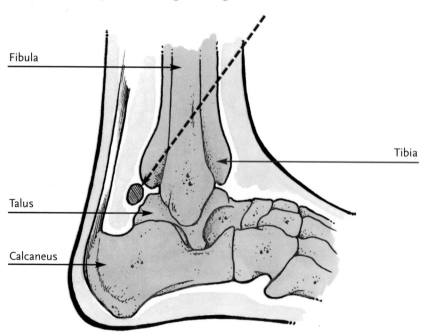

Fibula

Tibia

Talus

Calcaneus

**Figure 17.11** An accessory bone to the rear of the ankle bone (os trigonum) can give rise to pain when the ankle joint is bent downward. The bone is trapped between the talus and the tibia.

## Diagnosis

Diagnosis is clinical and is based on the pain in the rear of the ankle bone. Pain arises on stress, such as while running on uneven ground, when the ankle joint is placed under strain. Radiographic examination corroborates the diagnosis. Further examination such as by magnetic resonance imaging, is not necessary.

## Treatment

Initial treatment consists of correction of external training factors, such as soft insoles in footwear and changes in amount of training and training surface. Tape, which reduces movement of the ankle — especially on downward bending, can also be used. If the player has pronounced, persistent pain which prevents training or play, surgery is appropriate. During surgery, the bone is removed.

## Prognosis

Prognosis following surgery is generally good. The footballer can return to play after about 4 weeks. Immediate range of motion training is recommended after surgery.

# Footballer's ankle

Footballer's ankle (anterior impingement) occurs relatively often in footballers, especially at the end of their career (see Chapter 3).

## Injury mechanism

The injury occurs in association with repeated minor injuries to the front of the ankle. Following tearing of the joint capsule attachment to the tibia and talus, small bone fragments become detached. This is due to an outgrowth of bone fragments, which gradually builds up bone on the edges of the joint surface.

## Symptoms and signs

When over growth of bone increases in size, mobility decreases in the ankle joint and pain increases upon upwards movement of the joint (dorsal extension). The player experiences particular discomfort when running and jumping.

During examination there is soreness on palpation in the front of the ankle joint and soreness on provocation when the foot is bent upward, which is often reduced. Footballer's ankle is not uncommonly combined with chronic ligament instability.

## Treatment

Initially the injury can be treated with anti-inflammatory drugs and some sort of stabilizing ankle support such as tape, to prevent pain in the ankle. However, surgery is often necessary. During the operation, the bony over growth and cicatrization in the joint itself are removed. The surgery can very well be performed using athroscopy.

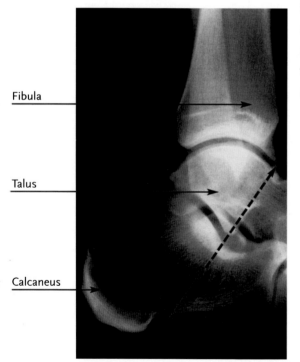

Fibula

Talus

Calcaneus

**Figure 17.12** In footballer's ankle, there is a build-up of bone on the anterior joint surfaces of the tibia and occasionally the talus, which leads to reduced mobility and pain.

### Prognosis

The damage is benign but often bothersome and painful. Results following surgery are generally good and the player can return to the same level of activity as before, after approximately 4 weeks.

# Osteochondritis dissecans

### Injury mechanism

The cause of osteochondritis dissecans is unknown. The damage is to the talus, generally on the medial corner (see Figure 17.13) and is sometimes related to ligament damage to the outside of the ankle joint. The condition is most common in young people, but does not often produce symptoms until adulthood. There is either fracture of a bone fragment covered by cartilage, or else this bone fragment has become detached and is floating free in the joint.

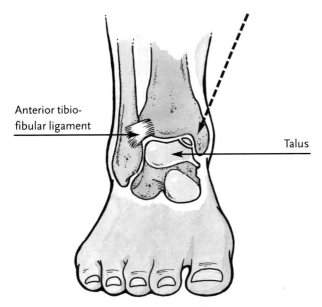

Anterior tibio-fibular ligament

Talus

**Figure 17.13** An osteochondral injury (osteochondritis dissecans) to the talus can occur in connection with ligament damage. A loose body can form and cause locking of the ankle joint.

## Diagnosis

Symptoms are either pain (generally triggered by exertion) or re-curring catching and/or locking, if a loose body has formed in the joint. The first symptoms are often pain on movement and reduced mobility.

In order to confirm diagnosis and differentiate this condition from, for example, footballer's ankle, radiographic examination is always necessary. In certain cases, arthroscopic inspection can be of great value in assessment, especially if surgical treatment be-comes necessary. In rare instances, osteochondritis dissecans is detected on radiographs which are taken for other reasons.

## Treatment

Treatment varies, more because of the findings made during ex-amination than what is seen on the radiographs. If there is a loose body, removal of this is recommended, if possible by arthroscopic surgery. There is then a bone surface which is not covered with cartilage in the joint. If, on the other hand, the surface of the carti-lage is intact, an attempt is made to promote healing by drilling or pinning.

## Prognosis

Prognosis is best in children and young people, especially if the surface of the cartilage is intact. If, however, a free body has formed in the joint, prognosis is worse. There is then a risk of damage from wear, particularly in the long term.

# 18. Injuries to the foot

Jon Karlsson

The foot is divided into three functional units — the forefoot, the metatarsus and the hindfoot. The foot is composed of 26 bones, not including the two sesamoid bones under the big toe. There are an additional ten or so named bones in different places. Some of these, such as the os trigonum in the rear of the ankle (see Chapter 17) can give rise to problems.

In all, there are 57 named joints in the foot and over 100 ligaments which hold these joints together.

Problems in the foot in connection with football are either acute injuries or overuse injuries. Fractures of the toes or bones in the metatarsus are the most common acute injuries. Many of these fractures do not involve any great malposition and can be treated relatively simply by temporarily taking weight off the foot or immobilization, and heal in 2–3 weeks. However, healing time, before full-scale footballing activity can be resumed, is generally roughly twice that. The prognosis for fractures of the toes and bones in the metatarsus is, with a few exceptions, good.

Serious injuries with fractures or dislocations in the foot are rare in football. On isolated occasions there are, however, compound fractures or dislocations in the metatarsus, for example in the joint between the forefoot and the metatarsus. Diagnosis can be difficult to make. If such an injury is suspected and there is soreness and pain on provocation, radiographic examination should be carried out. In certain cases, this must be complemented with computerized tomography. It is often revealed that the injury is more serious than was originally estimated.

Pain in the foot arises relatively often in football. Some of this is stress related and is also associated with tight football boots. Heels and toes are particularly vulnerable.

# Haglund's disease

Haglund's disease is a strain condition which arises in the upper part of the heel bone (calcaneus) and can be described by what is known as apophysitis. The condition is similar to Osgood-Schlatter's disease in the knee joint, as far as symptoms and changes in the bone are concerned.

### Injury mechanism

Haglund's disease occurs particularly in young people between the ages of 12 and 14. The problem disappears during late puberty. The

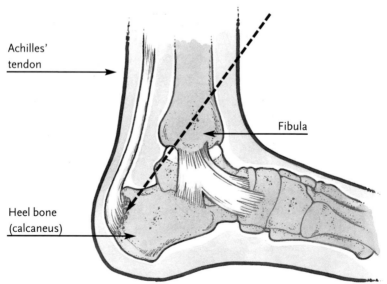

**Figure 18.1** Apophysitis. Due to fragmentation of the Achilles' tendon attachment to the heel bone, a painful protuberance forms.

Achilles' tendon attachment is strained where the tendon attaches to the heel bone, for example, probably after running a great deal on a hard surface, when the Achilles' tendon attachment is subject to repeated tension. Fragmentation of bone in the heel then occurs.

## Diagnosis

There is pain and a painful protuberance in the back of the heel, as well as soreness on palpation. The pain increases particularly during and after physical activity.

Diagnosis is made during clinical examination but on radiographs a fragmentation of the bone can be observed which confirms diagnosis.

## Treatment

Treatment is focused on symptoms. Footwear adjustment and a soft insole, such as a heel cup, with a slight heel lift, which reduces symptoms, can be appropriate. In certain cases temporary rest combined with alternative exercise can be necessary. It is completely safe to continue playing football despite the discomfort.

## Prognosis

Prognosis is always good and the condition is self-healing. A large, protruding lump can remain on the heel bone, which in isolated cases leads to later problems with exercise and sport.

Besides this, there are no known complications and young footballers can therefore continue physical activity without risk of future problems.

# Plantar fasciitis (calcaneal spur)

## Injury mechanism

This condition arises relatively often as an overuse injury in the tendon aponeurosis (plantar fascia) in the underside of the foot. Footballers are vulnerable to this, especially if training or playing on a hard surface, not least if they use football boots with insufficient shock absorption. Partial rupture with inflammation in the plantar fascia attachment to the calcaneus, or tendinitis (degenerative transformation), increases the pain.

Players with an unusually high (pes excavatus) or unusually low (pes planus) foot arch are considered more vulnerable than others.

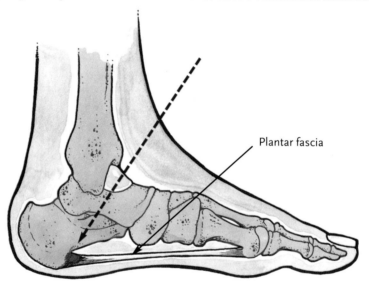

Plantar fascia

**Figure 18.2** Inflammation in the attachment of the plantar fascia to the calcaneus, which is caused by excessive stress, hard surfaces or poor footwear.

## Diagnosis

The most common symptom is pain, which correlates to strain, especially on running or jumping, particularly when the heel strikes the ground or on tension of the plantar fascia. There is generally pain after training and stiffness is relatively pronounced. The anterior edge of the calcaneus is sore during palpation, especially on the medial side of the foot.

Radiographs generally show no changes. In isolated instances, however, a "calcaneal spur" can be seen. The calcaneal spur, which is a protuberance on the bone, is not the cause of the problem, however, but rather a result of it.

Radiographic examination is recommended mainly to exclude or confirm other diagnoses, such as stress fractures in the calcaneus, which, however, is unusual.

## Treatment

Correction of external factors, such as unsuitable footwear, excessively hard training surface and internal factors, such as malalignment of the foot, is necessary.

Training should be altered, for example avoid running on the toes. Even running which involves a great deal of starting, stopping and/or changes in direction should be kept to a minimum. Temporary rest, combined with alternative exercise may be necessary. Stretching of the plantar fascia is recommended, along with an insole to correct foot malalignment, especially with an unusually high or low foot arch. Anti-inflammatory drugs in either tablet or gel form can produce good results in the acute phase. The latter is rubbed into the affected area morning and evening for around 10–14 days in this case.

Cortisone injections can also produce good results. Surgery is only appropriate in exceptional cases. If surgery is performed, a tenotomy, i.e. bisection of the plantar fascia at the calcaneus, is carried out.

## Prognosis

The healing period is often very long, but the prognosis is good and the condition normally heals on its own, although it can take several months until the player is completely free from pain.

# Stress fracture

A stress fracture can occur in several places in the foot, but is most common in the second metatarsal (known as a march fracture). This type of stress fracture generally occurs in long-distance runners rather than in footballers. A stress fracture also occurs to some extent in the fifth metatarsal and in rarer cases, in the navicular, talus and calcaneus. Women are more vulnerable than men.

### Injury mechanism

The injury mechanism in a stress fracture is always excessive strain, i.e. the strain is greater than the bone can stand. External factors, such as inappropriate footwear, too much training or excessively hard ground are often contributing factors.

### Diagnosis

In the initial stage, there is stress-related pain with every step, such as while running on a hard surface, but no pain while at rest. The pain increases gradually. Although training is possible in this phase, it eventually becomes too painful. On examination there is very localized pain when pressure is applied and on provocation. There is rarely any swelling.

Radiographs initially reveal no fracture. Radiographic examination should be repeated after 2–3 weeks. The fracture is then usually visible thanks to scar tissue in the bone (callus forma-

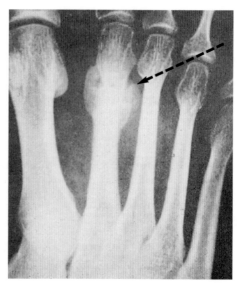

**Figure 18.3** Stress fracture to the second metatarsal.

tion). Where there are strong suspicions of a stress fracture, an isotope scan (scintigraphy) should be carried out. This shows the fracture within a day of the injury occurring.

Diagnosis of a stress fracture to the navicular, talus and calcaneus can be difficult. The fracture is often invisible on ordinary radiographs. When there is a suspected fracture of these bones, medical personnel should use isotope scans, computerized tomography or magnetic resonance imaging. Delayed diagnosis can lead to the results of treatment being impaired.

## Treatment

Treatment, including the length of immobilization, varies depending on which bone is damaged. Keeping weight off the foot, combined with alternative exercise, such as pool exercise, until the player is free from pain, is important. In certain cases immobilization, such as by means of plaster or a support can be necessary.

In the event of a stress fracture of a metatarsal (generally the second metatarsal), keeping weight off the foot for 3 weeks, either with or without a plaster, is sufficient. With other stress fractures, such as in the navicular, talus or calcaneus, lengthy immobilization is generally necessary (8–12 weeks). In spite of this, setbacks to healing can arise. Surgery is, however, rarely necessary.

## Prognosis

A stress fracture in the metatarsal generally heals with no persisting problems. However, the healing period varies. The healing period for a stress fracture in the navicular, talus and calcaneus is much longer. Rehabilitation can also be very long, as much as 6 months. However, with correct diagnosis, treatment and rehabilitation the prognosis for healing and the chances of being able to return to play are generally good.

# Jones' fracture

### Injury mechanism

Jones' fracture is a stress fracture to the fifth metatarsal. The fracture has a slightly worse prognosis than other stress fractures in the metatarsus. The reason for this is that the short peroneal tendon attaches to the upper part of the bone. On movement, a displacement of the fracture can occur, which entails a risk of setbacks to the healing process with delayed healing or a false joint (pseudo-arthrosis).

### Diagnosis

There is pain in the damaged area on direct pressure and provocation, and there is slight swelling. If there is suspected fracture, radiographic examination is recommended. If, for example, disturbances in healing and a false joint are suspected, computerized tomography may be necessary to confirm the diagnosis.

### Treatment

The fracture should be treated with immobilization, using plaster cast or a splint, for 4–6 weeks. Despite this, the risk of healing complications is relatively large. With delayed healing or development of a false joint, surgery is recommended. The safest option is then to screw the fracture together.

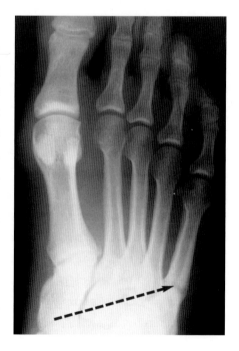

**Figure 18.4** Jones' fracture. Stress fracture to the fifth metatarsal.

## Prognosis

Healing complications are relatively common. Following surgery, however, prognosis is generally good. The fracture heals and the player can return to footballing activity (after usual rehabilitation) in approximately 6–8 weeks.

# Fracture of the sesamoid bone

Under the first metatarsal there are two sesamoid bones in the flexor tendon of the big toe. Damage to these bones is relatively common in football, especially when training on a hard surface. Fracture of the sesamoid bone can occur as a stress injury and a false joint can develop

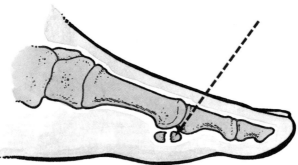

**Figure 18.5** Sesamoid bone. Fracture of a sesamoid bone under the metatarsophalangeal joint of the big toe.

## Diagnosis

Persistent, lingering problems and pain often arise. The damaged sesamoid bone causes pain when direct pressure is applied. In radiographs, which are not always necessary, however, it can be seen that the bone is in two pieces (false joint).

## Treatment

Treatment involving keeping weight off the foot, such as a cushioned insole and changes in the amount of training, weight bearing and alternative footwear are recommended. Surgery is resorted to only in exceptional cases. Surgery involves removal of the damaged sesamoid bone. This is especially appropriate when the damage is to the medial sesamoid bone.

### Prognosis
Prognosis is good in the majority of cases.

# Wear in the big toe (hallux rigidus)

### Injury mechanism
This is caused by wear-related transformation (arthrosis) in the metatarsophalangeal joint of the big toe, and is relatively common in slightly older players at the end of their career (after the age of 30 years).

### Diagnosis
There is pain and increasing stiffness in the metatarsophalangeal joint of the big toe. On examination movement is reduced and can eventually disappear completely, especially when the toe is bent upward (dorsal extension). In addition, there is a painful bony outgrowth, which is mainly felt on top of the metatarsophalangeal joint. Stress on the toe joint further increases while walking or running and wear-related changes can also arise as a result of this.

Radiographic examination aids diagnosis. It shows bony growths and wear with reduced joint space in the whole joint.

### Treatment
Taping of the big toe can reduce symptoms. A relatively stiff insole is often used, although with varying success. Cortisone injections in or around the damaged joint can provide effective, though short-lasting relief from symptoms.

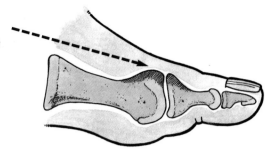

**Figure 18.6** Wear in the big toe. Wear changes (arthrosis) in the joint, which leads to reduced movement and pain.

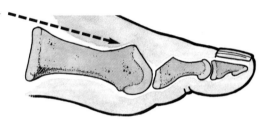

**Figure 18.7** Excision of bony out-growths where there is wear to increase movement in the joint.

Surgery often becomes necessary. Then excision of the bony growth on the top of the joint is recommended. Complete freedom from pain is achieved if movement can be restored. Other more drastic operations, such as creating a floating toe (Keller's operation) or fusion, are rarely successful in footballers.

### Prognosis

The condition can be very painful and lead to protracted problems. Surgery generally only gives temporary success.

## Turf toe

### Injury mechanism

The injury occurs as the result of severe overextension of the first joint of the big toe. The big toe can normally be bent upward to an angle of approximately 90° when walking on tiptoe or at the end of a step, such as is taken when running. The damage is associated with repeated minor injuries.

### Diagnosis

As a result of joint capsule damage, swelling and soreness arise in the joint, especially in the uppermost part. Diagnosis is made by means of clinical examination.

### Treatment

Acute treatment consists of compression, ice packs and possibly keeping the foot in a raised position for a short time. Once swelling has subsided for a few days, gradual range of motion training can be begun. Taping to reduce movement (especially upwards) can ease symptoms. A stiff sole can also be used, but is often found to be annoying by players.

### Prognosis

The condition is benign, but can be lingering and troublesome.

# Trapped nerves

The most common forms of trapped nerve which occur in football are in the forefoot, between the third and fourth metatarsals (Morton's metatarsalgia) and behind the inner anklebone (medial malleolus), known as tarsal tunnel syndrome.

### Morton's metatarsalgia (neuroma)

*Injury mechanism*

Morton's metatarsalgia occurs as a result of entrapment of a nerve in the forefoot, generally between the third and fourth metatarsals. The cause is probably tight football boots and excessive strain in training.

*Diagnosis*

With entrapment of a nerve between the third and fourth metatarsals (Morton's metatarsalgia) the player feels pain in the forefoot radiating out between the third and fourth toes. In isolated cases, nerve entrapment can occur between the other metatarsals but this is rare.

On examination, a characteristic cracking sound is noted with simultaneous pain when the foot is squeezed from the sides (Mulder's crack).

*Treatment*

With a confirmed trapped nerve in the forefoot, surgery involving excision of the nerve is the most definitive treatment. The operation is not performed, however, until correction of external and internal factors, such as footwear and the amount of training and using a cushioning insole, have not given sufficiently good results.

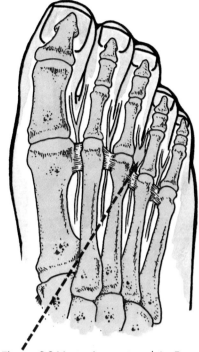

**Figure 18.8** Morton's metatarsalgia. Entrapment of a nerve between the third and fourth metatarsals.

*Prognosis*

Prognosis following surgery on Morton's metatarsalgia is generally good. The player is often free from pain and can return to footballing activity within 4–6 weeks.

**Tarsal tunnel syndrome**

*Injury mechanism*

The cause is probably bleeding which leads to inflammation behind the inner ankle bone (medila malleolus). The injury arises following a direct blow such as a kick to the inside of the foot.

*Diagnosis*

With tarsal tunnel syndrome, the player has altered, sometimes uncomfortable or reduced sensation in the sole of the foot and down

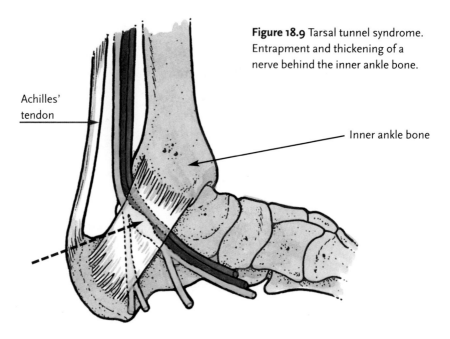

Achilles'
tendon

**Figure 18.9** Tarsal tunnel syndrome. Entrapment and thickening of a nerve behind the inner ankle bone.

Inner ankle bone

towards the inside of the heel. On direct pressure or light tapping over the nerve, a radiating pain, i.e., Tinel's sign is positive.

### Treatment

With a trapped nerve behind the inner ankle bone, correction of footwear and anti-inflammatory drugs are recommended. If this treatment does not give satisfactory results, bisection of the tarsal tunnel is considered. During surgery, the nerve is freed and any external pressure is removed. In rare cases, entrapment of the nerve occurs further down towards the sole of the foot. A more radical freeing of the nerve is recommended in these cases.

### Prognosis

Prognosis for tarsal tunnel syndrome is not as sure as for Morton's metatarsalgia. Trapped nerves can give rise to protracted problems.

# 19. Post-injury functional testing for return to competitive play

Alan Hodson

'Fitness testing' is an ambiguous term used in football to describe functional testing conducted as a means of determining whether or not a player can return to full training or competitive play. It is often taken to imply the last test before return to play. The decision should embrace all testing at the various stages of the rehabilitation process wherever possible rather than a 'one-off' decision-making test (see Figure 19.1). Given that the word fitness can be defined in many ways, the term 'fitness testing' would be better referred to as 'pre-competition functional testing'.

The primary aim of functional testing should be to confirm that a player has fully recovered from the injury and that the tissues that were damaged have now fully healed and possess the ability to cope with the functional stresses imposed on them by competitive play.

It should be recognized that injuries are multifaceted. The type and degree of injury will determine the length of time for healing, treatment and rehabilitation.

When considering functional testing, recovery from injury falls into short term (1–3 weeks) and medium to long term (4 weeks to 18 months or even more). In the case of short term injuries, the

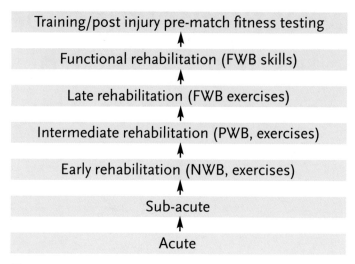

Training/post injury pre-match fitness testing

Functional rehabilitation (FWB skills)

Late rehabilitation (FWB exercises)

Intermediate rehabilitation (PWB, exercises)

Early rehabilitation (NWB, exercises)

Sub-acute

Acute

**Figure 19.1**

player will not have lost significant cardiovascular and 'match' fitness. However, players having sustained more serious injuries (long-term) will lose a significant degree of cardiovascular and 'match' fitness.

Many doctors and therapists argue that a dedicated functional test is not required for those players recovering from injury, particularly long-term injury. They also argue that the player's rehabilitation process into the late and functional phases would 'build in' activities and tests that in themselves would act as elements of a functional test.

Others argue that the functional test is of importance following short-term injuries (1–3 weeks) where time for functional rehabilitation has been limited and where the player has not lost significant cardiovascular and match fitness. Many therapists would comment that the functional test helps to confirm fitness to play to the player, manager and coaching staff, which is an important psychological confidence booster for all concerned.

It is important therefore to state the aims of functional testing.

## AIMS OF POST-INJURY FUNCTIONAL TESTING

- To confirm that a player is fully recovered from injury and able to return to competitive play.
- To boost player confidence.
- To demonstrate 'full fitness', to manager/senior coach/coaching staff.
- To prevent or reduce the danger of recurrence when participation is resumed.

# Factors to be considered before the performance of a functional test

When designing a functional test two key aspects should be considered. Knowledge and experience of the game by medical practitioners is of paramount importance.

- The demand of the game – aspects of physical functions required.
- Player position – specific demands and physical/physiological attributes required (see Table 19.1).

**Table 19.1** Factors to consider in performance of a functional test

| Player should be 'clinically functional' prior to test. Player should have normal: | |
|---|---|
| • strength | • weight-bearing control |
| • power | • speed |
| • endurance | • action time |
| • proprioception | • endurance |
| • balance/coordination | • no tenderness, pain or reactive |
| • full range of joint movement | signs and symptoms to |
| • full soft tissue extensibility | appropriate clinical testing. |

# Knowledge of demands of the game

Several studies have been conducted into the demands of the game. It should be realized that a functional test will usually last for 30–40 min and is specifically designed to test the previously injured structure. Thus the medical practitioner must not only make a decision as to whether a player is 'fit' to return to competitive play, but also whether in his or her opinion the player can play the full game or only a part of it. The practitioner should be knowledgeable about the general demands of the game i.e. metres covered per game, number of sprints, percentage of time spent running forwards, backwards, diagonally, jumping and landing episodes, sprints and recovery. In addition, they should be aware of the player's position and performance attributes. The use of player functional profiles outlined later in this section is advised.

# Player postition/functional profile

The functional attributes required for 90 minutes of play can be divided in general and specific terms and identified by studying player positions.

- Goalkeeper
- Wing back
- Centre back
- Midfielder
- Striker/midfielder

The practitioner must be fully aware of the specific demands required from each specific position.

These demands must be built into a well-directed functional test. The majority of activities in football involve short explosive episodes requiring strength and power with an overall need for endurance, given the length of the game. Without this knowledge, a practitioner is in a poor position to make a decision whether a player can not just start the game but also whether he/she can safely complete the game without recurrence of injury.

In addition to the player's technical skills the box on Page 400 shows activities that make up a player's requirements for play (see also Figure 19.2 and Table 19.2).

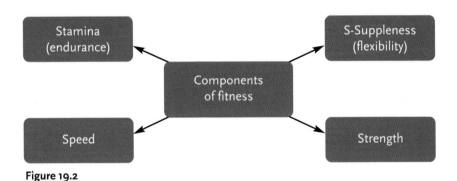

**Figure 19.2**

# Functional profiles

Specific clinical measurements for range of movement, muscle strength, muscle power, muscle girth etc. can be taken during the progressive phases of treatment and rehabilitation.

The concept of measurements of football function in the form of functional profiles is suggested as a method that can assist practitioners to assess progress or regression in the later functional phase prior to play.

It is suggested that following a comprehensive pre-season training programme, specific functional field tests can be performed by players to obtain objective measurements by repetition, time or distance using functional tests that are position specific i.e. contain activities that are linked to functional requirements of the player during competitive play.

**Table 19.2** Aspects of physical/functional fitness

| | |
|---|---|
| • Weight-bearing control | • Turning/'cutting' |
| • Balance | • Side stepping |
| • Proprioception | • Jumping (right foot/ left foot/both feet) |
| • Coordination | |
| • Reaction time | • Landing (left foot/right foot/ both feet) |
| • Transference of weight | |
| • Straight line running (all forms) | • Squatting |
| • Backward running | • Lunging/stretching |
| • Sideways running | • 'Rotational work' (weight-bearing turning) |
| • Diagonal running | |
| • Hopping (left leg/right leg) | • Tackling |
| • Bounding | • Being tackled |
| • Shooting | • Passing (long/short) |
|   – volley | • Kicking (stationary ball/ moving ball/volley) |
|   – half volley | |
|   – stationary ball | • 'Starting' |
|   – moving ball | • Stopping |

The functional profile measurements can be used as a guide for a player's functional ability when returning from a lay-off through injury (see Table 19.3).

The coach may use the functional profiles throughout the season to gauge maintenance of general fitness levels. The functional measurements are invaluable to the medical practitioner to assist the decision-making process for 'return to play'.

**Table 19.3** Functional profile – Functional assessments

- Designed and used on fit players.
- The measurements (time, reps, distance) can be used as a guide when repeated on players returning from injury or illness.

**Table 19.4** Advantages of functional profiles

- A measure of quality of physical attributes.
- For coach to ensure maintenance of standards through the season.
- For coach or player to instil competitive and achievement element into training.
- Objective guides for therapist or doctor of physical attributes against which achievement in functional rehabilitation stage can be compared.
- For player motivation.

There are several key points when devising functional profile tests. The designed test must be applicable to the players' position (position-specific). It must be safe, simple and repeatable. It must be measurable (time, distance, repetitions).

Please note it is *not a football drill* involving complex moves, several players and a ball being targeted at specific heights or lengths. Such drills are not simple and certainly not reproducible i.e. repeatable. As such the drill could *not* be used as a functional profile (see Table 19.5).

**Table 19.5** Functional profile assessments

- Applicable
- Specific (to playing position)
- Safe
- Simple
- Measurable (objective)
- Reproducible

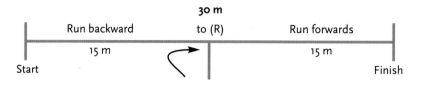

**Figure 19.3** Defender facing with back to run.

A simple example of a functional profile test is shown in Figure 19.3 above. It is a simple time measurement over 30 m involving backward running turning 180° to the left or right and sprinting forwards between a start and finish line. This simulates a defender or wing-back being attacked by a winger or attacker trying to go past him to deliver a cross into the box.

Following long-term injury, the treatment and rehabilitation phases should demonstrate steady progressive improvement through the stages where late phase specific gymnasium exercise rehabilitation decreases and functional gymnasium or field work increases.

## FUNCTIONAL TESTING – KEY RULES

- The player should only be subjected to a functional 'fitness' test when the doctor is certain that the player will pass the test.
- The test should be comprehensive and include specific activities that will stress the affected part and expose the player to specific functional patterns.
- The test should extend over a 30–40 min period involving several repetitions of each activity and expose the player to stress when 'comfortably tired'.
- Test should be conducted with player wearing boots on grass with a ball at the correct pressure.

It is important that the practitioner, player, manager and coaching staff do not let their 'hearts rule their heads' and allow a player to be exposed to testing when clinically and/or functionally they are not ready. Neither is it acceptable to conduct a modified fitness test where the player is not fully exposed to stress at the injury site or when a brief test (10–15 min) is conducted on the day of the game.

**IT IS UNWISE TO PERFORM A FUNCTIONAL TEST WHEN A PLAYER IS CLEARLY DYSFUNCTIONAL**

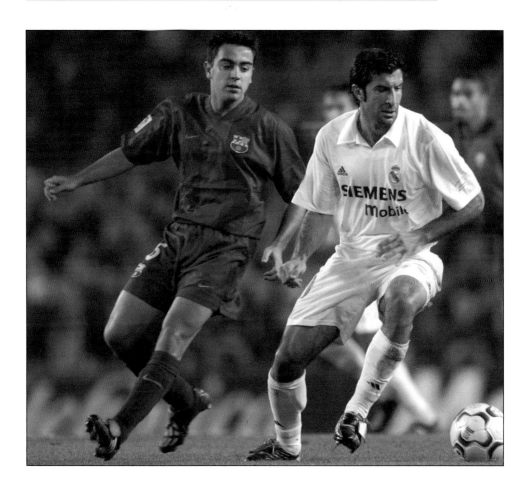

# Injury status – clinical and functional assessment protocol

A protocol for player 'fitness to play' assessment should begin with a 'cold' clinical assessment, Figure 19.4. When the medical practitioner is satisfied that the player's rehabilitation programme has achieved specific physical and physiological levels then and only then should a player be exposed to functional field testing.

Functional testing is carried out under normal playing conditions, subjecting the player to specific functional activities while weight bearing, stressing the player's previously injured structure(s).

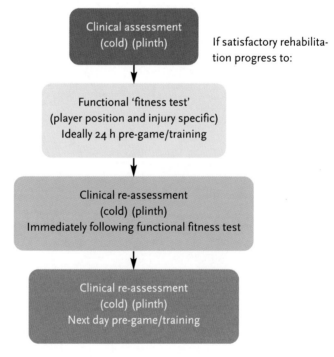

Injury status – clinical and functional assessment protocol
Procedure for 'fitness testing'
Making assessment/predictions

**Figure 19.4** Decision making process.

After the functional testing session the player should immediately be assessed for a reaction through 'cold' clinical assessment of his or her joint and soft tissue structures in the treatment room (see Figure 19.4).

This 'cold' clinical assessment should be repeated 24 hours later as a further test for possible reaction of the previously injured structure(s).

**Table 19.6** Clinical fitness vs functional fitness

| Clinical assessment | Functional assessment |
|---|---|
| • Muscle power<br>• Muscle stretch<br>• Soft tissue extensibility<br>• Range of movement of joint<br>• Normality:<br>  – Muscle<br>  – Joint<br>  – Tendon<br>  – Ligaments | • Will test muscle strength, joint range and soft tissue extensibility but also functional:<br>  – Weight-bearing control<br>  – Suppleness<br>  – Transference of weight<br>  – Muscle strength<br>  – Endurance<br>  – Muscle power<br>  – Speed<br>  – Reaction time<br>  – Skill factors<br>  – Player confidence |

During the functional testing observation of active range of movements, muscular control, balance, coordination and sensory feedback (proprioception) is important.

**Table 19.7** Functional assessment

- **Observe**
  1. **Active range of movement.**
  2. **Muscular control over this range.**
  3. **Performance of activities demonstrating good sensory feedback from all contractile and non-contractile structures.**
  4. **An ability of the body to integrate sensory input and respond with a quick and/or controlled motor response**
- **The qualities of:**
  - **speed**
  - **ability to change direction**
  - **acceleration/deceleration**
  **should be carried out in competition with other players and comparisons made.**
- **Profiles – comparisons can also be made if previous measurements of tests are avaliable.**

During functional testing the player's speed, power, acceleration, deceleration and the ability to change direction at speed should be observed (see Table 19.7).

## Progression of functional testing event

The player commences the functional testing session by a thorough warm-up involving 'pulse' raising activities, dynamic stretching, and range of movement activities. This prepares both body and mind for the more progressive functional work to follow.

The second phase should involve linear work i.e. running forward at half, three-quarter and full sprint speed. This will involve changes in running speed i.e. from half pace to sprint speed. In

**Table 19.8** Functional testing

- **Carried out in the following order:**
  1. Warm-up.
  2. Straight-line 'easy' introduction including rotational movement, jumping and landing.
  3. Progressive functional activities.
  4. Progressive functional activities related to specific anatomical area to be tested and should be position-specific.

addition, running backward, hopping, direction changes and jumping and landing should be included.

The player enters the third phase commencing specific activities designed to stress the anatomical structure(s) that are specific to his playing position. The FA's Professional Player Audit of Injuries Research Study has identified the following anatomical structures that are commonly injured, and for which a practitioner would need to plan 'stressing' activities namely:

- Hamstring muscles
- Rectus femoris muscle
- Hip adductor muscles
- Gastrocnemius muscles
- Medial collateral ligament of the knee
- Lateral ligaments of the ankle
- Achilles' tendon.

In general terms, stressing the hamstrings should involve football-specific activities of 'pushing off' with power (extensor thrust activities) i.e. sprinting and acceleration, and movements that will involve a changeover from concentric to eccentric muscle work and deceleration.

It should also involve functional ballistic stretching such as extensibility stress applied from follow through in kicking. All are in a linear (straight line) pattern.

Rectus femoris is the kicking muscle, therefore, progressive kicking increasing in length and power requirement — volley, half volley, moving ball and stationary ball, are important. The rectus femoris muscle is part of the 'extensor thrust' complex and therefore "pushing off", sprinting and jumping activities are important.

The hip adductor muscles and ankle ligament complex should be stressed by diagonal, side to side and rotational activities that are football specific. Activities in the frontal plane (sideways activity) involving pushing off, power and speed are required to apply correct functional stress to the area.

The gastrocnemius and Achilles tendon complex work primarily in the sagittal plane and are important structures for generating power when pushing off (extensor thrust) for sprinting, accelerating and jumping.

Repetition of activity is important. Following 30 to 40 min of testing all stresses should have been applied in a manner that mimics 'game' requirements.

**Table 19.9** Some inclusions for specific areas

## HIP ADDUCTORS

- Cutting/side stepping:
  - Affected leg leading
  - Affected leg trailing
- Sprinting
- Kicking – inswinger
- Block tackling
- Stretching for ball (lunging)
- Crossover sideways running (Cardiocas)
- Long ball kicking
- Long hopping sideways
  - Hard push offs
- Stretching for moving balls
  - Various heights
- Rotational movements

## HAMSTRINGS

- Backward running
- Sudden starts
- Follow through on kicking
- Getting up from ground to jump
- Pushing off
  - Extensor thrustle, sprinting
  - Acceleration/deceleration (straight line)
- Changeover from concentric eccentric muscle work/eccentric concentric
- Side tackling:
  - Leading leg

## RECTUS FEMORIS/QUADRICEPS COMPLEX

- Pushing off activities
- Sprinting
- Squat and spring
- Hard kicking stationary ball
- Kicking:
  - Sideways volleying
  - Long kicking
- Starting/stopping at speed
- Shooting
- Crossing
- Jumping (repetitive)

## MEDIAL LIGAMENT OF KNEE

- Side to side activities
- Cutting activities:
  - Foot fixed, turning outwards
- Block tackling
- Hopping activities
  - Round a marked square
- Kicking – inswinger
- Side stepping at full pace with direction on command
- Rotary activities
  - Rotation at the joint

## ANKLE LATERAL LIGAMENT COMPLEX

- Hopping:
  - Straight
  - Zig-zag
  - Figure of eight
  - Round square
  - Sideways
- Jumping/landing
  - 2 feet/left/right
- Side to side activities
- Rotary activities
- Kicking
  - Inswinger
  - Outswinger
- Driving low ball rolled towards player
- Chipping ball:
  - 10 m
  - 20 m
- Tackling

## ACHILLES' TENDON AND GASTROCNEMIUS

- Running backwards – pushing off on affected side
- Running forwards – pushing off on affected side
- Stride running —— pushing off (extended trot)
- Jumping/springing to head ball/landing:
  - Both feet
  - Left foot }  Plyometric type
  - Right foot
- Hard kicking – stationary ball
- Pushing off activities
- Jumping/landing – high/repetitive
- Sprinting

## Those present for testing

The manager and coach(es) should be present throughout the functional tests. Other players including a goalkeeper may participate to include a competitive element (see Figure 19.4).

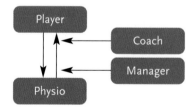

**Figure 19.5** Fitness testing. Use of 'similar profile' players and goalkeeper

# Timing of the test

This will vary from club to club. Ideally, managers would like to know 48 hours in advance of the game whether or not the player has been passed fit to play. In larger professional clubs where the squad size is large there is now less pressure for decisions to be made for 'late' fitness tests to be conducted. Clearly, a coach needs to know who can be selected in order to formulate his or her game plan (see Table 19.10).

**Table 19.10** Fitness testing assessment

It is important that there is standardization of the approach to offering management an coaching staff a medical opinion on individual fitness.
- Assessment of player fitness – feedback from medical staff to coaching staff:
  - Predication
  - Short term 0–7 days
  - Long term 23 days of game
  - Pre-game 0–24 hours.
- Assessment – doctor/physiotherapist feedback to coaching staff regarding player's medical condition:
  - Assessment
  - Monitoring
  - Prognosis
  - Prediction
  - Guidance/advice to manager or coach
  - Judgement
  - Justification.

**Table 19.11** Procedure for fitness testing: making assessment/predictions

1. • Warm-up
   • Stretching

   **Progress to:**

2. Straight line work

   • Jog
   • 1/4 Pace
   • 1/2 Pace
   • Hopping variations
     Transference of weight } straight line
     Space difference for | impact work
     hopping – horizontal | – forwards
     transfer | – backwards
   • 3/4 Pace | – start-stop
   • Sprint | – change pace
   | – stop quickly

   **Progress to:**

3. Advanced work

   • Side to side
   • Rotation/turning
   • Pushing off
   • Plyometrics
   • Diagonal/oblique work
   • 'Spinning' off a player
   • Receiving/shadowing
   • Direction change
   • Direction change (on command)

   **Progress to:**

4. Football-specific

   • Passing ball
     – Moving
     – Static
     – Volley
     – Half volley
   • Crossing
     – Outswing
     – Inswing
   • Shooting
     – Volley
     – Half volley
     – Moving
     – Static
   • Jumping
   • Heading

3. Training games

   4 v 4
   3 v 2
   3 v 1

Ultimately, the decision should rest with the player and the medical staff. The player should perform each test maximally and not reduce his or her efforts to 'guard' the area that was injured.

Whatever functional tests are conducted, there is no substitute for competitive play. If possible, the player should be involved in 3 v 3, 5 v 5 or 11 v 11 training games. Sometimes, time will not allow for this luxury. It therefore, becomes objective tests aimed at making as subjective less a decision as possible. It should be a black or white decision based on many objective tests and measurements. In practice it is not quite that simple. Table 19.11 offers an outline plan for the reader.

The practitioner should observe the psychological state of the player pre-, during and post-testing. Is he clinically functional fit? Objectively did the player appear in any difficulty during the session?

The testing must be thorough. It must be functionally searching and highly specific to the previously injured area and the-demands imposed by the player's playing position.

## Return to play

In ideal circumstances the player's rehabilitation will include time for late stage and functional work/testing. However, there will be times when a manager, player or coach may request a functional test prior to making a decision whether or not he is fit to play.

The practitioner must possess knowledge about player physical/-physiological attributes, the demands of the game and specific positional requirements. This knowledge must be integrated with an objective clinical approach embracing biomechanical, physiological, pathological and psychological considerations. To progress to a fitness test where there are still obvious limitations in terms of physical ability, is foolish. Don't let the heart rule the head! To do so, normally produces a predictable result of re-injury.

# 20. Football-specific injury rehabilitation

Stenove Ringborg

This chapter deals with the various mechanisms which give rise to muscle injuries, how they should be cared for when they are acute and how they should be rehabilitated.

## REHABILITATION OF MUSCLE INJURIES IN THE LOWER EXTREMITIES

Muscle injuries are common in football. There is a distinction between the two types of muscle rupture: contusion and distension.

---

**DIFFERENT TYPES OF MUSCLE INJURY**

**Contusion**
The muscle is pressed towards the underlying bone, which results in the blood vessels and muscle fibres rupturing. The injury is generally located deep inside.

**Distension**
The muscle ruptures as a result of excessive strain, such as while running or shooting. The injury is generally located superficially.

---

# Muscular bleeding

When a muscle is damaged there is bleeding. This causes swelling which then increases, leading to greater pressure in the tissues and pain. Haemorrhaging can be intramuscular (contained) or inter-muscular (dispersed). The type of haemorrhage is of great import-ance for the course of the healing process. It is therefore important to assess the extent of the injury after 2–3 days. When there is a large intramuscular haemorrhage, the muscle functions can cease completely. However, this is rare in association with football.

# Acute treatment (1–2 days)

Acute treatment should begin as soon as possible after the injury takes place, using pressure and cold, raising the affected area and avoiding strain.

### Pressure
- Pressure dressing, tightly applied for 15–20 minutes.
- Looser pressure dressing (compression dressing), two-thirds of the elasticity of the elastic bandage, for 1–2 days.

### Cold
- Cooling (ice-cubes, ice packs) for 20–45 min periods for the first 24 h (pain relief). Compression dressing between the periods of cooling.

### Raising
- The injured part of the body is raised at least 30 cm above the level of the heart.

### Avoiding strain
- Possibly crutches, though for as short a time as possible.

# Muscle damage to the anterior thigh muscle (quadriceps)

## SIGNS OF INTRAMUSCULAR BLEEDING IN THE ANTERIOR THIGH MUSCLES

- Sensitivity to palpation and pulsation in the thigh, even while at rest.
- Severely reduced movement — inability to bend the knee joint to more than 90° 2–3 days after the injury occurs.
- Difficulty in activating the muscle.
- Swelling in the area of the injury with no discoloration.

If these symptoms are still to be found after 2–3 days, a doctor should be consulted for a more thorough assessment of the injury. A large intramuscular haemorrhage can take up to 8–12 weeks to heal. An incorrectly treated intramuscular haemorrhage, or premature return to sporting activity can, in rare cases, develop into calcification or ossification of the muscle. This calcification results in impaired function with weakness, tightness and pain.

Distension rupture normally occurs while running, rapid deceleration or shooting and the player feels a 'stabbing' in the muscle. If the rupture is large, on examination a gap can be observed where the muscle fibres have broken. If the rupture occurs at the beginning of any activity, the cause can be a poor warm-up. If the injury occurs at the end of training or a match, it can be because the muscle is tired and cannot take the strain it is placed under.

It is not uncommon for a player to suffer repeated muscle ruptures in the same muscle, despite resting between injuries. Resting until the pain is gone is not enough; the muscle must be trained and stretched until it regains ist normal strength and normal length before the player can return to footballing activity.

417

# Rehabilitation schedule for muscle damage to the anterior thigh muscle (quadriceps)

## THE AIM OF REHABILITATION IS TO

1. Normalize range of movement.
2. Regain normal muscle control (coordination).
3. Restore muscle strength (power/stamina).

Rehabilitation is usually divided into three phases:
1) acute phase, 2) subacute phase and 3) rehabilitation phase.

### Acute phase (1–2 days)

With all recent muscle injuries, the principles for acute treatment of damage to the soft parts should be followed.

### Subacute phase (2–7 days)

A bleeding which occurs as part of an acute injury gives rise to inflammation. It is the inflammation which causes the swelling to abate.

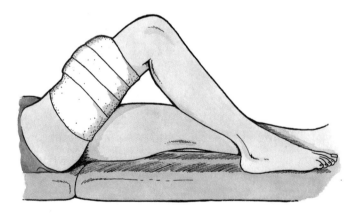

**Figure 20.1** Compressive dressing. Place a foam pad over the injured area and an elastic bandage on top of it.

The player should quickly (the day after the injury, if at all possible) begin range of motion training in a limited part of the exercise area. Initially this should be without putting pressure on the affected part of the body, such as lying on the floor and sliding the foot back and forth.

In the case of muscle damage, new collagen will start to rebuild within 2–21 days. This does not mean, however, that the muscle regains normal strength and length. As soon as the day after the injury, static (isometric) muscle activation should be started. This is done by contracting the muscle 20–30 times for a few seconds. This is repeated 3–4 times a day.

As soon as mobility permits, cycling exercise can begin, initially around 15 minutes, then increasing gradually. Careful stretching of the damaged muscle begins on day 2–3, such as with the player lying face-down, taking hold of the ankle and bending the knee. In this way the anterior thigh muscle is stretched. The muscle is held fully stretched for at least 30 sec and the exercise is repeated 2–5 times.

At the end of the subacute phase strength training is started using rubber tubing or an exercise machine. A suitable amount of training is three sets of 30 repetitions with light pressure at least once a day. To begin with, the movement should be performed slowly, gradually increasing in speed. All training should be reasonably painless — not more than grade 2 on the VAS scale (Page 78).

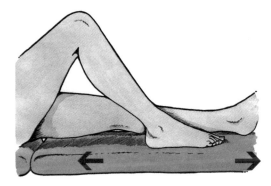

**Exercise 1.** Range of motion training without placing pressure on the affected part of the body should begin at an early stage after the injury. For example, lie on the floor and slide the foot back and forth. Gradually increase the flexion in the knee joint.

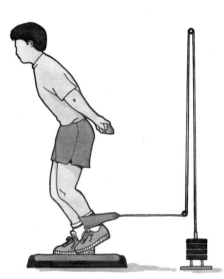

**Exercise 2.** Strength training using an exercise machine. Stand on the healthy leg, if possible on a raised platform, and pull the injured leg forward.

During both the subacute and rehabilitation phases, training, in the form of jogging, interval and speed training in water (if possible deep water) using a life-jacket or lifebelt, is excellent. It is important to know that pulse-rate is lower while training in water, and that during interval training rest periods should be shortened slightly. When training intervals are 2 min long, the rest period can be shortened to around 45 sec and when the intervals are 70 sec long, the rest period can be shortened to around 15 sec.

**Exercise 3.** Training in water with a life-jacket. The body should be held in the vertical position while running in water. Leaning forward reduces the resistance.

## Rehabilitation phase
### (>7 days — depending on the injury)

A player who has had a mild contusion in the thigh muscle is normally able to play within a week. A large contusion in the thigh with intramuscular bleeding must be treated properly. As these rarely occur in football, the rehabilitation described is intended for a distension rupture. During this phase, weight, coordination/speed and range of motion training take place. Cycling with gradually increased resistance is recommended. If the saddle is placed slightly lower than normal and the metatarsus in the middle of the pedal, the anterior thigh muscle receives a good workout.

The number of repetitions done during strength training can be gradually increased to 50 in 3–5 sets per day. As levels of stress are low, this type of training can be done every day.

Water training in this case can be changed to fitness training. Interval training is a suitable form of training in water. After approximately a week, the player can begin dynamic training with light resistance following the same principles as static training.

If training can be carried out without pain and swelling, the player can gradually change over to weight training with the emphasis on muscle growth. About 3–6 sets of 8–12 repetitions with 2–4 min rest between are suitable. The load can be 70–80 per cent of 1 RM (1 RM is the weight that can be lifted once).

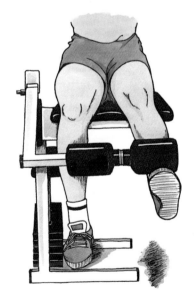

Weight training can be done every day. A principle in all rehabilitation training is that new exercises are begun slowly and then gradually increase in speed until they are as close to football as possible. After a further week or so, knee flexion exercises using a barbell can

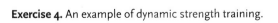

**Exercise 4.** An example of dynamic strength training.

be added. The load should be 70–80 per cent of 1 RM, with 3–6 sets of 8–12 repetitions and 2–4 min rest between.

Concentric strength training (i.e. the muscle works under contraction) can be done three times a week, while eccentric weight training requires longer rests between sessions and should therefore not be done more than twice a week. The eccentric training should be done directly after a thorough warm-up.

Running, in the form of jogging, can begin after approximately 14 days if movement in the damaged muscle is back to normal and strength training can take place without pain.

After about 3 weeks, it can be a good idea to begin coordination training in the form of jumping. Coordination training and speed exercises should be done early in the training session, before the muscles are tired out.

Damaged tissue is not rehabilitated before it has regained normal strength and movement and is well coordinated. It should be possible to perform all movements at as fast a pace as possible. A player who has had moderately large muscle rupture can generally return to the game after approximately 4–6 weeks. Muscle strength is, however, not fully restored until after 3–6 months. When the player returns to normal group training, it is therefore not advisable to take part completely in all sessions straight away.

This should be seen as a general schedule — in all rehabilitation, training must be adapted to each individual.

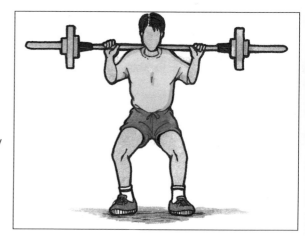

**Exercise 5.** Dynamic strength training using a barbell. In barbell training, it is important to keep the back curved and the head and upper body upright so as not to strain the back. The exercise should be performed slowly on the way down and more quickly on the way up.

# COORDINATION TRAINING

Coordination training is a very important part of rehabilitation. It is, of course, not enough simply to restore strength and mobility. The player must also be able to control all movements quickly enough to be able to avoid his or her ankle giving way. There now follow some examples of coordination exercises:

## Balance training following ankle injury

Exercises 6 and 7 can be started as soon as the pain allows. Coordination training should be performed for at least 5 min/day, 5 days a week for 2–3 months.

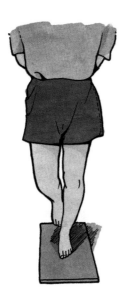

**Exercise 6.** Balance training using a soft mat. Stand barefoot with straight knee on a soft mat. Hold the arms against the chest or behind the back and stand as still as possible. To increase the degree of difficulty the mat can be folded in two and the eyes can be closed while doing the exercise.

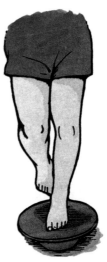

**Exercise 7.** Balance training on a balancing board. The same procedure as in Exercise 6 except that the balance board is used instead of a soft mat.

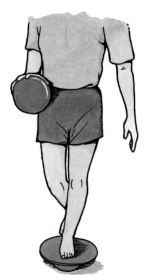

**Exercise 8.** To increase the degree of difficulty further, while standing on the balancing board, you can bounce a ball on the floor or against a wall or throw it up in the air and catch it.

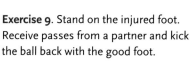

**Exercise 9.** Stand on the injured foot. Receive passes from a partner and kick the ball back with the good foot.

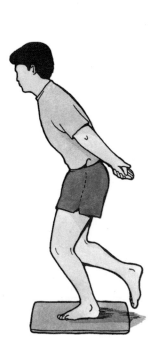

## Balance training following knee injury

Exercises 10 and 11 are similar to those for an ankle injury. The difference is that when training following a knee injury, the player should stand with the knee joint bent to an angle of approximately 60°. It is also important that the knee points straight forward over the foot. These exercises can be started as soon as the pain allows.

**Exercise 10.** Balance training using a soft mat.

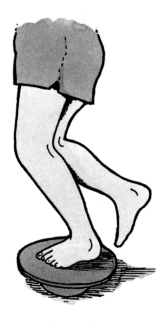

**Exercise 11.** Balance training on a balance board.

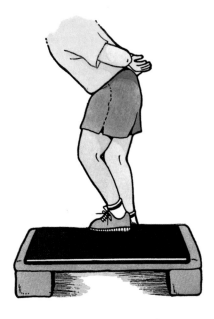

**Exercise 12.** Knee bends on one leg using a step platform. The exercise can also be performed using a step; 3–5 sets of 10–35 repetitions. This exercise can be started around 2 weeks after the injury occurred.

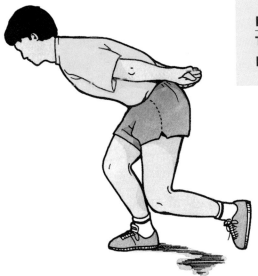

REPETITIONS =

THE NUMBER OF TIMES A MOVEMENT IS REPEATED IN A ROW, I.E. A SET.

**Exercise 13.** Sideways jump with the arms behind the back. Start with short jumps without going down too far. The exercise can be made more diffi- cult by increasing both the length of the jump and the depth of the flexion in the knee; 3–5 sets of 10–20 jumps/leg. This exercise can be started 3–4 weeks after the injury occurred.

**Exercise 14.** Different variations in jumping exercises. Lay out two ropes in a cross so that four squares are formed. The hop is performed forward, backward, sideways and diagonally on one foot or with both feet together. This exercise is performed for 30–60 sec and is repeated in 3–5 sets.

**Exercises 15 and 16.** Coordination and weight training using a Body-Bow, which is made from wood and works like a seesaw. Hold the arms behind the back and do not go over on the ankles. This exercise is performed for 30–60 sec and is repeated in 3–5 sets.

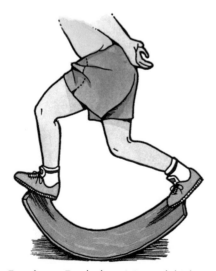

**Exercise 15.** For the knee joint and thigh muscles.

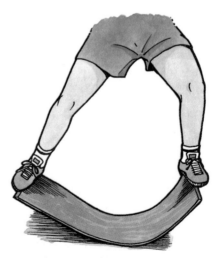

**Exercise 16.** For the hip joint and groin.

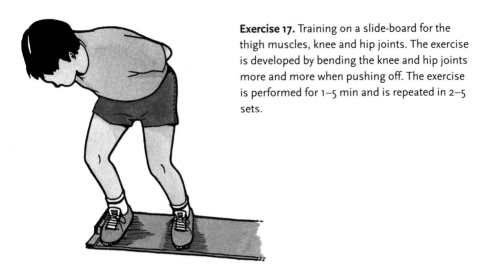

**Exercise 17.** Training on a slide-board for the thigh muscles, knee and hip joints. The exercise is developed by bending the knee and hip joints more and more when pushing off. The exercise is performed for 1–5 min and is repeated in 2–5 sets.

# AGILITY TRAINING (STRETCHING)

Agility training is an important part of football training, both when warming-up and cooling down. It is also an important part of rehabilitation. The exercises should be carried out for at least 30 sec with 2–5 repetitions.

## EFFECTS OF AGILITY TRAINING

- Counteracts muscle shortening and thus reducing the risk of muscle damage.
- Increases the length of shortened muscles.
- Maintains normal flexibility.
- Counteracts aches and pains from training.
- Improves circulation and produces speedier recovery after training or match play.

# The anterior thigh (quadriceps)

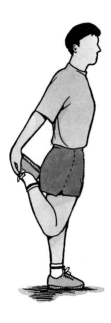

**Exercise 18.** A player with very stiff muscles in the front of the thigh can begin with a simpler variation: stand with the knees together and hips extended. Take hold of the ankle on the same leg the muscle is to be stretched. Pull the foot carefully towards the bottom. Hold for at least 30 sec.

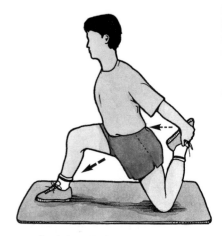

**Exercise 19.** This exercise requires great flexibility. The knee on the leg where the muscle is to be stretched rests on the floor. Let the upper body fall forward slightly. Take hold of the ankle on the back leg, extend the hip and pull the foot slowly towards the bottom. Hold for at least 30 seconds.

# The posterior thigh (hamstrings)

**Exercise 20.** The leg where the muscle is to be stretched is extended in front of the body. The heel rests on the floor and the knee on the other leg does the same. The knee joint on the front leg should be slightly flexed and the foot pointing forward. Let the upper body fall forward slightly. The stretching should be felt in the belly of the muscle in the middle of the rear of the thigh. Hold for at least 30 sec.

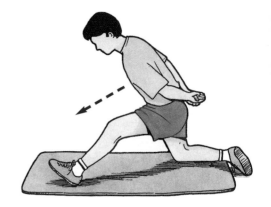

# The hip flexor (iliopsoas)

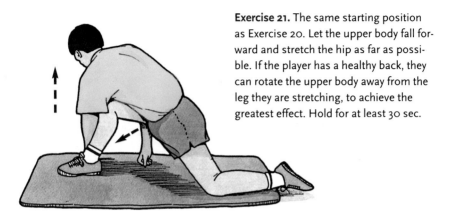

**Exercise 21.** The same starting position as Exercise 20. Let the upper body fall forward and stretch the hip as far as possible. If the player has a healthy back, they can rotate the upper body away from the leg they are stretching, to achieve the greatest effect. Hold for at least 30 sec.

# Groin muscles (adductors)

When stretching the groin muscles, a difference is made between the short muscles, which attach above the knee and the long muscles, which attach below the knee joint.

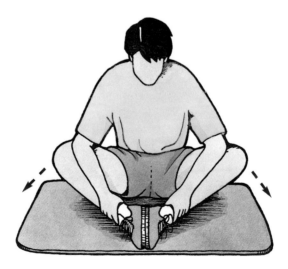

**Exercise 22.** Stretching of the short groin muscles. Sit with the legs apart and the soles of the feet together. Press the elbows against the knees. Hold for at least 30 sec.

**Exercise 23.** Stretching of the long groin muscles. The leg where the muscle is to be stretched is pushed straight out to the side, while the knee of the other leg rests on the floor. Lean the upper body against the leg where the muscle is to be stretched. Hold for at least 30 sec. Then move the leg backwards and repeat. Finish with the leg straight out behind the body and extend the hip. Hold for at least 30 sec in each new position.

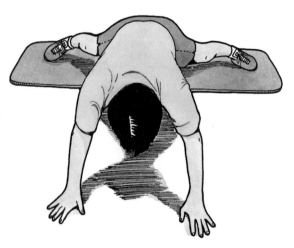

Starting position

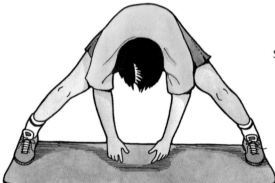

Outstretched position

**Exercise 24.** Stretching of the long groin muscles can be performed on both legs simultaneously. Stand with the legs as far apart as possible, let the upper body fall forward and very slowly slide the hands forwards on the floor. Stop for a few seconds when the hips are fully stretched and then go back very slowly to the starting position.

430

# The hip flexor (gluteus muscles)

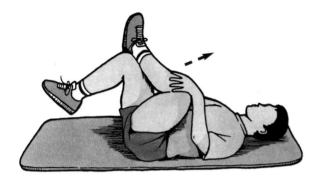

**Exercise 25.** Stretching of the hip rotators. Lie on your back, take hold of the ankle and knee on one leg. Using both hands, pull the leg towards the opposite shoulder. If necessary, use the other leg. Hold for at least 30 sec.

# Long and short calf muscles (gastrocnemius and soleus)

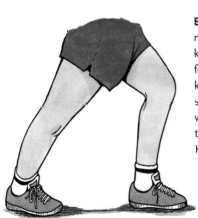

**Exercise 26.** The long calf muscle attaches above the knee joint and should therefore be stretched with the knee extended. For example, stand against a wall. Lean forward with knees extended and the entire foot on the floor. Hold for at least 30 sec.

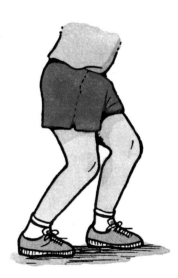

There are many further variations on stretching the same muscle groups. Those shown here should be seen as examples.

**Exercise 27.** In order to stretch the short calf muscle, move the rear leg forward a short step, and flex the knee joint. The entire foot should be in contact with the floor. Hold for at least 30 sec.

# TAPING

This section offers practical advice on taping. Further information can be found in Chapter 3.

## Basic principles of taping

**1** Never tape an injury which has just occurred with non-elastic tape. At this stage, bleeding and swelling often occur, and a tight, unyielding tape dressing can then lead to disturbances in circulation. In the acute phase, a compression dressing using an elastic bandage should be applied. Tape dressings with non-elastic tape are applied when the risk of bleeding and swelling have abated.

**2** Shave the skin to be taped to achieve the best adhesion.

**3** Wash the skin with surgical spirit if possible to remove skin cream and any other ointments.

**4** Tape adheres best directly to the skin. If base tape is used, apply adhesive spray to the skin first.

**5** The tape should be applied on top of the injured joint. Begin and end on healthy parts.

**6** No skin should be visible between the strips of tape. This can produce sores.

**7** Remove the tape using tape scissors or a tape knife. Follow the anatomical structure in question, for example immediately in front of or behind the malleolus in the case of taping of the ankle joint.

There are many different variations on taping of one and the same joint. A few examples are shown here.

## Taping of the ankle joint

There should be a 90° angle between the foot and lower leg. Urge the player to keep the foot in this position the whole time it is being taped up.

Start by placing 'anchors' on each side of the injured joint. These anchors only function as attachment points for the other layers of tape. The first anchor is placed on the lower leg, about a hand's width above the ankle bones. Place the ankle at a slight angle if possible as the lower leg is cone shaped. The other anchor is placed around the forefoot (see Figure 20.2). It is important not to pull the other anchor too tight — if this is done, there is a risk that the player will get a cramp in the foot.

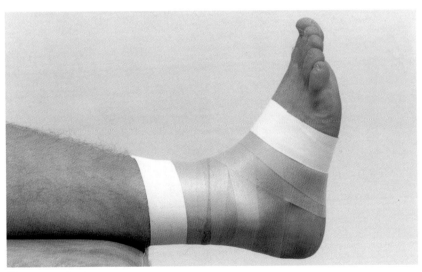

**Figure 20.2** Anchor.

Each new step in this and the following figures the taping is illustrated with white tape.

## Taping of the ligaments on the outside
## of the foot (lateral ligaments)

Starting from the anchor, three 'stirrups' are made. If the ligament on the outside of the foot is damaged, taping begins from the anchor on the inside of the lower leg.

**1.** Put the first strip of tape on the forward side of the inner ankle bone, under the heel, and finish on the back of the outer ankle bone.

**2.** The second strip of tape is centred on the ankle bones on top of the first strip of tape.

**3.** The third strip of tape is applied to the back of the inner ankle bone, on top of the other two strips under the talus and finishes on the forward side of the outer ankle bone. A fan-shape of tape is made on the inside and outside of the lower leg, and at the same time the strips of tape under the heel should lie one on top of the other. This makes the taping stable.

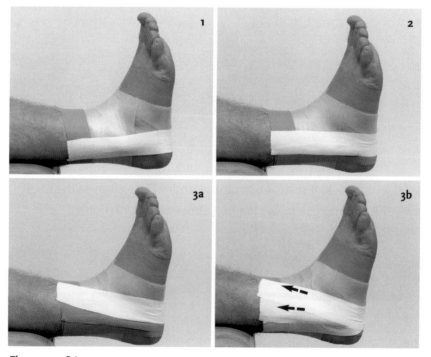

**Figure 20.3** Stirrups.

In the next phase of the taping, horseshoes are applied. A horseshoe consists of a strip of tape which begins on top of the anchor around the foot. Start at the bottom on the inside of the foot, go at right angles to the stirrups and end at the anchor on the outside of the foot. The horseshoes are then applied the whole way, half-overlapping, right up to the anchor on the lower leg.

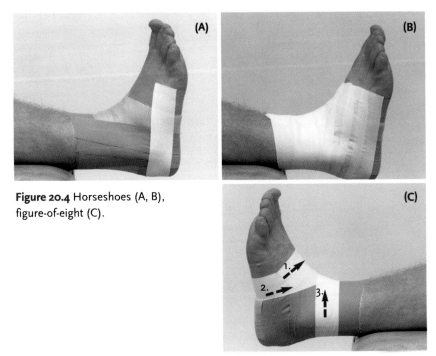

**Figure 20.4** Horseshoes (A, B), figure-of-eight (C).

The next step is a loop of tape in a figure-of-eight. It should start at the back of the foot, continue under the foot from the inside, and end around the lower leg just above the ankle bones.

Taping of the ankle finishes with a 'heel-lock' which is applied on top of the previous layers. The heel-lock starts on the outside of the lower leg and is applied diagonally over the ankle joint, continues under and around the heel and then goes one more turn around the lower leg to the inside. From there it runs diagonally over the ankle, under and around the heel and back to the lower leg. This way the heel is locked in both directions.

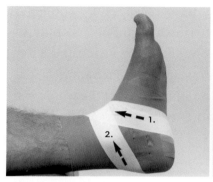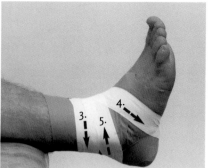

**Figure 20.5** Heel-lock.

Taping is then finished with two anchors. It is important to shape the tape to the foot. The tape is at its most adhesive when it is the same temperature as the skin.

### Taping of the ligaments on the inside of the foot (medial ligaments)

If the deltoid ligament is damaged, the tape is applied in the opposite direction, starting on the outside of the joint.

There is a simpler form of taping where only one anchor on the lower leg is used. A number of stirrups are then applied, some of them diagonally, to be then attached to the inside of the lower leg. End with another anchor.

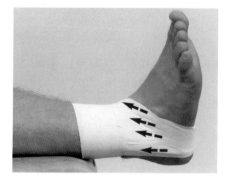

**Figure 20.6** Simplified taping of the ankle.

# Taping of the foot arch

## INDICATION FOR TAPING OF THE FOOT ARCH

Taping of the foot arch is appropriate if the falling arch is under excessive strain.

The foot should be in a relaxed position while being taped. Apply an anchor around the heel and one around the foot. It is important not to overtighten the anchor around the foot.

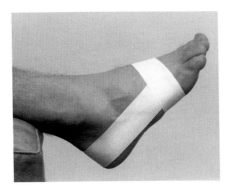

**Figure 20.7** Anchors around the heel and foot.

**Figure 20.8** Fan.

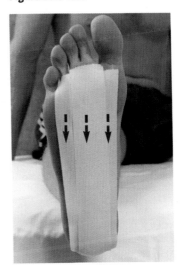

Starting just below the toes, three strips of tape are applied covering the forefoot like a fan and meeting under the heel. The strips are attached to the anchor on the heel.

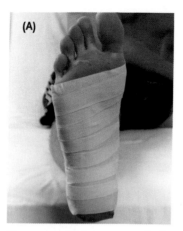 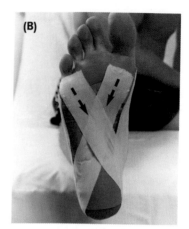

**Figure 20.9** (A)Strips are applied at right angles to the previous ones. (B) Diagonal strips.

The strips of tape are applied at right angles to the previous ones starting right at the back of the heel and ending at the anchor around the forefoot. The strips are applied half overlapping each other.

The next step is two diagonal strips of tape. The first strip starts at the base of the big toe, runs diagonally over the foot arch, around the heel and back to its starting point. The second strip starts at the base of the big toe, runs diagonally across the foot arch, around the heel and back to its starting point.

Tape ends with two new anchors.

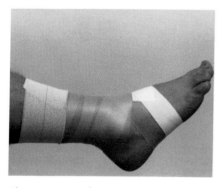

**Figure 20.10** Anchors.

## Taping of the Achilles' tendon

Start with an anchor of elastic sticking plaster on the lower leg, just under the belly of the muscle. The second anchor should be made of non-elastic tape, and is applied around the foot as shown (Figure 20.10). Do not overtighten the anchor to avoid cramp in the foot. Then measure out

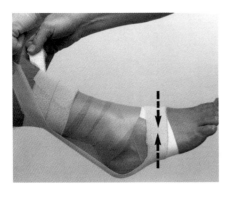

**Figure 20.11** The two ends of the tape are first fastened around the foot.

a piece of elastic sticking plaster, which stretches from the foot arch, around the heel, up to where the calf muscle crosses over into Achilles' tendon. The sticking plaster is divided in two at both ends. First fasten the ends around the foot, then stretch the foot to the desired extent and attach both the other ends around the lower leg, exactly where the calf muscle ends and the Achilles' tendon begins. The more the foot is stretched before the ends are fastened around the lower leg, the harder it is to bend the foot and thus stretch the Achilles' tendon.

Taping can be finished off with about a 1 cm wedge-shaped heel-lift in the shoe. This prevents the Achilles' tendon being stretched to its full extent.

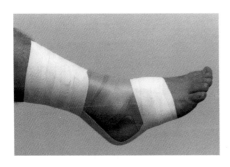

**Figure 20.12** Finish taping by applying some anchors to the lower leg, starting from the top.

## Pressure-relieving taping of the patellar tendon

Use Leukotape P, which has better adhesive qualities. When this tape is used, there should be a layer of Fixomull underneath to avoid injury to the skin. Fixomull is self-adhesive and elastic and made of a material that is not harmful to the skin.

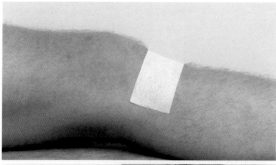

**Figure 20.13** Fixomull is used to avoid injury to the skin.

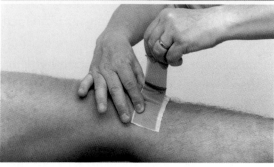

**Figure 20.14** The strong tape is applied over the Fixomull.

Tear off a relatively short piece of tape to be applied to one side of the knee. On the other side of the knee a longer piece of tape is applied. These ends are then stuck together, in such a way that on the longer strip there is still a surface that has adhesive to attach to the lower leg. Lift the tape straight up. Move a little tissue with one hand and fasten the longer piece of tape to the skin.

The same type of taping can be used for excessive strain on the insertion of the patellor tendon to the tibia (Osgood-Schlatter's disease, see Page 339). The difference is that the tape must be moved a few centimetres and fixed on top of the Achilles' tendon attachment.

## Taping of the ligaments between the scapula and clavicle

Stretching of the ligaments and the joint capsule between the clavicle and the scapula can occur following a shoulder charge or a fall on the shoulder.

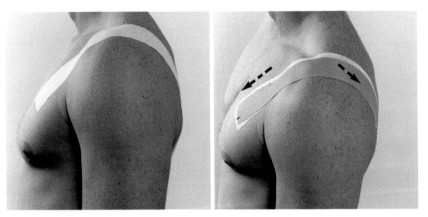

**Figure 20.15** Taping of ligaments between the scapula and clavicle.

Use a stronger kind of tape and first apply a layer of Fixomull to protect the skin, starting at the shoulder blade, passing over the damaged ligament and ending on the front of the shoulder.

Then the tape is applied upwards and down over the front and back of the shoulder, so that the tape ends up right over the joint and relieves pressure on the damaged ligament.

For further relief from pressure, a length of tape can be fixed from the middle of the upper arm on top of the first tape. First of all, apply a strip of Fixomull to protect the skin. When the tape is applied the upper arm should be at an angle of 45° to the body.

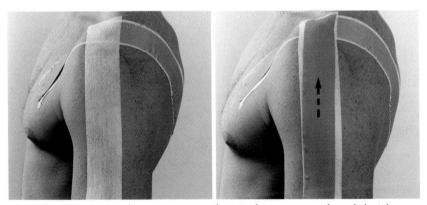

**Figure 20.16** Taping to relieve pressure on the joint between scapula and clavicle (acromioclavicular joint).

441

# 21. Disease and medication

Mats Börjesson

There are a number of diseases which, thanks to efficacious medication, need not present an obstacle to playing football, even at the highest level. The player must know how the disease is to be treated and how the body reacts to physical activity. Other conditions, such as various infections, are more temporary in nature and require that the player refrain from activity for a short time.

This chapter gives an overview of the most common diseases and their treatment.

## Diabetes (diabetes mellitus)

Diabetes is a common chronic disease. Generally speaking, there are examples of active sportsmen and women in all kinds of sport, including football, who have diabetes.

The symptoms are caused by a lack of having too little of the hormone insulin. The illness is divided into insulin-dependent diabetes (juvenile-onset diabetes) and the more common non-insulin dependent diabetes (adult-onset diabetes or NIDDM), which most commonly makes its first appearance in adulthood.

### Background and symptoms

When we eat, blood sugar increases. The carbohydrates are taken up by the body's cells and used as energy or stored as glycogen. As insulin is required for sugar to be taken up in the cells (especially muscle and fat cells), a lack of insulin leads to an increase in the blood sugar (glucose) levels in the blood.

The first symptoms of diabetes are an increase in the volume of urine, thirst, hunger and a reduction in weight. If the condition is not detected in time, the blood sugar levels may be very high with a resulting risk of coma (diabetic coma) with redness in the face, dehydration and unconsciousness. Such cases must receive immediate hospital care.

Blood sugar can also become too low due to a high dose of insulin, reduced food intake or increased physical activity without correction of the insulin dosage. Low blood sugar manifests itself as irritability, anxiety or restlessness, dizziness, hunger but sometimes also as unconsciousness and cramps (insulin coma). It is then important to raise the blood sugar level quickly. A diabetic should always have readily accessible sugar, such as chocolate or dextrose

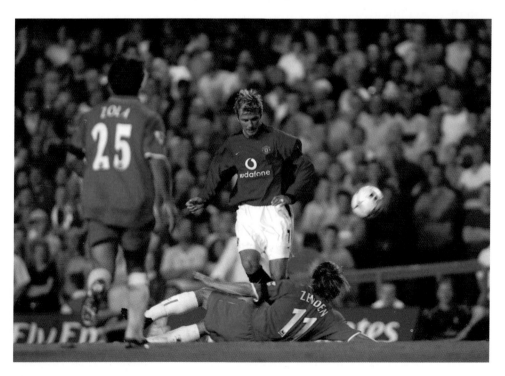

with him or her. If a diabetic player becomes unconsciousness, transport to a hospital must take place as quickly as possible.

During match play, the match doctor, if there is one, should be informed, so that in an acute situation he or she can give an injection which rapidly raises the player's blood sugar (glucagon).

## Too high or too low blood sugar?

It can be very difficult to determine why a diabetic is unconscious. The most common problem in the case of an athlete is low blood sugar level. Giving sugar to someone who has high sugar level is not harmful, but on the other hand, can be extremely important if the blood sugar level is low. So if in doubt, give the person sugar!

## Treatment

The objective in treating diabetes is to try to correct the metabolism, so that the sugar content in the blood is kept as normal as possible. This can be done by:

1. Diet; regular, well put-together meals — avoid pure sugar, eat a lot of fibre and little fat.
2. Administration of insulin by injection 1–4 times a day.
3. Regular physical activity in equal amounts each time is ideal but difficult to carry out in practice.

## The benefits of physical activity

Exercise is an important part of the treatment of NIDDM. In the case of insulin-dependent diabetes, the evidence for the benefits of physical activity is not as strong. Physical activity increases sensitivity to the insulin level in the body, which is good for proper blood sugar control. Research shows that blood sugar level also improves with regular activity in insulin-dependent diabetics.

## Diabetes in footballers

The metabolism of a diabetic differs from that of others as the externally administered insulin can never completely imitate the body's own insulin production. It is therefore necessary to plan food, liquid and insulin intake carefully before every physical activity (such as a game) depending on the length and intensity of the activity and also on the body's present blood sugar level. Different people react in different ways. A diabetic should have tested her or himself for a relatively long time how she or he reacts to different activities (training or matches), different match times (early or late), etc. The blood glucose can theoretically react in three different ways during a football match, of which only the first is desirable:

1. If the blood sugar is well under control approximately 30 min before the match, the player can normally manage around an hour of play with the energy reserves in the muscles and liver. If the insulin intake has been planned so that the highest effect does not coincide with the middle of the game, the blood sugar drops slowly and steadily. Liquids containing sugar should be supplied, especially during the second half.

2. If the blood sugar is low approximately 30 min before the game or if the insulin level peaks during the match, the player risks having too low blood sugar. Sugar must then be supplied before, during or after the game.

3. If the blood sugar is high approximately 30 min before the match, the player should avoid physical activity and instead correct the sugar level by resting, taking liquids and administering insulin.

## Conditions for sporting activity

There are no organized sports in which a diabetic cannot take part, irrespective of the level. The following conditions should be observed, however:

- Proper care of the disease is important, for example adjustment of insulin doses, diet and more frequent blood glucose checks.
- Assessment of the individual's physical condition and the demands the activity in question will place upon him or her.
- There should be none of the following complications (contraindications):
  - Poorly controlled diabetes
  - Visual defects (proliferative retinopathy)
  - Damage to the kidneys and nerves
  - Vascular disease.

**Strategy for good sugar control during activity**

*Mealtimes*

The player should eat 1–3 h before any activity. The amount of food is determined by the length and intensity of the planned activity.

*Blood sugar*

The player should perform regular controls of blood glucose with a portable test kit. However, it should be noted that precise values as to what is a high and what is a low blood sugar level are very hard to give (approximately 15–16 mmol/l and 5–6 mmol/l). The most important indication of high blood glucose is when the urine stick gives a reading for ketones.

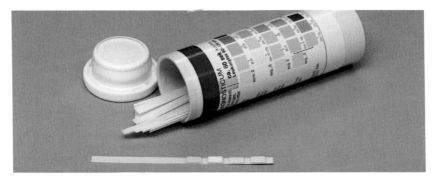

**Figure 21.1** Using a urine stick the player can easily and regularly check their blood sugar level by her or himself.

- Measure blood glucose 30 min before a game. If blood glucose is high — put off the activity and correct the sugar level. If blood sugar is low, take extra carbohydrates before, during and after the match.
- Check blood sugar after activity. There can be a risk of low blood sugar up to 12 h or more after activity due to carbohydrate stores in the muscles and liver being replenished after activity and this exhausts the glucose in the blood.
- Avoid activity late in the evening (risk of low blood glucose during the night). Some people also need to check their blood glucose during the night, particularly if they have competed in a late game.
- If the planned activity lasts longer than 30 min (football match/ training), supplement with carbohydrate drinks during the activity.
- Be prepared for possible low blood glucose, i.e. have sugar tablets ready. Inform the team management.

*Insulin*

- Avoid matches when insulin activity is at its highest (time the insulin). Short-acting insulin reaches its maximum effect after 2–4 h, medium-long acting after 6–12 h and long-acting after 14–24 h.
- Do not inject insulin into muscles which are going to be exerted within 1 h. This can increase insulin uptake and result in low blood glucose.
- Reduce the insulin doses: medium-long acting insulin — reduce the dose before training and competition by 30–35 per cent. Medium-long and short-acting insulin — skip short-acting insulin just before the start of training or a game. Multiple doses of short-acting insulin — reduce the dose by 30–35 per cent before activity and take extra carbohydrates.

# Infections in footballers

Infectious diseases in association with sport and football should be taken seriously. The infections can both affect performance and the infections themselves can be aggravated by the activity with potentially grave consequences. When the infection has been properly treated, the question arises of when the footballer can return to play.

## Background

Infections are caused by three main groups of micro-organisms: viruses, bacteria and fungi.

The body defends itself by means of our immune system. The first line of defence, however, is the skin and mucous membrane, which act as 'armour'. The immune system, which consists of many different components, can attack intruding micro-organisms, such as viruses, and can often prevent an infection from breaking out.

## Are athletes more prone to illness?

Does sporting activity give increased protection against infection? Top sportsmen and women, such as marathon runners, have shown that they have a higher number of infections, for example colds after intense competition.

It seems as if sport and regular physical activity to some extent improve the body's own defences against infection. It is also believed that prolonged intensive physical exertion, such as marathons, triathlons and possibly also intensive periods of training such as those of training camps without sufficient recovery, can lead to temporary inhibition of the immune system following activity.

It is this sensitive period which could account for sportsmen and women having a higher number of infections after a very active period. The theory has been put forward that the length and intensity of the physical activity determine whether the immune system is inhibited or stimulated. What is known, however, is that an in-creased number of infections occur following over-training. Normal recreational sport seems to offer protection from infections. Except during intensive periods of training, such as long tournaments with no recovery time, playing football does not result in an increased risk of infection.

### Should one play football with a high temperature?

Our immune defence protects against attacking micro-organisms by means of a series of reactions. These reactions manifest them-selves as inflammation with redness, soreness, raised temperature and swelling. The general body temperature also rises, i.e. there is a fever. Many organisms are destroyed in this way because they cannot survive in high temperatures.

It is usually inadvisable to train or compete with a high body temperature. It is best to set a limit which can be adhered to. Infection spreads more easily during physical activity and can also become more serious. Body temperature is individual, but stable for a healthy person — between 36.5 and 37.5°C. For some individuals 38°C can signify a nasty infection. But as important as checking the body temperature is listening to the body's signals — if the player is feel-ing weak, cold or achy, they should refrain from any intense activity.

A possible complication of viral infection is myocarditis, some-thing which can occur following exercise with an ongoing infection. There are even some reported deaths related to this. Recommenda-tion: common sense! If a player is feeling tired, out of sorts, or sore anywhere, they should refrain from any sporting activity.

### When can you go back to playing following an infection?

Generally it is important that the player should no longer have a high temperature, any remaining soreness or feel ill, before re-turning to sporting activity. A return to play should be made grad-ually. A good basic rule is to stay away from playing until any course of antibiotics is finished. *Before deviating from this basic rule, a doctor must be consulted.*

# Examples of infection

### Infection of the respiratory passages
*Viral cold*

The most common infection which affects athletes is generally caused by a virus ('the common cold'). The infection leads to swelling of the mucous membrane in the respiratory tract, particularly the nose and throat with watery secretion, a sore throat, mild coughing and hoarseness. Other symptoms include aching muscles, tiredness and feeling ill, but generally no high temperature is present. This infection itself cannot be treated with antibiotics, only the symptoms. Nasal congestion can be relieved with nose drops and a high temperature can be brought down with anti-febrile preparations. Generally, it is important to refrain from sport while the infection is ongoing.

A return to sporting activity is normally possible after about a week. The course of the illness cannot be shortened but can sometimes be lengthened if a proper break from sport is not taken. The player should be careful with cough medicines which can contain ephedrine as this substance is included on the doping list. Viral infections are generally very contagious via direct contact in the changing room.

## AVOID SPREADING INFECTIONS

- Do not share a same water bottle with a team-mate.
- Do not use the same towel as a team-mate.
- Avoid direct contact with ill people.
- Cover verrucae, herpes blisters, etc.

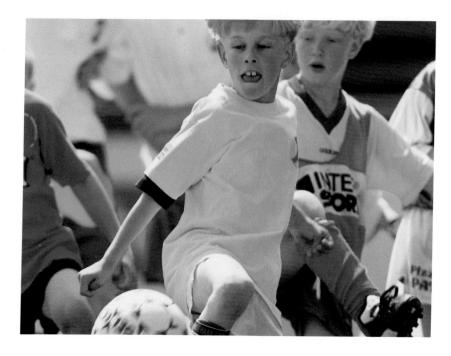

Other viruses can cause more pronounced infections of the respiratory tract. Some of these viruses can also result in myocarditis. In the case of infections with persistent high temperature lasting more than 5 days, pronounced muscle ache or stomach intestinal symptoms, a longer break from training can sometimes be necessary once a doctor has been consulted.

*Bacterial infection of the respiratory tract*
A bacterial infection, for example tonsillitis, ear inflammation or sinusitis, often arises as a complication of a viral infection. If someone has a cold and is on the way to recovery, but instead deteriorates and has thick, yellowish-green nasal mucus, a high temperature and feels worse, a bacterial infection has probably taken over. Treatment with antibiotics, generally penicillin, is then appropriate, after which the infection becomes markedly better after 2–3 days. A return to sport can then be made after full recovery. In this case infection occurs via direct person-to-person contact.

### Tonsillitis

Tonsillitis is generally caused by streptococci, but can also be caused by a virus. Tonsillitis manifests itself as a very sore throat with yellow coating on the tonsils and, as a result, swallowing becomes difficult. There are often no typical cold symptoms, except occasionally a high temperature (up to 39°C and more). Tonsillitis is treated with antibiotics.

### Bronchitis

Bronchitis is generally caused by bacteria and is often a sequela of viral cold with yellowish-green phlegm being coughed up. Varying results are obtained from expectorant medicine. Otherwise, bronchitis is treated with antibiotics.

### Pneumonia

Pneumonia can be caused by bacteria, such as pneumococci and produces serious symptoms including high temperature, coughing up of phlegm and extreme tiredness. Intense physical activity is out of the question. Pneumonia is treated primarily with antibiotics. However, a relatively long convalescence time should be expected.

In young people, pneumonia can be caused by a micro-organism called mycoplasma. This infection of the respiratory tract has influenza-like, protracted symptoms.

## Infections of the urinary tract

Infections of the urinary tract are the second most common type of infection and most often occur in women.

### Infections of the lower urinary tract (cystitis)

Cystitis is caused by bacteria. The infection manifests itself as pain when passing water, soreness of the bladder and sometimes even high temperature. It is treated with antibiotics.

*Infections of the upper urinary tract*

An infection of the lower urinary tract can spread to the kidneys. A renal pelvic infection often results in strong feeling of sickness, a high temperature (over 39°C) and backache. Symptoms from the lower urinary tract including burning pain when passing water and soreness in the bladder can also occur. The condition is treated with antibiotics for approximately 14 days.

## Skin infections

The skin protects the body from all forms of external influence, such as infections, heat, cold and the sun, but also from physical injury from kicks and falls. The skin acts as a 'shield' against the environment. If the skin is damaged, such as when a player is grazed or cut, an infection can set in.

Infection can be prevented by washing the wound properly. If it is badly contaminated — scrub it with a brush. During the first few hours there can be a clear discharge from the wound. Cover it with a clean dressing. As soon as there is no discharge from the wound it should be uncovered as much as possible to aid healing (cover during training and matchplay).

## Infection of cuts

If a cut remains red and irritated and there is a discharge of yellowish pus, infection of the cut should be suspected. Soreness, redness and swelling increase around the cut. A high temperature may also develop. The cause is bacteria, generally staphylococci, which are treated with antibiotics. The player should refrain from sporting activity for the duration of the infection and during treatment with antibiotics. Occasionally the infection spreads deeper and is called cellulitis. If the infection spreads via the lymphatic system to the neighbouring lymph glands, lymphangitis and/or lymphadenitis can develop, which appears as a 'red line' on the skin. In everyday speech this is sometimes called 'blood poisoning'. A graze on the knee which becomes infected can lead to complications including high temperature, red line on the thigh and swollen lymph glands in the groin. The condition is treated most quickly with antibiotics. Vaccination against tetanus is also recommended.

### Fungal infections in the skin

Athlete's foot is a common problem in sportsmen and women. It is caused by a fungal infection and manifests itself as redness, flaking skin and itching between the toes. The cause is the warm, damp environment in shoes. It is treated with regular washing and careful

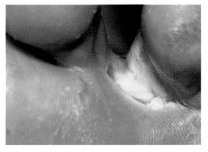

drying of the area between the toes. An over-the-counter anti-fungal ointment can usually be used. A doctor should be consulted if the problem continues.

**Figure 21.2** "Athlete's foot", a fungal infection which results in redness, flaking skin and itching between the toes, is common among sportsmen and women. Photo: *Håkan Mobacken.*

### Groin fungus

Fungal infection in the groin area manifests itself as redness, often in combination with bothersome itching, and is treated with fungal ointment which is applied for at least a week.

### Fungal infection of the nails

Fungal infection of the nails, usually on the toes, manifests itself as yellowed, disintegrating nails and is very difficult to treat. It is treated with anti-fungal medicine in tablet form for a lengthy time.

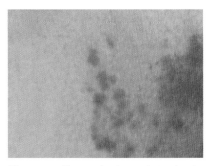

**Figure 21.3** Fungus in the groin region is an example of another common infection among sportsmen and women. It manifests itself as redness combined with bothersome itching. Photo: *Håkan Mobacken.*

### Infections of the stomach and intestines
#### *Gastroenteritis*

Different viruses can cause gastric 'flu', which entails diarrhoea, vomiting, stomach pains, high temperature and loss of appetite. Antibiotics are ineffective. It is treated by replacing lost liquids, preferably with drinks containing sugar and salt. Avoid milk.

#### *Food poisoning*

Food poisoning can occur after eating contaminated food and manifests itself as vomiting and diarrhoea approximately an hour after the meal. The symptoms usually pass quickly.

#### *Traveller's diarrhoea*

Traveller's diarrhoea can arise on trips to some hot exotic countries and is thought to be the result of being exposed to new forms of intestinal bacteria, which can cause diarrhoea for a few days. One should therefore only drink bottled or canned liquids, not eat ice cream or salad and avoid ice-cubes. If the diarrhoea is still there after returning home, bacterially transmitted infection should be suspected. A doctor should then be contacted for examination, taking a bacterial culture and possibly antibiotic treatment.

### Other infections
#### *Glandular fever (infectious mononucleosis)*

This disease is caused by a virus and affects mainly young adults in the 15–25 years age group. It cannot be treated but instead most often heals up on its own after 2–4 weeks. Transmission is via direct contact. The incubation period is long, up to 50 days. The first symptoms are headache, high temperature (often very high), sore throat, loss of appetite and extreme tiredness. Enlarged lymph glands (hence the name) are observed in the armpits, groin, on the neck and by an often enlarged spleen.

456

The player can return to sporting activity when he or she feels fit, has normal blood test results and no longer has a high temperature. If the spleen has been enlarged, it must return to normal size. The required rest from sport is calculated at least 4 weeks from the outbreak of the disease.

## Asthma and exercise-included asthma

Asthma is one of the most common disorders of the respiratory tract. It is characterized by a varying degree of obstruction of the respiratory tract for a short time, known as an asthma attack. There are several causes:

1. Contraction of the muscles in the bronchi.
2. Swelling of the mucous membrane in the bronchial tubes due to inflammation
3. Increased production of viscous phlegm in the bronchi.

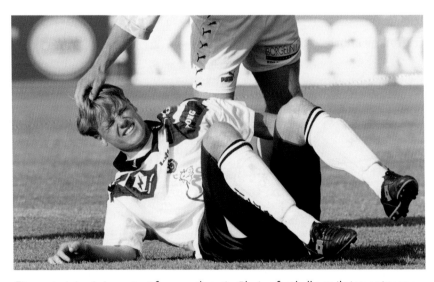

Fitness training is important for an asthmatic. Playing football entails intermittent exertion and is therefore suitable for asthmatics, as the risk of asthma attacks is lower.

Hyperreactivity of the bronchi to various irritating factors such as cold, smoke and dust — known as hyperreactivity — is often seen.

### Sport and asthma

Intense physical activity can trigger acute attacks of asthmatic problems. It is now known that an asthmatic can benefit from physical activity, because of improved oxygen uptake among other things. Well-supervised and controlled asthma represents no obstacle to playing football.

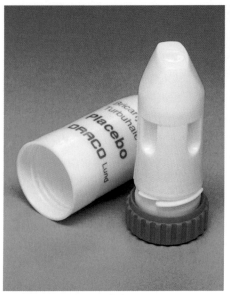

**Figure 21.4** Asthma inhaler.

### Treatment of common asthma

Mild asthma is treated with inhaled medication, which dilates the bronchi (e.g. Bricanyl, Ventoline). This is taken as required when the air passages 'tighten', normally in association with allergy, infection or sporting activity.

Chronic asthma requires treatment with 'bronchodilators' and inhaled medication to alleviate the inflammation in the bronchi (cortisone preparations).

### Exercise-included asthma (EIA)

This refers to the temporary obstruction of the airways which can occur in association with intense exertion.

### How can exercise-included asthma be avoided/treated?

Some 80–95 per cent of all asthma sufferers have EIA, i.e. an asthma attack in connection with sport. Three phases are typically described:

**1. Acute phase:** After 5–10 min of exercise at 75–85 per cent of maximum heart rate, contraction of the air passages is produced, which leads to a reduction in breathing capacity by at least 15 per cent (by definition). After approximately 8 min, breathing capacity is at its lowest and returns to normal after an hour or so.

**2. 'Protected period':** Within 1–3 h after an EIA attack, the sufferer is more resistant to new attacks. Thus an asthmatic should warm up for 15–30 min at a relatively high intensity before a game to trigger an obstruction. The player then rests for 15 min before the game starts and is then less prone to bronchial contractions.

**3. Delayed reaction:** Some 40–50 per cent of people with EIA can have a similar but less pronounced, temporary reduction in breathing capacity 4–8 h after the initial physical exertion.

### What aggravates or triggers asthma in sport?

Some types of physical activity trigger asthma attacks more easily than others. The symptoms increase proportionally with the degree of exertion, i.e. they depend on the intensity of the activity. The length of the activity is also significant. Doing sport in cold, dry air increases the problems, while a warm, damp climate reduces them.

Other factors which increase the problems are infections of the respiratory tract (airways), stress, excessive training and irritants such as pollen and dust.

### How can asthma problems be avoided?

*Non-pharmacological*

- An activity with varying intensity and rest periods in between (such as football) gives fewer problems than long, continuous endurance sports such as skiing and running.

- Breathing through the nose increases the moisture content in the air and reduces the problems compared with breathing through the mouth.
- Avoid being cold. A warm shower and warm clothes are recommended after training.
- If the sufferer warms up for around 10–15 min at a high intensity level, he or she can have a period during the game when an attack is difficult to trigger (a 'protected' period).
- Training regularly is an advantage — it increases fitness and reduces both the need for medicine and reactivity to irritants.
- Colds and allergies should be treated.

*Medicine*

Common 'bronchodilators' in the form of inhalers are used most often. Two inhalations 10–15 min before doing any sport is effective in about 90 per cent of cases against EIA, lasting for several hours. The other alternative is cortisone in the form of inhalers or a recently registered inhaled medication — leukotrienantagonist.

# Vascular problems and sport

### The benefits of exercise

The benefits of sport are well known. In recent years it has been possible to show that physical inactivity is an important risk factor for vascular disease along with high blood pressure, smoking, high lev-

---

### ATHLETE'S HEART

- Slow heart rate at rest.
- ECG variations.
- Enlarged heart.

els of blood lipids and diabetes. Generally speaking, sport has a positive effect on most other risk factors by lowering body weight, reducing blood lipids, the lowering the blood pressure, increasing insulin-sensitivity and increasing fitness.

### The effects of exercise — athlete's heart

The heart normally beats around 70 times/min at rest and approximately 75 ml of blood are pumped with every heartbeat. This means that roughly 5 l of blood pass through the heart per minute (cardiac output). In fit individuals, up to 40 l can pass through the heart per minute. Increasing cardiac output, i.e. the effect of exercise, practically consists of the increased volume of each heartbeat increasing by up to approximately 200 ml. The heart's way of adapting physiologically to long, intensive training is manifested in what is known as athlete's heart. It is important to know about this physiological adaption to exercise in order to be able to distinguish it from dangerous conditions and not to misinterpret it as a disease.

### High blood pressure (hypertension)

When the heart pumps blood through the body's blood vessels, these dilate and the blood forms a pulse-wave where the highest pressure constitutes the systolic pressure and the lowest pressure constitutes the diastolic pressure, normally around 120/70 mmHg.

During physical activity blood pressure often increases but this is partly counteracted by reduced resistance in the blood vessels to muscles, which results in an increase in blood pressure to roughly 170 mmHg (in fit athletes often at least 200 mmHg).

With high blood pressure, initially there is an increase in cardiac output. Left untreated, high blood pressure leads to heart failure and changes in the blood vessel walls together with increased risk of cardiovascular disease such as stroke, heart attacks, kidney damage or visual impairment.

## Recommendations regarding physical activity with high blood pressure

Physical activity generally results in better-controlled blood pressure and reduced risk of cardiovascular disease. Exercise of moderate intensity such as walking for 30–60 min, 5 times/week is considered optimal. High-intensity exercising, in a top athlete, can increase resting blood pressure, and heavy strength training with few repetitions is not recommended in a person with high blood pressure, although light strength training may be of benefit.

## High blood pressure and football

Well-regulated blood pressure represents no obstacle to taking part in sports, for example football. However, a doctor must have excluded underlying kidney disease, and signs of any blood pressure-related damage to the eyes, kidneys, heart or nerves. Within football these questions are most relevant among older players in, for example, inter-company and veteran leagues.

If the first step in the treatment of high blood pressure, i.e. increased physical activity, smoking cessation, weight loss and reduced salt intake, have not produced any results, medicines must, of course, be used as additional treatment.

# 22. Late sequelae of football – osteoarthrosis

Harald Roos

This chapter deals with the consequences of injuries, particularly those affecting the knee, in the long term. In addition, it discusses how the joints are affected by playing football without any specific injury having occurred. The possible consequence of this is what in everyday language is called aching joints or arthrosis.

## Arthrosis

For a joint to work well, normal joint cartilage is required. Cartilage is a shiny, white layer, a few millimetres thick, which covers the ends of both bones in a joint. The movement is smooth when the surfaces of the cartilage rub together and the friction is extremely low, which is facilitated by the synovial fluid in the joint.

By varying its water content, joint cartilage can become more or less resistant to compression forces. Cartilage therefore acts as a shock absorber and distributes even pressure over the whole joint. The cartilage is maintained continually so that function is preserved and if for any reason it loses its shock-absorbing properties or if the surface becomes less smooth and even, damage occurs to the surface of the cartilage. This can be a stage in the normal ageing process, where the ability to maintain and repair the cartilage diminishes, but can also occur following injuries or extreme strain. The joint's functions then deteriorate gradually and symptoms such as pain, swelling and reduced movement appear. Initially the symptoms are noticed only when the joint is placed under strain, but as the process continues, it can also involve pain when at rest.

It is this reduction of the joint cartilage's normal function with subsequent loss of cartilage which is called arthrosis.

## Symptoms of arthrosis

In a footballer, the first symptoms of arthrosis can be pain after playing on a hard surface or after shooting practice. On radiographic examination signs of cartilage loss are visible in the joint. When the effects on the cartilage or cartilage loss are visible on a radiograph, the process is advanced and the general opinion is that it is no longer possible for the body to repair the changes in the cartilage. In early stages, changes in the cartilage and minor cartilage loss are detected by means of magnetic resonance imaging or by arthroscopy of the joint.

## Treatment

Treatment of arthrosis in the early stages is with analgesic drugs, reduced activity and physiotherapy. A properly functioning musculature around the joint can have a positive effect on the problem. This is the reason why a very fit person can continue doing sport even with damaged cartilage. A footballer can often play relatively unhindered, with temporary swelling or stiffness at the end of training or a match as the only problem. Gradually, as the extent of the cartilage damage increases, pain also occurs while doing any activity and the functions of the joint deteriorate.

In later stages of arthrosis, when there is a reduction in the ability to walk and also pain when resting, surgical treatment is often required. In younger people strain is alleviated on the poorly functioning parts of the joint by changing the angle of the joint and thus transferring weight to healthier parts of the joint (wedge surgery osteotomy). In older people, the problem is solved by replacing the

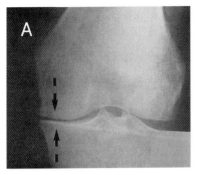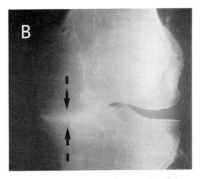

**Figure 22.1** (A) Moderate wear with a reduction in the joint space on the inside of the knee joint. (B) Pronounced wear with disappearance of the joint space. The cartilage is completely worn down.

damaged joint surfaces with artificial surfaces made from plastic or metal (joint prosthesis).

It is important to be aware that those changes in the joint which are detected by magnetic resonance imaging, arthroscopy or radiographs and is termed arthrosis, are not automatically associated with pain or other symptoms. Therefore, what may look like seriously affected cartilage does not necessarily result in great problems. When discussing arthrosis, for example as a consequence of playing football, the reason behind this is nearly always based on the existence of changes in the joint, generally visible on radiographs, and not on any experience of symptoms. However, it should not be ignored that the risk of symptoms from a joint is greater if there are visible changes on radiographs, compared with if the joint looks healthy.

### Risk factors

There are many risk factors for arthrosis, of which ageing is the most significant. Other risk factors are gender, hereditary factors, overweight, overuse and injuries. Wrist, knee and hip joints are most often affected by arthrosis. Arthrosis of the wrist and knee affects women more often while arthrosis of the hip is more evenly divided between the sexes.

It is thought that football may increase the risk of arthrosis in two different ways: through injuries primarily in the knee joint and through the high strain football places on the joints.

Injuries to the joints are a well-known, significant risk factor. Bone damage in a joint can mean that the surfaces of the joint become uneven with increased strain as a consequence. Even following the occurrence of an injury where the bone is not affected, such as when the joint is subjected to twisting with damage to the ligaments and the menisci, there is an increased future risk of arthrosis.

# Arthrosis following knee injuries

Arthrosis is a natural consequence of the ageing process and normally occurs in one's 60s and 70s. It is well known, however, that a knee injury can lead to arthrosis at a relatively young age. This is probably not because the course of arthrosis is more rapid following an injury, but rather it is thought to be a result of the process of arthrosis beginning earlier after an injury than in someone who has not suffered an injury. It is possible that a continued high level of activity, such as continuing to play football, following an injury further increases the risk of arthrosis, although there is no definite proof of this.

### Anterior cruciate ligament damage

Anterior cruciate ligament damage is thought to result in more rapid development of arthrosis than isolated meniscus damage. Fifteen years after anterior ligament damage, approximately half of those affected present changes which are characteristic of arthrosis. The reason for cruciate ligament damage leading to a higher risk of arthrosis is probably that the greater forces acting on the joint as a result the injury involve associated damage to the other parts of the joint, such as menisci, collateral ligaments and cartilage surfaces. The risk of developing arthrosis in the joint increases with time after the injury, which means that an injury as a teenager involves the risk of arthrosis as early as in one's 40s.

### Meniscus damage

The risk of arthrosis following meniscus damage is well documented. A study has shown that in 75 per cent of those who underwent surgery for meniscus damage 20 years ago there was some form of change in the knee joint visible on radiographs. At that time the entire meniscus was removed by opening the knee (arthrotomy), which is different from the surgical technique of today (arthroscopy). Changes on radiographs had no clear link with ex-

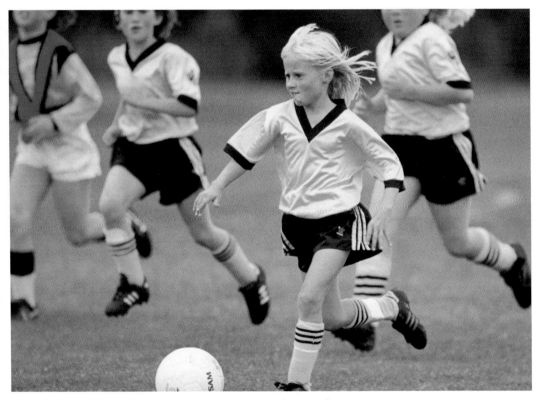

The risk of developing arthrosis in the joint increases with time after the injury, which means that an injury at an early age involves the risk of arthrosis as early as in one's 40s.

perience of symptoms, but those who were operated on revealed that the incidence of knee-related symptoms was more than twice that of the control group.

It seems, therefore, as if symptoms have a greater significance than changes observed on radiographs for meniscal damage. It is therefore possible that meniscus surgery following today's modern principles, where only the damaged part of the meniscus is removed, results in fewer permanent problems with continued playing of football.

## Can treatment of knee injuries affect the development of arthrosis?

There is no definite evidence that cruciate ligament surgery can reduce the future risk of arthrosis. As stabilizing the knee joint reduces the risk of meniscus damage in the long run, it can be assumed that this indirectly reduces the risk of arthrosis. However, paradoxically, return to play following successful cruciate ligament surgery increases the risk of arthrosis as a consequence of more footballing activity. If the player with cruciate ligament damage finds that his knee is stable enough to make playing football possible once again, which is generally the case with modern surgical techniques, the player then returns to a sport, which at the same time involves an increased risk of arthrosis.

There is a study which, perhaps for this very reason, suggests that those who have undergone cruciate ligament surgery really have a higher incidence of arthrosis than those who have not been operated on. Any joint damage caused by surgery itself or altered mechanics of the knee joint following cruciate ligament surgery can also contribute to this negative effect. There is still, however, a lack of scientifically correctly performed studies of this important question.

With meniscus damage, the aim nowadays is to save as much of the meniscus as is possible and to remove only the damaged parts, which can be done by means of arthroscopic surgery. In younger people, an attempt is made to preserve the whole meniscus by sewing it back in place instead of removing the damaged parts. This is a more demanding operation, with a significantly longer rehabilitation period and generally up to 4–5 months' absence from football. Unfortunately, there is no convincing evidence for surgery which aims to preserve the meniscus thereby reducing the risk of arthrosis. It seems to be a definite advantage, in any case for the function of the knee, to preserve as much of the meniscus as possible during surgery.

## Strain and arthrosis

Running as exercise for many years, even relatively long distances, has not been shown to produce any damaging effect on the joint cartilage, while running for training purposes at a high level can result in an increased risk of arthrosis in the hip joint in particular.

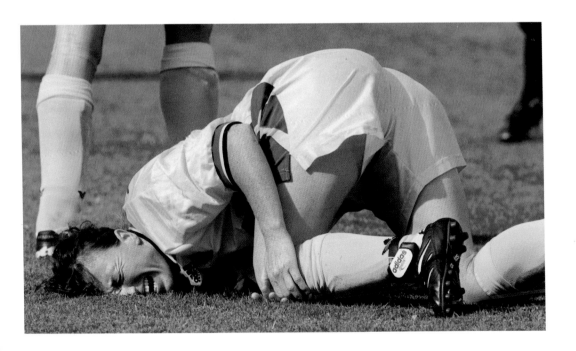

Also, there is probably an increased risk of arthrosis in the knee joint when there is extremely high strain.

Playing football at lower levels, even for many years, does not result in any increased risk of arthrosis in either the hip or knee. Arthrosis in the ankle only occurs if there has been previous bone damage. Those changes which are seen in the ankle in the form of bony out-growths (osteophytes) on the front of the lower leg sometimes called 'footballer's ankle', are not considered to be arthrosis.

High-level football has, on the other hand, been shown to result in a clearly increased risk of arthrosis of both the hip and knee joints. It has been shown that in former top-level footballers in their 60s, changes due to arthrosis in the hip joint are found in 15 per cent of cases, while the percentage in the rest of the population in this age group is around 3 per cent. There is an increased risk of arthrosis of the hip occurring in top-level players as early as in their 40s.

As for arthrosis of the knee joint among former top-level players in their 60s, the situation is the same as for the hip, or around 15 per cent, compared with 4 per cent for the remainder of the population. If players with previously known knee injuries are excluded, there are still 11 per cent who have arthrosis of the knee joint. Among players around 40 years old, there are very few who have signs of arthrosis of the knee joints. These results indicate that football at a high level involves great strain on the joint cartilage, which in the long term can result in arthrosis.

Women who have played football were also shown to have an increased incidence of arthrosis in the knee joint. Those women who were examined were on average 43 years old and had played high-level football for an average of 13 years. It can therefore be assumed that women develop arthrosis to a larger extent, or at least earlier in life, after playing football, than men. The opposite seems to be the case for the hip joint, as there was no increased incidence of arthrosis of the hip joint in the women examined.

# Can football-related arthrosis be prevented?

That football at a high level results in an increased risk of arthrosis in the hip and knee joints is considered obvious, due to both the risk of knee injuries with subsequent risk of arthrosis and due to increased strain on the joints. Injuries result in an increased risk of arthrosis developing after 15 years in approximately 50 per cent of cases. In the earliest stages of arthrosis, there are no symptoms in the joint to any real extent but it is worth noting that over half of those under the age of 50 years who underwent surgery in the knee had a serious knee injury.

One reason why arthrosis is difficult to prevent following a knee injury may be that its course is perhaps already decided at the moment of the injury and cannot then be changed. Cartilage damage of the joint surface often occurs together with an acute cruciate ligament injury, which can only be detected by means of magnetic resonance imaging. Cartilage damage like this can mean that the subsequent course of the problem will be unfavourable irrespective of treatment.

With cruciate ligament damage, the player feels that the knee is more or less unstable and on examination increased laxity can be felt in the knee. If the knee joint is stabilized by means of cruciate ligament surgery, the risk of arthrosis should decrease, especially as stabilization means that the risk of meniscus damage diminishes. There is, however, no definite proof that cruciate ligament surgery really entails any advantage as regards the future development of arthrosis.

With today's surgical techniques, where, in technical terms, cruciate ligament surgery is relatively uncomplicated, it is possible for the player to undergo fast and almost painless rehabilitation. It is therefore easy to see the injury only in the short term with a rapid return to football as the main objective. The cartilage is probably more sensitive to high levels of strain at this stage, partly due to the force which is necessary for the cruciate ligament to be damaged

## ARTHROSIS – FACTS

- Arthrosis involves a reduction in the normal functions of the joint cartilage with subsequent loss of cartilage.
- Arthrosis generally affects the wrist, knee and hip joints.
- The risk factors for arthrosis are increasing age, hereditary factors, overweight, overuse and traumatic injuries.
- It is thought that playing football increases the risk of arthrosis, partly due to injuries to the knee in particular and partly due to the large amount of strain football per se places on the joints.
- An early sign of arthrosis in footballers can be pain after playing on a hard surface or after shooting practice.

and partly due to the effect that surgery probably has. In both cases an inflammatory reaction is brought about with increased water content in the cartilage, which probably results in lower resistance.

### Risk factors

The safest way to reduce the risk of arthrosis in football would be to reduce the number of knee injuries. It is felt to be especially urgent to address the high number of cruciate ligament injuries among women footballers, not least those injuries which occur in childhood and adolescence. The earlier a knee injury occurs, the greater is the risk of early appearance of symptoms of arthrosis. It is therefore important to define the risk factors which lead to a knee injury so that these can be avoided.

To date, it has not been possible to determine for sure whether low muscle strength or an insufficient level of general fitness might be risk factors. However, there is a connection between limited movement in the knee and cruciate ligament damage, as the latter then risks being trapped when the knee is twisted. There is also a connection with increased general laxity of the knee joint. Both these factors are over-represented in women and can partly explain the higher risk of injury among them. Unfortunately, neither of these factors can be affected by preventative exercises.

As the risk of knee injury is also related to what level the footballer plays at (the higher the level, the greater the risk of injury), it has been discussed whether an age limit might have any influence on the risk of cruciate ligament damage in young players. It has also been put forward that changes in the rules to prevent rough play and tackling from behind might be one way to reduce the number of injuries. Bearing in mind that the majority of cruciate ligament injuries, at least among women, occur without any contact with an opponent, it would probably not have any preventative effect for knee injuries.

Reducing strain on the hip and knee joints is not possible in football, as the increased amount of training and greater intensity of modern football put more strain on the joint cartilage. The evidence for a footballer suffering from arthrosis in the hip or knee joints, especially after a career at top level, paints a negative picture but cannot be ignored. It must be pointed out, however, that most studies in this area have dealt with radiographs only and not patients. The relationship between changes observed on radiographs and actual symptoms is, as has been stated, not clear. In addition, good musculature is one way to reduce symptoms in the case of early arthrosis. There is good reason to believe that a former active sportsman or woman has good chances of retaining good musculature in later life.

The normal course of slight changes in the hip or knee due to arthrosis is not clear. Furthermore, it has been shown that only a small number of those who were found to have slight changes in the cartilage developed problems which required surgical treatment in the long term.

# 23. Children and football

Åke Andrén-Sandberg

There has been some concern that early training of children might, in some respects, be harmful. Primarily, the thinking is that the body's growth might be disturbed or that the child would suffer permanent effects from sports injuries. Both these problems occur in isolated cases, but in all likelihood are not of much significance.

Football belongs to that group of sports which children become involved in from an early age. In many countries, football is the largest children's sport and its organizers have a great responsibility. It is important that everyone knows how children's training should differ from adults', and be aware of what injuries children can suffer.

## Special training for children

Many football coaches believe that children and adults should train in the same way. Therefore it should be emphasized that children are not small versions of adults and the type of training for adults is not always suitable for children. There are certain conditions that make children unique from a training point of view and coaches and other team personnel must take these into consideration.

In terms of the effects of training, the dividing line between children and adolescents can be drawn at puberty. This chapter primarily describes the characteristics of children's football training, i.e. before they reach puberty.

# Growing and maturation or the effects of training?

One problem for those who train children is being able to distinguish between the effects of training from normal growth and maturation. From the time when children start school until they are adults, their bodies will more than treble in size, while their muscle strength increases even more and the brain and nerves change the child's clumsy movements into the precise, quick, calculated movements of an adult footballer.

A certain degree of training is necessary for children to grow and develop normally, but it is not easy to say what the limit is. There is, for example, nothing to indicate if normal football training affects the bone growth, either positively or negatively. On the other hand, extreme training can have a negative influence on the development of bones and muscles in isolated cases.

Coaches of pre-pubescent adolescents would like to think that increased strength and speed are dependent on training, but this is only true to a small extent. The chief benefits of children's training lie in the technical side and in developing an understanding of the game.

# Development of fitness

In everyday terms, capacity for oxygen uptake is normally used as a measurement of fitness. Training of children and adolescents has been shown, in scientific studies, however, to contribute to only around 30 per cent of the individual's fitness (maximum capacity for oxygen uptake) — the same being true for speed and strength. A significant amount of what children are capable of is due to innate factors.

Inactivity or lack of training affect children's fitness in the same way or slightly less than that of adults. However, fitness is recovered more quickly, for example, following an injury in a child.

Children's fitness can be developed through training but the effect is small. It can be compared to different rates of interest in a bank — if an adult gets 25 or 40 per cent 'interest' from training hard, a child gets 5 or at most 10 per cent. In addition, fitness is something that disappears quickly. Fitness is lost approximately three times faster than it is built up, which means that even a child who is in very good shape for a number of years will lose the fitness he or she has acquired if training does not continue. There is, therefore, never any reason to train children so that they will be fit later in life. The only reason to train young players for fitness is because they need that extra addition of oxygen uptake capacity at that age. It may also be possible to justify fitness training by saying that later in life it will be useful for children to have learned the basics of how to train.

## RELATIVE DIFFERENCES OF TRAINING EFFECTS FOR CHILDREN AND ADULTS

|  | Before puberty | During puberty | After puberty |
|---|---|---|---|
| Fitness | + | + | +++ |
| Lactic acid | o | + | ++ |
| Joint flexibility | o | + | +++ |
| Strength | + | ++ | +++ |
| Technique | +++ | ++ | + |
| Need for immediate fun | +++ | ++ | + |

# Lactic acid and training

Children never have levels of lactic acid in the blood as high as adults after doing high intensity sporting activity, but this is not due to the fact that they are fitter but rather that the metabolism of the muscles works differently. They do not have as large a number of those enzymes which form lactic acid upon exertion. An absence of oxygen is made up more quickly early in childhood than later on. Therefore, there is no reason to try to train children to get used to the effects of lactic acid. This ability increases with age whether they train or not. When they first reach puberty, lactic acid training can be positive but even then it is almost always easier to improve technique than to train in this very strenuous way.

# Weight training

Muscles can be trained in several different ways; for example, the muscles' speed, stamina and 'brute force', can be increased. Children can try to develop muscle strength before puberty in all these respects but do not achieve as good results from training as adults. For muscles to develop, testosterone is required, and this hormone is not formed in large quantities in the body until puberty (in girls, too, but not in as large quantities as in boys). Muscle training can, however, to a certain extent improve muscle strength in both boys and girls before puberty. This occurs without any appreciable increase in muscle mass, and is primarily due to the fact that the heart has learned to make better use of the muscles.

As muscle strength — both in terms of speed, stamina and ability to lift heavy weights — just like fitness is something which quickly disappears if one stops training, there is no reason to try to develop children's strength. Weight training for young players should therefore be primarily aimed at speed and stamina.

# Joint and muscle flexibility

A problem for adult players is often reduced joint and muscle flexibility, which can lead to both acute injuries and overuse injuries. This is not a problem for children — in principle they do not have shortened muscles or reduced joint flexibility. In addition, their flexibility can be improved somewhat by training, but this is not an advantage — rather it is a disadvantage as the muscles' insertion on the skeletal structure renders the joints more unprotected and the risk of injury increases in both the short and long term.

Before children have reached adult proportions, there is no reason to do any training which involves stretching and flexibility. This should be reserved for children who have had muscle injuries of such a nature that they needed to seek medical help.

# Technique training

Skill in moving is worse in children than in adults — they are clumsy and find it difficult to perform different movements in quick succession. In all sports, not least in football, it is necessary to be able to move both quickly and precisely. During a fairly easy movement for adults, such as kicking a football, almost all the large muscles in the body must be able to contract and relax again or vice-versa. A certain skill and training both are required. It is therefore difficult for a little child to kick a ball.

A normal child's rate of maturation cannot be accelerated through exercise. Therefore it is of no use to do cycling exercise before the brain is ready for it. In the same way a child cannot train in footballing technique before it has reached a certain degree of maturity. When the brain has matured enough for a movement to be performed, it is easy — and fun — to learn, and the knowledge is saved forever in the brain's memory for automatic movement.

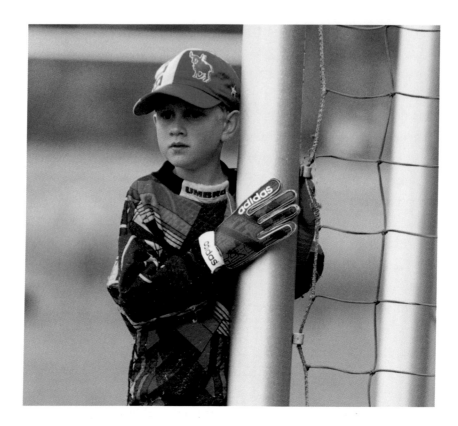

This type of knowledge can be compared to a computer program in the cerebellum. It takes a certain amount of time to install the program, but when it has been done well it often works smoothly. Incorrect patterns of movement can also be learned through training and they are just as permanent. Changing an incorrect pattern is, however, significantly more difficult than learning a new one — the incorrect behaviour must first be erased, which is difficult and time-consuming.

It is therefore important that even the youngest players learn good technique. This means that there should be a well-qualified or even the best technical coaches at this level.

It is, however, not only nerve impulses to a specific muscle which must go where they are supposed to, but the brain must also mature in order to be able to deal correctly with all the impulses

## TRAINING FOR CHILDREN

- Children's fitness and muscle strength can be developed, but not with as good results as in adults.
- Children nearly always have normal joint flexibility and therefore do not need to develop this specially.
- Lactic acid training is almost impossible to do with children.
- Technique training is important for children.
- Children should have fun when they train and play football!

from different sensory organs. Therefore, there is a gradual refinement of movement in the brain and technique becomes gradually more and more accomplished.

It takes a longer time for children's brains to receive and send out impulses, which means that movements take longer and are perceived as awkward or clumsy. In the same way a certain maturity is required for them to acquire an understanding of the game and to be able to learn its tactical aspects.

# Over-training

Over-training can also occur in children, although in principle they are less prone to it than adults. Over-training results in a feeling of the whole body being 'tired and heavy'. In addition, the player becomes depressed and occasionally develops increased sensitivity to infection. Often a child who trains hard goes to see a doctor about recurrent infections, which can be a symptom of excessive or incorrect training. It is quite uncommon that neither the child nor the parents have thought that the various symptoms might be due to too much

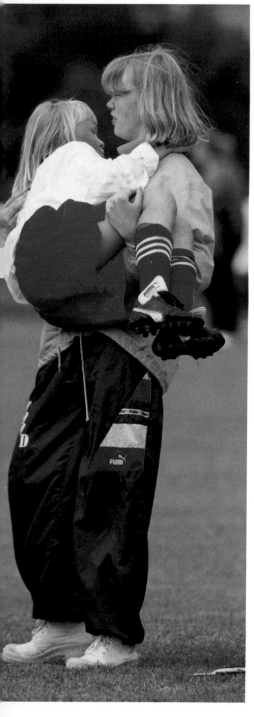

training, but rather are worried that it might be some kind of physical problem.

There is also a corresponding mental phenomenon, where prolonged training can result in exhaustion. It is quite simply not as much fun to play football any more! Coaches must understand that poor performance on the pitch can be due to over-training, which means that children who are not in good form perhaps need to rest instead of training more.

## Particular problems in girls

Intensive training for young girls can lead to delayed puberty. In extreme cases this can affect the development of the body in a permanent, negative fashion. In particular, if failure to menstruate is combined with inappropriate diet, impaired growth of the bones can be a possible consequence.

In the event of a girl showing a tendency to want to train more and harder than the rest of the team, especially hard fitness training, and in addition, wants to train on her own, one should be attentive to the risk of anorexia. For some girls sport can be an excuse to be able to train in order to lose weight. Indications that things are not all right are if the girl loses weight and refuses food and sweets even when it is obvious that she should be hungry. If the coach notices any such tendency, either a doctor or the school nurse should be contacted to obtain professional help. Early treatment gives better results than when the illness is revealed by clear symptoms. Eating disorders are, however, a lesser problem in football than in endurance and artistic sports (see Chapter 24). Boys can also suffer from anorexia, but it is much less common.

## Sports injuries in children

A minority of sports injuries in children are due to congenital weaknesses, such as congenital excessive laxity in the joints. A slightly larger number are due to improper training while the majority cannot be explained by anything other than the inherent risks of playing football.

The risk of injury in footballing activity is much less for children than for adults, and even if they are injured, the injury heals more quickly and with less risk of permanent damage.

During the spurt in growth in puberty it is thought that adolescents are especially susceptible to certain injuries. Excessive stress injuries may be due to the fact that strength and

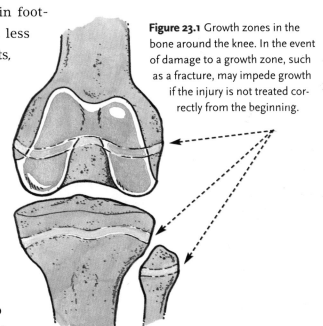

**Figure 23.1** Growth zones in the bone around the knee. In the event of damage to a growth zone, such as a fracture, may impede growth if the injury is not treated correctly from the beginning.

## INJURIES IN CHILDREN

- The most serious injuries are those which result in damage to the growth zones in the bone or cartilage. This can lead to lasting and, in time, aggravated injuries.
- Normal strain from training has a positive effect on the development of the joints and bones – too much strain is detrimental.
- In children, ligaments are two to five times stronger than cartilage and the bone's growth zones, which leads to broken bones and fractures affecting these sensitive growth plates. On the other hand, ligament damage is unusual in children.

flexibility do not develop at the same rate, and stereotyped movements from adult training may result in undue stress. At the same time, the amount of training at this age dramatically increases for those who decide to put a great deal into their sport. Competition becomes more and more important, which further increases the risk of injury. At the same time, the pattern of injury changes from that of a child to that of an adult.

### Overuse injuries

Overuse injuries can be characterized as inflammations which are caused by minor but frequent injuries. The typical place for young footballers to be affected is the heel (Haglund's disease) and the patellar tendon's attachment to the front of the lower leg (Errand-boy's disease or Osgood-Schlatter's disease).

Around 60 per cent of all overuse injuries in children can probably be attributed to improper training, with excessive intensity and insufficient variety being the most significant factors. In all cases of strain injuries, a reduction in the amount of training is the first and most important step. The next most important step is to try to explain why the injury occurred, in order to be able to prevent it recurring. In the meantime, there is nothing to stop the child being part of the social group around training, and becoming involved in something which does not place strain on the injured part — if anything, the case is the opposite.

### Fracture of the clavicle

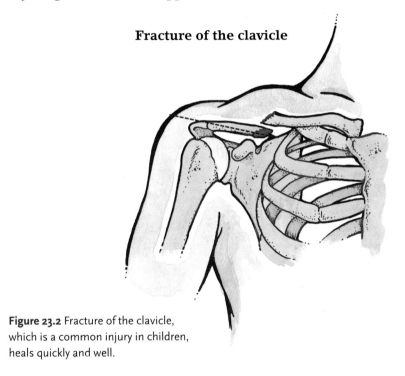

**Figure 23.2** Fracture of the clavicle, which is a common injury in children, heals quickly and well.

This is the most common sports injury of significance in children, especially younger children. The injury can be diagnosed by means of examination by a doctor and usually does not need to be radiographed. Clavicle injuries heal without any particular treatment and the child is generally back playing football again after 3–4 weeks. A small bump at the point where the fracture occurred may remain for a few months or more, but has no importance other than cosmetic.

## Dislocation of the shoulder

Dislocation results in a complete inability to move the shoulder, but causes no pain as long as it is held still. The articular head must be put back in place as soon as possible, for which the child should be taken to the nearest casualty department. Adolescents who have dislocated a shoulder have a high risk of recurring dislocations and should discuss continuing doing sport and training with a sports doctor or a specialist physiotherapist. The risk of recurring dislocation is greatest in young players aged between 16 and 20 years, around 60–70 per cent. In the case of repeated recurrence, surgery is often necessary.

## Fracture of the elbow
## (supracondylar fracture of the humerus)

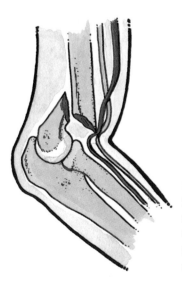

**Figure 23.3** In the event of fracture of the humerus there is a great risk of damage to the nerves and blood vessels from the sharp ends of the fracture. The injury must always be treated with the highest priority.

Fracture of the elbow is a treacherous injury which can occur in children before puberty when they fall with their arms under them. If there is pain in the elbow when it is moved following an injury of this type, the child should be examined as soon as possible, as there is a risk of damage to the nerves and blood vessels. Emergency surgery is often necessary.

### Fracture of the wrist and lower arm

This is a relatively common football injury in children (but uncommon in adult footballers), which heals quickly and without any residual problems, although the fracture sometimes affects the growth plate of the radius. The injury must always be examined by a doctor and radiographs should be taken. If there is any malposition, the fracture must be reduced and then placed in a cast for 3–6 weeks, depending on where the fracture is.

### Inflammation of the hip joint (coxitis)

Inflammation of the hip joint can affect boys of pre-school age. They cannot say exactly where it hurts, but usually complain that their 'leg hurts'. An otherwise healthy child who, for more than a day, does not want to run because their leg hurts should be examined by a doctor.

### Coxa plana (Perthes disease)

This is a disorder of the hip which mostly affects boys in their early years at school. The symptoms are that the hip and leg hurt when they try to run and they may limp slightly. These boys must be examined by a doctor and radiographs taken, among other things. Unlike in the case of simple coxitis, they cannot play football for many months. These boys often visit a doctor complaining of pain in the knee.

The problem lies in the hip joint, but even so, the pain is sometimes located in the knee area. The hip joint should therefore always be examined in children who start to limp and/or suffer from pain in the knee.

### Fracture of the femur

Fracture of the femur occurs in isolated cases in football. It can seem very dramatic, but heals well with the right treatment and football can normally be fully resumed in 4–6 months.

### Loose cartilage fragments in the knee (osteochondritis)

Loose fragments of cartilage in the knee can affect children in their early years at school. Simple examination cannot distinguish this from meniscus damage. If cartilage damage is suspected (locking of the knee, recurrent and stabbing pain) the child should be sent to an orthopaedic surgeon for examination. Children and adolescents with swelling in the knee joint should always undergo radiographic examination. In certain cases, arthroscopy may be necessary to remove loose fragments of cartilage.

### Meniscus damage

Meniscus damage is rare in children, but the injury becomes more common in puberty. If a child cannot straighten the knee or it locks in certain positions, meniscus damage must be suspected. With suspected meniscus damage, arthroscopic inspection is recommended. A secure diagnosis can then be made and any meniscus damage can be treated. Generally, a damaged part of the meniscus is removed, but in certain cases the meniscus can be repaired. A specific complaint is discoid meniscus, which gives rise to painful cracking and locking, generally related to the lateral (outer) meniscus. Treatment is surgical. Assessment should be made by a specialist orthopaedic surgeon.

### Cruciate and collateral ligament damage in the knee

These injuries are, as with meniscus damage, uncommon among children, but occur more often with increasing age. On twisting of the knee — but not following a direct blow — cruciate ligament and collateral ligament injuries can arise. Diagnosis can be made by any doctor trained in sports medicine, but should be treated by a specialist orthopaedic surgeon.

Surgery on a cruciate ligament injury can be performed even on children with open growth plates. This is true either if a fragment of bone has become detached from the tibia (the cruciate

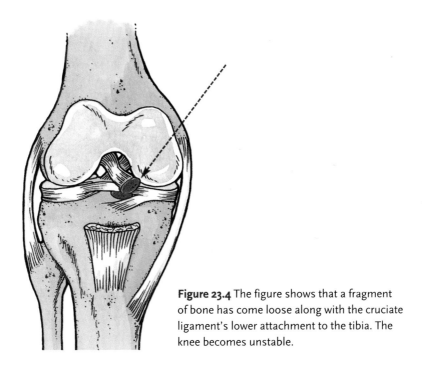

**Figure 23.4** The figure shows that a fragment of bone has come loose along with the cruciate ligament's lower attachment to the tibia. The knee becomes unstable.

ligament can be reattached to the bone) or if the cruciate ligament itself is damaged and cruciate ligament reconstruction has to be carried out. New studies show that surgery on adolescents, who have reached puberty, involving the drilling of small channels through the growth plates does not impede growth or result in risk of complications in the future. Treated correctly, the injury heals without permanent damage, while incorrectly treated injuries can give problems throughout one's life.

### Osgood-Schlatter's disease

This is one of the most common reasons for a child to seek help for a sports injury. It is an overuse injury in the area where the patellar tendon attaches to the lower leg. Diagnosis is simple: typical age, bilateral problem and pain precisely in the bony protuberance in the upper part of the front of the lower leg. Treatment consists of communicating the information effectively: the less the child runs, the less the pain will be. Previously, children with Osgood-Schlatter's disease were recommended to refrain from playing football, but to-day the child is advised to continue playing on condition that the coach is informed and can give special training advice. There are many activities, such as technique training, which can be carried out with no problems and there is absolutely no risk of playing sport, even with the pain. However, if the pain persists, even after the above changes have been made to training, help should be sought from a sports doctor.

### Patello-femoral pain

This is a condition which affects teenagers. Treatment is almost always similar to that for Osgood-Schlatter's disease in its first phase, but if the problem persists for a relatively long time, or is very intense, it is advisable to seek help from a sports doctor or a sports physiotherapist. With a specially designed rehabilitation programme, lasting relief is often achieved.

### Dislocation of the patella

Dislocation of the patella is a typical childhood sporting injury, which principally affects girls. The patella often spontaneously moves back into place when the knee is straightened. After any dislocation, help should be sought from an orthopaedic surgeon within a few days to discuss treatment which can prevent re-dislocation initially rehabilitation. In certain cases surgery becomes necessary.

### Periostitis

Periostitis affects mainly older adolescents and is caused by excessive training or poor technique. Occasionally better football boots, temporary use of running shoes or taping can reduce the problems but generally the most important action is to reduce the level of activity for a few weeks. Thereafter, the type of training which resulted in the problem should be avoided and strength should gradually be built up in the leg over the long term.

## Sprained ankles

Sprained ankles occur less frequently in children than in adults. With a sprained ankle, it is important to reduce the tendency to swelling by promptly applying an elastic bandage. A child who cannot support himself on his foot and who walks slowly should be examined by a doctor within 24 h. Radiographs are rarely needed if the swelling is minor and a fracture is not suspected. Unlike the case of adults, it is important not to force rehabilitation, but rather give the injury time to heal. Generally taping of sprained ankles in children should not be advised.

## Heel pain

Pain in the heel is not unusual in children in their first years at school. Unlike in adults, it is not the Achilles' tendon itself which is affected but rather the tendon's attachment to the bone, i.e. called the apophysis. This is a specific injury in children, which is treated by reducing activity and changing to football boots with good shock absorption. Children can, without risk of future problems, continue to take part in football training, but should avoid running activities and concentrate more on, for example technique training.

# 24. Specific aspects of women's football

Peter Adolfsson, Harald Roos and Anna Östenberg

There are certain fundamentals which are the same for both men and women football players, but there are also large differences which coaches and other team personnel must consider. Besides anatomical and physiological differences between the sexes, there are also differences in behaviour, for example in attitude to team-mates and the sport, and also in motivation and perception of themselves. Girls' social intercourse is often characterized by closeness and feelings of solidarity while activity and performance come first with boys. Performance on the pitch can, as far as boys are concerned, have a direct bearing on their placing in the team, which is not common among girls.

When a boy moves up from a junior team to a senior team, he generally sees it as something positive. He receives more respect from players in the junior and senior teams and that is looked on as a real achievement. For a girl, a similar change might be more prob-lematic, as she must then form new relationships and find new con-fidence.

If coaches and other team personnel understand and are aware of these differences, training for girls and women can develop further.

# Female training physiology

Until puberty the physical and psychological differences between girls and boys are small. Puberty starts on average 2 years earlier in girls (10–11 years of age) than boys (12–13 years of age). This means that girls develop earlier, physically and psychologically, which leads to their being able to tolerate higher training loads at an earlier age. Individual differences are, however, large within each sex. During growth girls develop greater stamina and better coordination than boys, while boys, on the other hand, develop more 'brute strength'.

Aerobic working capacity is lower in women. Women have approximately 70 per cent of men's maximum capacity for oxygen absorption. This is due, to a large extent, to differences in body size and composition. If working capacity is given in relation to body weight, the difference is 15 per cent and in relation to body weight without

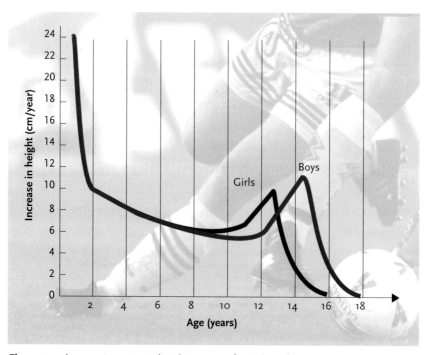

**Figure 24.1** Average increase in height per year for girls and boys.

fat only 10–15 per cent. Any remaining differences are due largely to differences in heart size and blood levels.

Although men have a higher maximum working capacity, they have a shorter time to exhaustion with a rate of work at 70–80 per cent of maximum capacity for oxygen absorption. It is believed that this is due to women's ability to utilize fat burning during exertion. Oestrogen has been shown to increase the ability to burn fat and reduce the usage of carbohydrates. Women generally have a higher proportion of fat in the composition of their bodies. In the 15–30 year-old age range, 26 per cent of average weight consists of fat, while the corresponding figure for men is 15 per cent. A high proportion of body fat is negative from the point of view of performance when the body is moving vertically, such as when running, but is positive if one has to swim long distances.

Women have approximately 70 per cent of men's muscle strength in the lower body and 50 per cent in the upper body. The difference is partly due to women being smaller than men. An examination of strength in proportion to area of a cross-section of muscle reveals that there is, however, no difference. Nor has it been possible to demonstrate any difference in the relative development of fatigue or feeling of tiredness between the sexes.

## Blood haemoglobin concentration (Hb level)

Haemoglobin in the red blood cells has two important functions. It transports oxygen from the lungs throughout the body, and also waste products, such as carbon dioxide, back to the lungs where they are removed in exhaled air. Haemoglobin contains iron compounds, which bond to oxygen.

Women generally have a lower Hb level than men. Because haemoglobin transports oxygen, a reduction in this level therefore leads to a reduction in performance. Women footballers have a greater iron requirement than male players. Iron deficiency is more common in female players, but the effects of iron supplements have not produced unequivocally positive results.

### Sources of iron in food

Iron in food exists as both 'haem' (in blood products and meat) and non-haem (in cereals and vegetables).

The volume and duration of blood loss affect both blood and iron levels. One in five pre-menopausal women has iron deficiency due to losses resulting from menstruation and around 10 per cent of sportswomen suffer from iron deficiency. However, with iron deficiency the body's ability to absorb iron increases, which can be taken advantage of by eating especially iron-rich food. Iron supplements in tablet form should be taken and monitored by a doctor.

# Menstruation and performance

A woman's first menstruation normally occurs between the ages of 12 and 15 years. Menstruation then normally lasts 3–8 days and recurs after 23–25 days. There are large individual variations.

For most women there does not seem to be any reduction in performance associated with menstruation. Variation in performance has been shown to be marginal during the menstrual cycle. There are, however, studies which point to greater hand-strength

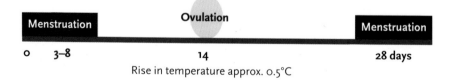

**Figure 24.2** Menstruation cycle.

and an ability to jump further in a standing long jump during menstruation. An increase in performance during certain times of the menstrual cycle means that training during different times of the menstrual cycle could be adapted to suit this. Research is in progress in this area.

One study has shown an increased incidence of injuries just before and during menstruation. Women who took the contraceptive pill presented fewer injuries. This may be due to the fact that the contraceptive pill affects a woman's psychological state during menstruation, which in itself can affect performance and risk of injury.

There can occasionally be a desire to postpone menstruation, such as before a tournament or an important play-off, linked to the fact that the woman suffers from period pains. Contact a doctor in good time for consultation and planning.

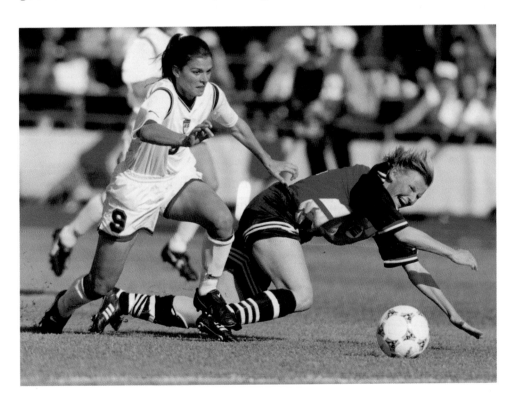

## Menstrual disturbances

### *Dysmenorrhea (period pains)*

Some women suffer heavy, painful periods. It is important that these women receive suitable treatment. There are several alternative forms of this. Regular exercise at whatever level has been shown to reduce pain during menstruation.

### *Amenorrhea (absence of menstruation)*

Primary amenorrhoea is the name given to the condition where menstruation has not begun by the age of 16. Secondary amenorrhoea is the condition where a woman has interrupted menstruation for more than 3 months.

An increased incidence of menstrual disturbances has been observed in very fit women, especially with intense physical exercise. Extremely intense exercise before the beginning of menstruation entails an increased risk of later disturbances. There can be a number of causes of menstrual disturbances in very fit women — even factors such as insufficient food intake, low body fat and stress can have an influence.

Increased fibre intake in food for a long time can lead to a lower level of the female hormone oestrogen. Vegetarian food contains a great deal of fibre and a greater frequency of menstrual disturbances has been observed among vegetarians.

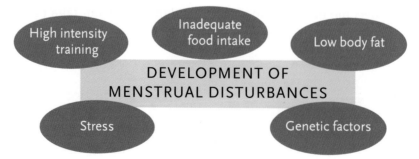

**Figure 24.3** Significant factors for the development of menstrual disturbances in sportswomen.

# Stress fractures

The skeleton develops at an early age and reaches its maximum strength between 18 and 25 years of age. Physical activity has a positive effect on bone strength and young girls who play football have been shown to develop stronger bones in the back and legs. Brittle bones are more subject to injuries, such as stress fractures. There are several causes of stress fracture:

- Repeated overuse during training.
- Brittle bones – menstrual disturbances, insufficient food intake, low body fat.

### Overuse during training

Overuse injuries can be due to high levels of strain at individual moments during training or the total volume of exercise being too high. Changes in the quality and amount of training, surface also have an influence.

### Menstrual disturbances

Hard physical exercise can periodically lead to failure to ovulate and menstruate. Women then have a relatively low level of the female sex hormone oestrogen, as this is mainly formed in the cells surrounding the egg. Osseous tissue is dependent on oestrogen and bones become more brittle if this stimulation does not take place. Oestrogen has positive effects on bone.

- It reduces bone resorption.
- It stimulates the absorption of calcium from the intestine, which is required to build stronger bones.
- It stimulates the formation of vitamin D, which is of benefit to the bones.

499

*Inadequate energy intake*

Excessively low energy intake results in an increased risk of menstrual disturbances and thus the importance of food. Oestrogen supplements in the form of contraceptive pills have a positive influence on bone mass, especially among women with amenorrhoea or anorexia.

*Low body fat*

Low body fat also contributes to a decline in female sex hormones. If, in addition to failure to ovulate and menstruate, body fat is low, this leads to a greater decline in oestrogen. Normalization of body fat and menstrual cycle, on the other hand, leads to an improvement in bone mass.

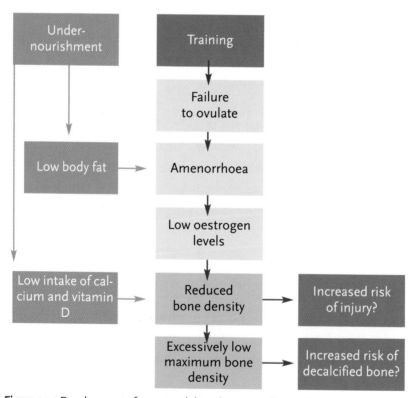

**Figure 24.4** Development of menstrual disturbances and possible consequences.

Insufficient energy intake in relation to the energy consumption that training entails has an effect on body fat. A negative balance of energy may also have an influence on central hormone regulation. It is unclear whether it is fat content or balance of energy which has the greatest influence. The influence of food is, however, very great.

## Food, nourishment and eating disorders

To achieve maximum performance and keep the body free from injury, it is important to eat the right food. Several studies have shown that some sportswomen have too low an energy intake in relation to the energy they consume. Dieting is therefore a health risk for anyone who trains a great deal. There is a very fine line between what is intended to be dieting and illnesses such as anorexia nervosa and bulimia nervosa.

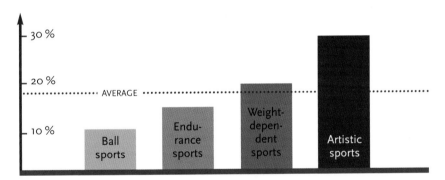

**Figure 24.5** Occurrence of eating disorders in different sports.

### Anorexia nervosa

Eating disorders are more common among top-level sportsmen and women than others. The occurrence of anorexia in ball sports is somewhat lower than in endurance and artistic sports. The basic cause of sports anorexia is a high level of physical activity combined with difficulty to eat enough to redress the balance between

## SIGNS OF ANOREXIA

- Increased interest in food, weight and physical activity. Weight loss and growth disturbances.
- Dissatisfaction with performance and appearance, disturbed feelings about one's body.
- Psychological changes such as self-centredness, restlessness, depression, irritability and social isolation.
- Menstrual disorders.

## SIGNS OF BULIMIA

- Tooth decay, sores in the corners of the mouth.
- Laryngitis, swelling of the salivary glands.
- Hair loss, sores on hands, dry skin.
- Coronary dysrhythmia.
- Stomach aches, intestinal problems (constipation and diarrhoea).
- Menstrual disturbances.

energy requirement and energy intake. Another casual factor is a strong desire to achieve good results. Many young sportswomen also have insufficient understanding of general nutrition.

Sports anorexia appears less serious than 'normal' anorexia. Weight loss is not as great and perception of one's own body is not disturbed to the same extent.

### Bulimia nervosa (compulsive eating)

For some, the solution can be to throw up what they have eaten or to use laxatives to rid themselves more quickly of food. This can in turn lead to bouts of compulsive eating followed by renewed vomiting and so on. Repeated vomiting means that the mucous membrane, throat, mouth and teeth are exposed to the hydrochloric acid which is normally to be found in the stomach and one of the consequences is erosion of tooth enamel.

An anorectic or bulimic needs the support of others, but generally also professional help. It is important for coaches and other team personnel to be on the lookout for signs of eating disorders, as well as not making apparently innocent comments about weight and physical appearance. At the 'wrong' time, this can have very negative consequences.

# Pregnancy

A pregnancy involves great changes in a woman's body and among other things blood pressure drops and heart rate increases. The hormonal effect makes the flexibility of connective tissue and ligaments increase, which in itself results in an increased risk of ligament damage. Every pregnancy is unique and it is therefore difficult to give general advice. Each woman must make her own decisions based on her own specific situation.

### Training during pregnancy

Being physically active during pregnancy has only advantages, as the capacity to cope with both physical and psychological stress is greater at this time. Most studies show a number of advantages with exercise.

- The exertion involved in childbirth feels less severe.
- The mother can cope better with pain.
- Childbirth takes less time.
- Children exhibit less stress during birth.

Negative effects of physical activity during pregnancy such as miscarriage or stillbirth have not been proved. The newborn child, however, weighs less and women who train during pregnancy put on less weight. As always, it is important to listen to the body's signals. If anything abnormal is felt, one should stop training and see a doctor for a check-up. Pregnant women with the following conditions should, however, not train without first having a medical examination:

- Medical illnesses
- Twin pregnancy
- Pregnancy complications involving haemorrhages, rise in blood pressure, stunted growth of the fetus, premature labour.

## GENERAL ADVICE

- Training should be low-intensity with heart rate <140/min, especially during the last 3 months.
- Avoid training in warm, damp weather.
- Avoid training with very heavy loading (anaerobic exercise).
- Avoid intensive weight training.
- Avoid abdominal muscle exercises and exercising in a lying position during the last 3 months.
- Non-weight carrying exercise such as swimming has a positive effect, because among other things it also counteracts swelling in the legs.

### Training after pregnancy

Training can be resumed when the woman feels ready. The length of time it takes to go back to full-scale activity cannot be predicted. The woman must decide herself if training feels right. If she has continued training during pregnancy, however, returning to it is made easier. When training after pregnancy, it is important to include pelvic floor exercises. Certain studies show a kind of 'doping effect' from pregnancy in moderately fit individuals, with improved maximum capacity for oxygen absorption for several weeks following childbirth. There are no general studies to indicate any such positive effect on performance.

## Increased risk of knee injuries among women

In football, the risk of anterior cruciate ligament injury is greater in women players than in men. This is true for all age groups but the greatest difference is in the younger age group.

Many attempts have been made to identify the reason for these differences in injury risk between the sexes with the aim of being able to prevent these injuries. A reduction in cruciate ligament injuries would not only be positive in the short term, but would also mean that the risk of any premature joint wear might also be reduced (see Chapter 22).

**Why do women footballers have more knee injuries?**
It has been argued that cruciate ligament injuries at an early age among women may be the result of the fact that there is less competition to play in A-teams in women's football. The consequence of this can be that a good junior player has a chance to play A-team football as early as the age of 16. The faster pace, greater intensity and the physically stronger and perhaps heavier players which the girl has to face, can lead to an increased risk of injury. As a consequence of this reasoning, the suggestion has been put forward that a lower age limit be set for women to play in an A-team. Against this, on the one hand, there is evidence that most cruciate ligament injuries in women's football occur without any physical contact, and on the other hand, that there is also a significantly increased risk of

cruciate ligament injury in junior football among girls. There are more factors which are of significance including strain due to training and coordination.

Most cruciate ligament injuries in women occur without any contact with opponents. One injury mechanism which has been described is that the player lands with the knee outstretched after jumping. The increased susceptibility to injury among women in situations where there is contact with opponents has been considered the result of inferior muscle strength to men. No absolutely conclusive evidence for this has emerged, but it has been shown that women have relatively stronger quadriceps muscles on the front of the thigh than the hamstring muscles on the back of the thigh. The hamstring muscles reinforce the function of the anterior cruciate ligament, while the quadriceps are antagonistic to the function of the cruciate ligament. Studies indicate that the balance between muscle strength in the front and back of the thigh is different in male and female players. Women have an excess of strength in the front muscles and also activate the muscles in the front first to a greater extent in the course of a twist. There is no controlled study, however, to show how intensive training of the thigh muscles to achieve the right muscle balance and energy pattern might prevent anterior cruciate ligament damage.

In a joint, there is normally a certain amount of play which is limited

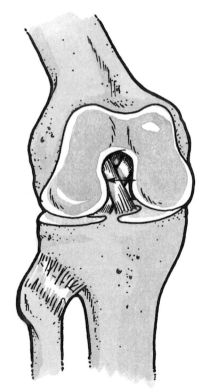

**Figure 24.6** Limited space in the centre of the knee (the intercondylar notch) could be a cause of susceptibility to cruciate ligament damage among women.

by the joint capsule and ligaments. This play is called laxity and there are specific assessments to determine the degree of laxity. Generally greater laxity in women has also been put forward as an explanation. In a recent study of women footballers an increased general risk of injury for female players with increased joint laxity was observed. The study did not show, however, whether that was true especially for knee injuries or only injuries in general. There are also other studies which show that there is an over-representation of individuals with increased laxity among women who were injured playing football. It was not clear whether this is also the case among men.

Limited space (compared with men) in the centre of the knee (the intercondylar notch) has also been discussed as a cause of increased susceptibility to cruciate ligament damage among women.

The anterior cruciate ligament can probably become trapped in this central space and snap against the edge of the bone when the knee is twisted. This relative tightness often occurs in both knee joints. Surgically widening the corresponding space in the healthy knee has been discussed as a preventive measure. However, there is no evidence to justify any such operation. The narrower space in the centre of the knee may also be an indication that the cruciate ligament is narrower and thus weaker, with an increased risk of being damaged upon twisting.

### What are the consequences of an increased risk of cruciate ligament damage among women?

Anterior cruciate ligament damage is relatively uncommon, but even so, a senior team in the women's premier division anticipates one such injury a season. For any one individual this is a large setback in her career and entails an absence from football of at least 6 months and often up to a year. Not all players return to the game even with surgery and the best possible rehabilitation. There are reports of women having less chance of returning after anterior cruciate ligament injury than men. There may be many reasons for this other than purely physical ones, such as social factors, insufficient motivation, etc.

Furthermore, there may be long-term negative effects involving a risk of joint wear (arthrosis). The dominant mechanism of injury in women, that is no contact with an opponent, can be viewed favourably from another aspect. With an anterior cruciate ligament injury which occurs without contact, further injuries to the knee such as meniscus and cruciate ligament damage occur less often. An isolated cruciate ligament injury has in all likelihood a better long-term prognosis. With anterior cruciate ligament damage in male players on the other hand, there is often damage also to other tissues in the knee.

# 25. The role of the referee

Lars-Åke Björck and Jan Ekstrand

## Why are rules and referees needed?

According to the Federation of International Football Association (FIFA) the rules of football are designed to:

- Safeguard the game
- Safeguard the players
- Safeguard the spectators.

The rules are there to safeguard the players from dirty, violent play where injuries can occur. They also safeguard the individual player by enforcing requirements for equipment design.

The rules are also intended to safeguard the game and the spectators and are formulated in such a way that makes football attractive and interesting. Technical players should not, for example, be eliminated by means of rough, violent play. This results in, among other things, fewer goals and fewer exciting situations, which in the long term can result in the spectators being disappointed.

Football is a competitive game where there must be a neutral person, the referee, to see that the rules are followed. In other words, the referee has an important job to do in applying the rules to safeguard the game, the players and the spectators.

# Which rules might be associated with risk of injury?

The referee's tool is the Laws of the Game. The decision-making body in charge of formulating rules for football throughout the world is the IFAB (International Football Association Board) which comprises eight members, one each from England, Scotland, Wales and Northern Ireland and four from FIFA. The IFAB was formed in 1896 by the four British football associations and since then has had 'sole right' to draw up rules (FIFA started to take part in IFAB's work in 1913).

It was not until the 1990s that the rules were changed in any tangible way — not only to make the game faster and more attractive, but also to prevent rough, violent play. Stricter interpretation of the rules was introduced particularly with the aim of preventing injury. The following rules have some bearing on the risk of injury.

### Rule 1 — The pitch

The referee should check the pitch before the match. The goals must be constructed in such a way that players cannot be injured due to them being badly constructed or insufficiently anchored in the ground.

In international matches there are also regulations regarding how close advertising signs may be placed to the pitch, and how close behind the goal photographers may get. The aim is to prevent injuries if a player unintentionally ends up off the pitch.

### Rule 2 — The ball

This rule regulates the dimensions and weight of the ball. Here the emphasis is on the fact that no part of the ball should be a danger to the players.

### Rule 4 — The players' equipment

This is the fundamental rule for safeguarding the individual player and his or her opponents. A player may not use equipment or wear

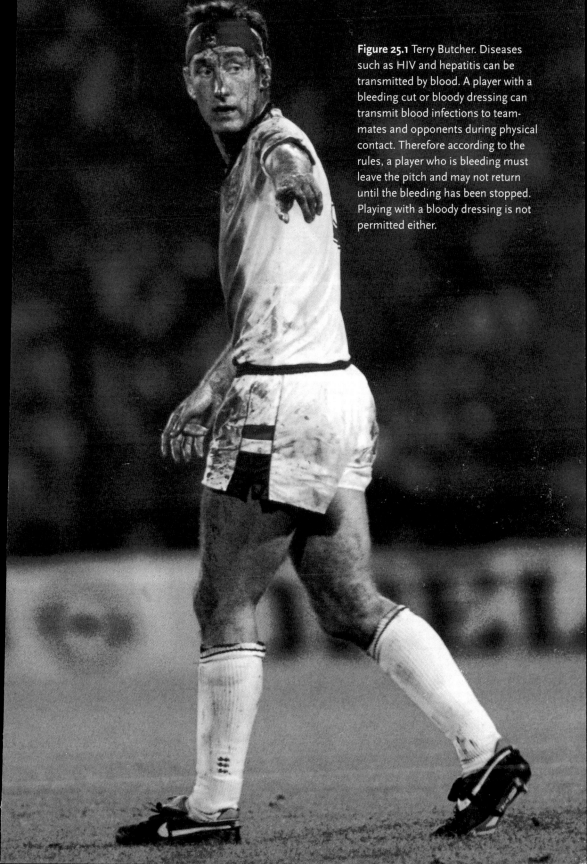

**Figure 25.1** Terry Butcher. Diseases such as HIV and hepatitis can be transmitted by blood. A player with a bleeding cut or bloody dressing can transmit blood infections to team-mates and opponents during physical contact. Therefore according to the rules, a player who is bleeding must leave the pitch and may not return until the bleeding has been stopped. Playing with a bloody dressing is not permitted either.

anything which is dangerous to him or herself or to another player (also includes all forms of jewellery).

A player who wants to use any protection or dressing made of plastic, plaster, or comprising metallic parts or any other hard material, must pad any such dressing so that it is not dangerous to his or her team-mates and opponents. Padding means that the hard parts of the dressing should be covered with foam rubber, elastic bandages or any other soft material. The referee must approve the dressing before play is permitted.

What is most important and nowadays obligatory in all football matches, is the use of shin pads. The rule clearly states that the shin pads should be completely covered by the socks, be produced of suitable material and offer satisfactory protection (see Chapter 3). The referee should check the players' boots and other equipment before the match.

As far as boots and their studs are concerned, the rules no longer state what size they should be – it is the referee who has the final say as to whether someone can play or not, basing his or her decision on the grounds 'if it is a danger to him or herself or another player'.

### Rule 5 — The referee

This rule deals with the referee's authority on the pitch. Here it is clearly stated that the referee must stop the match if, in his or her opinion, a player is seriously injured and then ensure that they quickly receive medical attention or is taken off the pitch.

Furthermore, the referee should make sure that any player bleeding from a cut leaves the pitch. The player may only return following a signal from the referee, who must then be convinced that the bleeding has stopped.

### Rule 12 — Unlawful play and unsuitable conduct

This rule refers to the referee's duty to safeguard players from injury by awarding free kicks (penalty kicks for the attacking team inside the penalty area) for unlawful play. The following are examples of offences which are considered as unlawful play: knocking down, kicking, punching, pushing and similar attacks or attempts at attacks on opponents. Slide tackles on opponents where the tackler hits the player but not the ball, tackling from behind and kicks aimed at the head also constitute unlawful play. Unsuitable behaviour, such as spitting at opponents or deliberately handling the ball, also come under this rule.

What is important in Rule 12 is the increasing enforcement (interpretation) of the direct sending-off rule. The referee should show the red card when he or she considers that a player has been guilty of violent or uncontrolled behaviour or unlawful play.

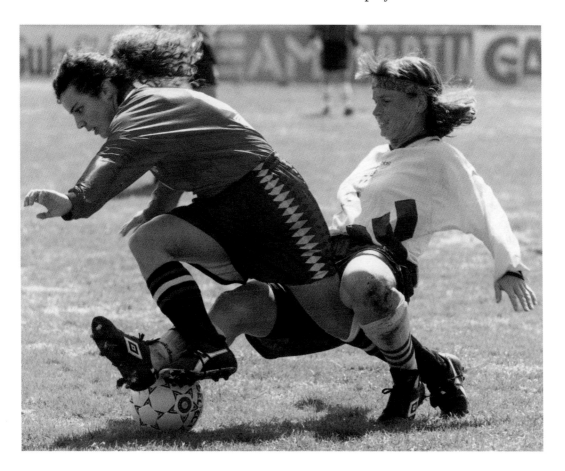

The most common example of this is play with the studs first, regardless of whether the attacking player does this from the front, behind or from the sides. Any player who goes into a situation is obliged to do it in such a way that there is no risk of injuring an opponent or themselves. Note that a dirty tackle can lead to the offender themselves being injured.

In any situation where an injury occurs or where a tackle is performed incorrectly, it is the referee who decides on disciplinary action.

# Application of the rules

In all large football tournaments, the referees and assistant referees meet before the start of the tournament to draw up a common standard for decision making. Before every season, a similar process takes place in all countries. If everyone follows FIFA's referee committee's recommendation, there will be a uniform interpretation of the rules and thus significantly fewer injuries.

### Injuries should be assessed on the pitch
### but treated off the pitch

Proper cooperation between medical personnel and the referee is important for the referees to be able to fulfil their obligation to prevent an injury being aggravated. It is therefore important that the referees receive certain medical information during their training. It is the referee who must decide whether an injured player needs medical attention or not.

The rules say that the team's medical personnel may only come on to the pitch if the referee considers that an injury is serious and requires medical attention. In the case of unconsciousness or other injury which the referee judges to be serious, medical personnel are called in immediately. If there is any doubt, the basic rule is that

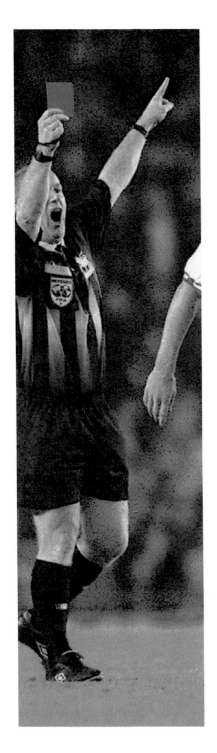

the referee asks the player: 'Do you need medical attention?' If the player then answers that they do, help is called for. As a rule no more than two people can come on to the pitch and then only after being called by the referee.

The referee's reason for calling medical personnel is that the nature and the degree of severity of the injury can be assessed. So as not to delay the game, this assessment should be performed in the quickest possible way. Treatment of the injury and a more comprehensive assessment of whether the player can or cannot continue should, on the other hand, take place off the pitch. Treatment on the pitch should be limited to serious injuries, such as unconsciousness, severe bleeding and shock or a broken bone where rash movement could aggravate the injury.

Competition regulations state that all grounds must be equipped with stretchers and in international matches a stretcher is often used to transport an injured player off the pitch

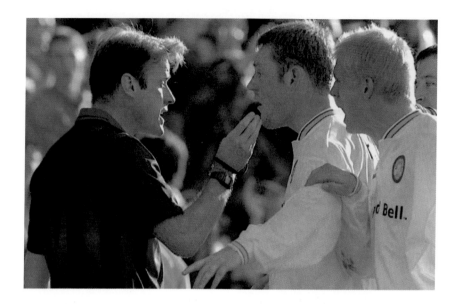

quickly. FIFA dictates that a doctor must accompany the stretcher on and that the player must leave the pitch either on or alongside the stretcher. Players who refuse to do so are penalized with a yellow card. In less serious situations it is up to the referee to decide how the player should leave the pitch. However, it is still required that any treatment should take place off the pitch.

Faking an injury also leads to showing the yellow card. A player should consider that faking injuries can lead to the wrong decision being taken in the event of 'real' injuries, where the referee wrongly suspects faking.

A player who leaves the pitch for treatment or closer examination must have a clear sign from the referee before he or she can return to play.

**Who is responsible for preventing injuries during a match?**
It is the referee's job to prevent dirty play by being in the right place on the pitch, interpreting a player's behaviour and body language (e.g. seeing if a player is on his way to 'get his own back') and taking decisive action if a player is guilty of rough, violent play.

A great deal happens during a match and the referee is subject to great psychological pressure. Referees nowadays have a deep understanding of the theory behind the rules and generally also the necessary ability to apply the rules properly. The referee should also be in good physical shape. However, sometimes wrong decisions are made. Often the referee's incorrect decisions or failure to act can be seen as a result of the fact that no one is always mentally and physically prepared or sufficiently fit.

The referee's most important task, is by means of correct application of the rules, to contribute to making football more attractive with no elements of violent, rough play and to prevent injuries occurring. The players and coaches, of course, also have a responsibility to act within the bounds of the rules so that football is overall fairer and more attractive to everyone. To achieve this, there must be cooperation between all parties involved in football and respect must be shown for each other's work and authority.

# 26. Travelling abroad with the team

Jan Ekstrand and John Crane

This chapter gives practical advice prior to travelling abroad. Running a training camp abroad is a considerable financial investment and it is therefore important that all squad members are able to participate from beginning to end.

## Vaccinations

The squad's vaccination cover should be reviewed thoroughly in good time before a trip abroad and the club's medical director should also check which vaccinations or other measures are recommended for the country of destination.

### Tetanus and diphtheria

A football player should be vaccinated against tetanus as spores of the disease can be normally found in soil and a player who has a cut or graze risks being infected.

Diphtheria is a common disease in many developing countries and an increasing number of cases have been reported in recent years from East European countries. When travelling to these countries, the players' vaccination cover for diphtheria should be reviewed.

### Polio

Polio is a viral disease that causes paralysis and is primarily spread through water. Its occurrence is related to the general hygiene and vaccination status of a country. Even if polio does not occur in the player's home country, they should be vaccinated when travelling abroad. The vaccine is administered into the arm.

## Hepatitis

Hepatitis is the collective name for inflammatory diseases of the liver. If contracted, hepatitis restricts the flow of bile, which leads to the pigment from the bile collecting in the blood causing yellowing of the skin and the whites of the eyes. The distinction is made between hepatitis A (epidemic hepatitis) and hepatitis B (serum hepatitis).

Hepatitis A is caused by a virus spread via human excrement which contaminates water or food. The disease occurs most commonly in tropical and subtropical regions. The better the water and food hygiene is in a country, the less likelihood there is of infection. When travelling around Europe, the risk is low. Passive immunization in the form of a gamma globulin injection or active immunization in the form of a vaccine such as Havrix© (a hepatitis A antigen) will provide protection against hepatitis A.

An injection of gamma globulin provides temporary protection for a period of 3 months. The substance is injected into a muscle, either in the buttock or (for outfield players) in the arm and should be administered as close to departure as possible.

For those who travel abroad often and who do not want to take gamma globulin prior to every trip, there is the option of being vaccinated (for example with Havrix©). The vaccination should be repeated after about 1 year. Protection is then provided for 20 years and the risk of side effects from the vaccination is minimal.

Hepatitis B is caused by a virus that is spread via contact with blood, saliva and other body fluids. Vaccination against hepatitis B is in the form of three injections where the second and third injections are given 1 and 6 months respectively, after the first. After this process is complete, a blood test should be carried out to ensure the presence of antibodies.

# Jet-lag

Flights across several time zones either in an east-to-west or west-to-east direction affect a person's diurnal rhythm and disturb the body's biological clock. Jet-lag itself does not affect performance but can cause a number of mental symptoms, leading to fatigue, sleep disturbance and reduced concentration, which in turn can impair performance.

The effect of jet-lag increases with the number of time zones crossed. The time difference between Europe and the United States, for example, is 6 (in Florida) to 9 (in California) hours, which means six to nine time zones have been crossed. Travelling east has less of an effect. Jet-lag affects every individual differently and to what extent each individual is affected varies from trip to trip. Younger, better-trained individuals are less affected. It takes about 1 day/time zone crossed for an individual to recuperate from jet-lag symptoms when travelling in a westerly direction.

# Match-time training

Performance is affected by a player's diurnal rhythm even without having been on an aeroplane. This varies considerably from player to player. A person who is at their best in the mornings performs to their maximum potential at about 11.00 am and already begins to tire at 3.00 pm. People who prefer evenings reach their maximum performance capacity at about 4.00 pm. This can be affected by a variety of things.

Prior to an important match, it may be worthwhile adjusting the diurnal rhythm so that the body gets used to performing at its best at a particular time of the day. This is accomplished by having training sessions at the same time of day as a match to be played a few days ahead.

## THE FOLLOWING MEASURES MAY ALLEVIATE JET-LAG

1. **Shift the diurnal rhythm backwards or forwards 1 hour/day a day or so before departure.**

   When travelling west, the day should be prolonged. Get up 1 h later than usual in the morning and go to bed 1 h later in the evening. Sometimes this is difficult to implement in practice and a compromise may be necessary. When travelling east, the day should be shortened. Try to get up 1 h earlier in the morning and retire 1 h later in the evening.

2. **Start eating an adjusted diet a few days before departure.**

   Breakfast and lunch should contain a lot of protein (eggs, meat, fish, etc.), which causes increased secretion of adrenaline, thereby heightening alertness. The evening meal should contain a lot of carbohydrate (bread, pasta, rice, potato, etc.) which increases secretion of serotonin, causing increased drowsiness and facilitating sleep.

3. **Adjust the diurnal rhythm according to the destination.**

   Put clocks forward or back to show the time of day in the destination country on the plane and try to adjust sleeping and meal times accordingly.

4. **Drink mineral water on the plane.**

   The air pressure in a plane is low (equivalent to the air pressure at 1500–2000 metres above sea level). The air is dry and passengers lose fluid and become dehydrated. Travelling by plane may therefore have a negative effect on a footballer's performance. It is important for players to drink a lot of water during a long-haul flight. Take bottles of mineral water and drink at least 1 l on a long trip. Alcohol consumption produces the opposite effect and should definitely be avoided.

5. **Eat small meals and try to sleep on the plane.**

**6. Do some light training on arrival.**

After arriving, try to adapt to the local diurnal rhythm as quickly as possible. If arriving during the day, try to keep awake until the normal bedtime. Light training is recommended.

For the first 24 h after a long-haul flight, urine production usually increases, which means one needs to go to the toilet more often. This is perfectly normal but can disturb sleep. Do not be overly worried if it is difficult to sleep the first few nights. This has no negative effect on performance. Rest by itself provides adequate recuperation.

# Location and accommodation

The team's location must be carefully chosen. It is beneficial to stay close to the training facilities, thereby avoiding long travelling distances. Hotels situated in the centre of a large city should be avoided because of the risk of traffic noise and poor air quality.

The players' rooms should also be chosen with great care. Try to accommodate all the team on the same floor as this facilitates contact between team members. Players staying in rooms that look out on to roads with heavy traffic may be disturbed by noise. A lack of air-conditioning may result in the room temperature being overtly high, making the players sweat and lose fluid and causing them to lose sleep and rest. It is therefore prudent to choose rooms that are in the shade when players are resting prior to a match.

The treatment room should be close to the lift and stairs and be easily accessible to the players. Medical personnel should have their rooms close by. If possible, book an extra room as a reserve in case a player needs to be isolated due to a cold or stomach flu.

When staying abroad for a long time, opportunities for alternative training are of considerable value. If the weather is poor, if a player has injuries that need rehabilitation, for recuperation training or simply to break with normal training routines, it is useful to have access to green areas for running, a gym and a swimming pool for water-running.

Be careful with powerful air-conditioning in hotel rooms and assembly rooms. If a player is sensitive, the dry air can cause respiratory tract problems and give him or her a cold.

# Climate, fluids and sunbathing

Chapter 5 discusses training and playing matches in hot and cold climates. During the World Cup Finals in the USA in 1994, many matches were played in the middle of the day at temperatures of 40°C and air humidity of 80–90 per cent. From a medical point of view, playing football in these conditions can represent a problem, since players lose a great deal of fluid and their performance is negatively affected.

Members of one national team were weighed before and after training sessions and matches. Weight loss was on average 1.2 l (variation 0–2.7 kg) per training session and 2.9 l (variation 1.3 –4.3 kg) per match, despite the fact that players were encouraged to drink more than just to quench their thirst. The players drank about 2 l during each training session or match, which meant that their fluid loss was about 3 l during a training session and 5 l during a match. When being tested for illegal substances, some players had to drink 7–8 l of mineral water before they could give a urine sample.

Usually, water bottles are placed around the pitch in such circumstances. Those playing in the wings were closer to the bottles and therefore drank more often, and were less affected by fluid loss than other players.

Players should be encouraged to use breaks in the game to replenish their fluid levels.

In extremely hot climates, training should be avoided at the hottest time of the day. Players should train early in the morning rather than late in the evening. If it is necessary to train at such a time (for example at the same time of the day as a forthcoming match), it should take place a few days before the match itself. Sometimes it can be a question of weighing up the advantages of match-time training against the disadvantages of subjecting the players to excessive sun and heat.

Make sure the players — especially those who are sensitive to the sun — are sufficiently protected against sunburn (sun cream with a high protection factor, sufficient covering of clothes etc.) during training sessions and when out in the sun at other times. Sunbathing or similarly subjecting the body to direct sunlight may easily lead to dehydration and fatigue. Therefore avoid staying in direct sunlight for long periods of time and sunbathing more than 15 min/day.

# Diet

If possible, a menu should be sent to the hotel where the team is going stay prior to departure. For example, many national teams use a 'framework' menu, developed and analysed by a group of nutrition experts made up of dieticians, chefs and doctors. Every meal consists of 1300 Kcal, made up of 55 per cent carbohydrate, 15–18 per cent protein and 30–32 per cent fat. Together with sports drinks, these meals give a daily intake of about 4000 Kcal. The menu includes fish or pasta on the day of the match, and a special high-carbohydrate meal the evening before.

When travelling to countries where the risk of stomach infections is high, it may be useful to take the team's own chef, drinks and ready-prepared food. If this is done, make sure the customs and import regulations for the country of your destination allow this.

The most important task of an accompanying chef is not to cook all the food him or herself, but to supervise the standards of hygiene when the food is being prepared. If the team does not have its own chef, the team doctor should be made responsible for diet and hygiene. The standards of hygiene in the kitchen should be assessed on site by the doctor.

## AVOIDING STOMACH INFECTIONS

- Never drink tap water.
- Make sure mineral water is served at meal times.
- Do not put ice in drinks — it is often made from tap water.
- Many hotels put ice in guests' drinks. Inform the kitchen/restaurant personnel not to do this.
- Do not drink juice that has been diluted with tap water.
- Do not eat salad that has been rinsed in tap water. Freshly boiled vegetables are fine, as are fresh, uncooked ones that have been peeled and rinsed in clean water just before eating.
- Only eat well done meat (fried or boiled).
- Avoid shellfish and mayonnaise.
- Do not eat ice-cream or other unpacked food whilst out in the town. Hamburger/hot-dog stalls and the like are not renowned for their hygiene.
- Peel all fruit.
- Avoid buffets that may have been laid out some time in advance and where many people come into contact with the different foodstuffs on the table.

**IMPORTANT FACTORS WHEN ASSESSING
THE STANDARDS OF HYGIENE IN A HOTEL KITCHEN**

- The chefs' hygiene. Are their clothes, nails etc. clean? Is their hair covered? Are there sores on their hands?
- What standard of hygiene are the hotel's cold-storage room and its other raw ingredient storage facilities?
- Are the staff toilets clean? Is there clean water, soap and paper?

# Getting medical help abroad

It might be useful for a team doctor to try to establish contact with doctors and hospitals in the country of destination prior to departure, in case emergency medical care, radiographs are needed. Addresses of clubs and club doctors in the country of destination can be obtained by contacting the home country's own football association, UEFA or FIFA.

Taking a doctor's bag through customs is not normally a problem as long as it is being carried by a doctor (having a doctor's ID card in English does help). For a doctor, it is not normally a problem to take the doctor's bag into the plane as hand luggage. On the contrary, flight personnel normally appreciate having a doctor on board with a medical bag — it may turn out to be very useful.

Make sure that crutches are packed along with the other luggage. Travelling home might otherwise be difficult for a player with a leg injury.

## CHECK LIST

### PRIOR TO DEPARTURE

- Contact the hotel where the team is going to stay.
- Send a menu to the hotel. Take a copy with the team.
- Contact the vaccination centre.
- Tell the squad both verbally and in writing about vaccination requirements, how to avoid jet-lag, traveller's diarrhoea and other infectious diseases, fluid loss, etc.
- Check the medical equipment. Do not forget crutches.
- Contact a doctor/hospital at the destination if it is necessary.

### WHEN TRAVELLING

- Take a doctor's bag on the plane as hand luggage.
- Adjust clocks/watches to the local time of the destination.
- Make sure all the players drink plenty of mineral water.

### ON ARRIVAL

- Check the facilities (distribution of rooms, facilities for alternative training, etc.).
- Go through the menu with the head chef.
- Go through other requirements, e.g. no ice in drinks, well-cooked food, no juice diluted with tap water, mineral water in the rooms, etc.
- Check the hygiene in the kitchen.

# 27. Doping

Sverker Nilsson

## Definition

The Doping Commission publishes an up-to-date list at least once a year, which is based on the International Olympic Committee's (IOC's) medical council's list, of classes of banned substances and banned procedures.

General rules apply to all sports, including football, and there are, in addition, special regulations within certain sports. For international football competitions, FIFA/UEFA's (the world and European football associations) rules apply to the respective competitions, which are based on the IOC's rules.

## Classes of banned substances

Before any medicine is used, it should be checked that the substance is not included on the list of banned doping pharmaceuticals. The list, which is always current and comprehensive, is updated at regular intervals. Substances which are included on the list may not be used, unless the player can be granted an exemption from the rules due to special circumstances, such as asthma. If a footballer is tested in association with national training or competition, at the time of the test or subsequently he or she must be able to prove that the medicine was prescribed by a doctor or by a doctor's certificate (not older than 3 years).

The medicine can also be used in international competitions, but in this case the player must apply for authorization in advance. Exemption is granted by the competition organizers and is then valid for the whole competition. In the case of national teams, this is dealt with by the UEFA/FIFA inspector or by a special doping inspector.

## Accidental doping

Use of those substances which are included on the banned list is forbidden. In each main group, the forbidden substances are listed. At the end of the groups, the phrase 'and related substances' appears, so that the player cannot use a similar substance which has a doping effect. At the same time this unfortunately leads to other related compounds, which have no doping effect, also being classed as doping substances. This creates a risk of accidental doping, which can result in penalization of both the individual and the whole team.

The risk of accidental doping can be avoided if all medicines are checked against the list of banned substances and if all players are careful with medication. Medicines bought at a chemist's have a detailed list of contents, which is not the case for natural remedies bought in health shops. These can contain doping substances, although this is not stated on the packaging, and the player risks penalization. For this reason, it is important not to use natural remedies without first checking that the medicine is free from doping ingredients.

## Stimulants

This group includes drugs that stimulate the central nervous system, such as amphetamines, cocaine, bromantan, ephedrine and caffeine. For all banned substances, except caffeine, the limit is zero in tests. This means that even a trace of a substance is tantamount to doping. For caffeine the limit is 12 µg/ml, a value which is not possible to exceed even with very high coffee consumption.

Also included in this group are asthma medicines which can produce stimulating effects in high doses and are therefore banned except for treatment of asthma. An asthmatic can inhale (but not take tablets or inject pharmaceuticals intravenously) usual medicines such as Ventoline, Bricanyl and Serevent. Another stimulant substance which is permitted for local use is adrenaline, which may be used together with a local anaesthetic when required. The team doctor, in these cases, submits a report to the competition organizers.

## Strong analgesics

This group comprises principally morphine and related substances and includes medicines which have similar effects. The group previously caused concern as for example, codeine, was banned but this is no longer the case.

## Substances with anabolic effects

This group contains the compounds most sportsmen who have been caught for doping have used, i.e. male sex hormones. Use of the male sex hormone, testosterone, and other anabolic steroids is banned. In men, use of hormone preparations can accelerate muscle build-up after intensive strength training. This can be of advantage in certain sports, although not in football. A footballer improves his or her performance by means of many different types of training, and technical and tactical skill is particularly important.

A doping test reveals the use of anabolic steroids and analyses the quotient between male sex hormones and the products of their degradation. The quotient cannot be higher than 6. If higher, there is suspicion of doping, which is proved by repeated tests.

## Diuretic medicines

Diuretic drugs are banned as they can hide intake of other banned substances and lead to cheating when combined with dieting to lose weight. This is not a problem in football.

**Other hormones**

This class consists of banned substances such as growth hormones and the blood-producing hormone erythropoietin (EPO). Increasing the body's ability to transport oxygen by training at high altitudes or in high-altitude chambers is permitted, but obtaining the same effect with EPO is forbidden.

# Banned techniques

Besides introducing the substances which have been described into the body, it is also forbidden to use doping techniques. One such technique is blood doping. Regardless of whether one's own blood is removed and then replaced, or if blood products from another individual are transfused, this is not permitted. The effects of blood doping are similar to what happens when taking erythropoietin. To uncover this doping technique, blood tests are being done during some competitions.

In addition to manipulation of blood volume, all other forms of medical, chemical or physical manipulation are banned. Irrespective of whether the manipulation was successful or not, an individual who is caught, for example during a doping test, is punished for attempting to gain an unfair advantage.

# Classes of restricted pharmaceuticals

**Alcohol and marijuana**

In certain sports, there are special regulations regarding alcohol and marijuana. FIFA and UEFA have the right to draw up rules regarding the use of these during competitions.

## Local anaesthetics and cortisone

Injection of local anaesthetic and cortisone locally or into a joint is permitted but must be reported to the competition organizers by the team doctor during international competitions. In national competitions, use of these pharmaceuticals (in the last weeks) must be supported by a doctor's certificate if a doping test is performed. The use must be medically authorized.

Use of cortisone is also permitted locally on the skin, auditory meatus, the eyes and for inhalation for asthma. On the other hand, use of cortisone in tablet form or intravenous injection is banned. The same rules of exemption apply for spraying cortisone into the respiratory passages for the treatment of asthma as for other asthma medicines.

## Heart medicine

Certain sports, such as shooting, prohibit the use of the type of medicine which reduces palpitations and a tendency towards muscle tremors. This is not the case in football, as this preparation only impairs performance.

# Testing process

The tests are done without warning during training and competition and during larger competitions the best in each section are tested as well as a few who are chosen at random.

Training tests are performed without prior warning in order to uncover and prevent hormone doping. Urine tests are analysed only for hormone doping or an attempt to conceal it. During sampling in the course of a competition, all banned substances and techniques are tested for according to the IOC's list of prohibited substances. Tests in football have mainly been carried out in connection with matches.

In the course of a test, the specimen collector selects the players to be tested. When they have been informed, they must report to give a urine sample within 60 min after the end of the match. Failure to report for the sampling after being selected results in penalization.

The player in question may, if he or she wishes, and indeed should, have their doctor and another member of the medical staff or team management with them to check that everything is carried out correctly. It is not permitted to take one's own drinks along to the test centre; instead the player is provided with drinks by the specimen collector. It is important that the player being tested does not drink out of any bottles which have already been opened, or which can be resealed with a screw cap etc.

The individual being tested provides his or her urine sample under supervision of the specimen collector, pours the urine into the sample bottle which they themselves have chosen and checks that the same number is on the sample bottle and all the forms. The player then closes the receptacle and sees to it that it ends up in the right place for transport to the laboratory for analysis.

The procedures concerning sampling, transport and analysis at the laboratory take place according to strict rules. Only the specimen collector and the player know whose identity lies behind the number on a particular urine sample. The results of the analysis are reported to the inspector who in turn informs the player. If the doping test should turn out positive, the player her or himself decides whether the analysis should be performed on the other half of the urine sample which was sent in. If he or she chooses not to do so, the results of the first test count.

In the case of a positive result, the relevant association decides on disciplinary action. It is the Football Association and its competition committee who make the decision regarding disciplinary action. Disciplinary action can be a maximum of 2-year suspension from all sporting activities in all sports.

# Drug-free football

All footballers should be provided with a list of banned substances and a sound knowledge of why it is prohibited to use the pharmaceuticals which are included on the list. Gaining an unfair advantage by means of different substances can not only lead to penalization for the individual involved and the team — it is also in the vast majority of cases completely ineffective.

The greatest risk for future doping cases in football is a player, who for example takes anabolic steroids, for reasons other than improving his or her footballing performance, is tested in connection with a match. The most common reason for taking anabolic steroids among teenage boys today is not sporting ambition but rather is to do with today's ideals of physical perfection.

Over the years, there have been very few incidences of drug-taking in football. Recently, however, there have been a number of doping cases which have attracted a great deal of attention.

## FACTS ABOUT DOPING

- You do not become a better footballer by taking drugs.
- Taking drugs is cheating.
- Medicines can result in a risk of accidental drug taking.
- All footballers should be provided with a list of banned substances.

# BIBLIOGRAPHY

## Chapter 1 – The risk of injury and injury distribution

**Ekstrand J, Gillquist.** Soccer injuries and their mechanisms: a prospective study. *Med Sci Sports Exerc* 1983; **15**: 267–70.

**Ekstrand J, Gillquist, Möller M et al.** Incidence of soccer injuries and their relation to training and team success. *Am J Sports Med* 1983; **11**: 63–7.

**Ekstrand J, Topp H.** The incidence of ankle sprains in soccer. *Foot Ankle* 1990; **11**: 41–4.

**Hawkins RD, Fuller CW.** An examination of the frequency and severity of injuries and incidents at three levels of professional football. *Br J Sports Med* 1998; **32**: 326–32.

**Hawkins RD, Fuller CW.** A prospective epidemiological study of injuries in four English professional football clubs. *Br J Sports Med* 1999; **33**: 196–203.

**Hawkins RD, Hulse MA, Wilkinson C et al.** The association football medical research programme: an audit of injuries in professional football. *Br J Sports Med* 2001; **35**: 43–7.

**Inklaar H.** The epidemiology of soccer injuries in a new perspective. Thesis. University of Utrecht, 1995.

**Inklaar H.** Soccer injuries. I: incidence and severity. *Sports Med* 1994; **18**: 55–73.

**Junge A, Chomiak J, Dvorak J.** Incidence of football injuries in youth players. Comparison of players from two European regions. *Am J Sports Med* 2000; **28** (Suppl 5): S47–50.

**Söderman K, Adolphson J, Lorentzon J et al.** Injuries in adolescent female players in European football: a prospective study over one outdoor season. *Scand J Med Sci Sports* 2001; **11**: 299–304.

## Chapter 3 – Preventing injury

**Caraffa A, Cerulli G, Projetti M et al.** Prevention of anterior cruciate ligament injuries in soccer. A prospective controlled study of proprioceptive training. *Knee Surg Sports Traumatol Arthrosc* 1996; **4**: 19–21.

**Cerulli G, Benoit DL, Caraffa, A, Ponteggia, F.** Proprioceptive training and prevention of anterior cruciate ligament injuries in soccer. *J Orthop Sports Phys Ther* 2001; **31**: 655–60; discussion 661.

**Dvorak J, Junge A, Chomiak J et al.** Risk factor analysis for injuries in football players. Possibilities for a prevention program. *Am J Sports Med* 2000; **28** (Suppl 5): S69–74.

**Ekstrand J.** Injury prevention. In: Ekblom B (ed). *Football (soccer)* Oxford: Blackwell Scientific Publications, 1994, Pp. 209–15.

**Ekstrand J.** Soccer injuries and their prevention. In *Department of Surgery*. Edited, Linköping, Sweden, Linköping University, 1982.

**Ekstrand J, Gillquist J.** The avoidability of soccer injuries. *Int J Sports Med* 1983; **4**: 124–8.

# BIBLIOGRAPHY

**Ekstrand J, Gillquist J.** Soccer injuries and their mechanisms: a prospective study. *Med Sci Sports Exerc* 1983;**15**: 267–70.

**Ekstrand J, Gillquist J, Liljedahl SO.** Prevention of soccer injuries. Supervision by doctor and physiotherapist. *Am J Sports Med* 1983; **11**: 116–20.

**Ekstrand J, Nigg BM.** Surface-related injuries in soccer. *Sports Med* 1989; **8**: 56–62.

**Ekstrand J, Wiktorsson M, Öberg B, Gillquist J.** Lower extremity goniometric measurements: a study to determine their reliability. *Arch Phys Med Rehabil* 1982; **63**: 171–5.

**Garrett WE, Kirkendall DT, Contiguglia SR.** (eds) *The US Soccer Sports Medicine Book.* Baltimore: Williams & Williams, 1996.

**Inklaar H.** The epidemiology of soccer injuries in a new perspective. *Department of Medical Physiology and Sports Medicine.* Edited, Utrecht, University of Utrecht, 1995.

**Lysens R, Auweele Y W, Ostyn M.** The relationship between psychosocial factors and sports injuries. *J Sports Med* 1986; **26**: 77–84.

**Möller M, Ekstrand J, Öberg B, Gillquist J.** Duration of stretching effect on range of motion in lower extremities. *Arch Phys Med Rehabil* 1985; **66**: 171–3.

**Östenberg A, Roos H.** Injury risk factors in female European football. A prospective study of 123 players during one season. *Scand J Med Sci Sports,* 2000; **10**: 279–85.

**Parkkari J, Kujala UM, Kannus P.** Is it possible to prevent sports injuries? Review of controlled clinical trials and recommendations for future work. *Sports Med* 2001; **31**: 985–95.

**Reid DC.** *Sports Injury Assessment and Rehabilitation.* Edited, New York: Churchill Livingstone, 1992.

**Sitler MR, Horodyski M.** Effectiveness of prophylactic ankle stabilisers for prevention of ankle injuries. *Sports Med* 1995; **20**: 53–7.

**Söderman K, Werner S, Pietila T et al.** Balance board training: prevention of traumatic injuries of the lower extremities in female soccer players? A prospective randomized intervention study. *Knee Surg Sports Traumatol Arthrosc* 2000; **8**: 356–63.

**Tropp H, Askling C, Gillquist J.** Prevention of ankle sprains. *Am J Sports Med* 1985; **13**: 259–62.

**Wiktorsson-Möller M, Öberg B, Ekstrand J, Gillquist J.** Effects of warming up, massage, and stretching on range of motion and muscle strength in the lower extremity. *Am J Sports Med* 1983; **11**: 249–52.

# BIBLIOGRAPHY

## Chapter 4 – The biomechanics of football

**Besier TF, Lloyd DG, Cochrane JL et al.** External loading of the knee joint during running and cutting maneuvers. *Med Sci Sports Exerc* 2001; **33**: 1168–75.

**Davids K, Lees A, Burwitz L.** Understanding and measuring coordination and control in kicking skills in soccer: implications for talent identification and skill acquisition. *J Sports Sci* 2001; **31**: 211–34.

**Kirkendall DT, Jordan SE, Garrett WE.** Heading and head injuries in soccer. *Sports Med*; 2001: **31**: 369–86.

**Lees A, Nolan L.** The biomechanics of soccer: a review. *J Sports Sci* 1998; **16**: 211–34.

**Levanon J, Dapena J.** Comparison of the kinematics of the full instep and pass kicks in soccer. *Med Sci Sports Exerc* 1998; **30**: 917–27.

**Orchard J.** Is there a relationship between ground and climatic conditions and injuries in football? *Sports Med* 2002; **32**: 419–32.

## Chapter 5 – The physiology of football

**Ekblom B.** Applied physiology of soccer. *Sports Med* 1986; **3**: 50–60.

**Ekblom B** (ed) *Handbook of Sports Medicine and Science: Soccer.* Oxford: Blackwell Scientific Publications, 1994.

## Chapter 6 – Nutrition and football

**Balsom PD, Söderlund K, Ekblom B.** Creatine in humans with special reference to creatine supplementation. *Sports Med* 1994; **18**: 268–80.

**Balsom PD, Wood K, Olsson P, Ekblom B.** Carbohydrate intake and multiple sprint sports: with special reference to football (soccer). *Int J Sports Med* 1999; **20**: 48–52.

**Blomstrand E, Andersson S, Hassmen P et al.** Effect of branched chain amino acid and carbohydrate supplementation on the exercise-induced change in plasma and muscle concentration of amino acids in human subjects. *Acta Physiol Scand* 1995; **153**: 87–96.

**Ekblom B.** Applied physiology of soccer. *Sports Med* 1986; **3**: 50–60.

**Ekblom B** (ed) *Handbook of Sports Medicine and Science: Soccer.* Oxford: Blackwell Scientific, 1994.

**Malm C, Svensson M, Ekblom B et al.** Effects of ubiquinone-10 supplementation and high intensity training on physical performance in humans. *Acta Physiol Scand* 1997; **161**: 379–84.

**Maughan RJ.** Energy and macronutrient intakes of professional football (soccer) players. *Br J Sports Med* 1997; **31**: 45–7.

# BIBLIOGRAPHY

## Chapter 7 – The use of nutritional supplements in football

**Bangsbo J.** Energy demands in competitive soccer. *J Sports Sci* 1994; 12 (Suppl): S5–S12.

**Clarkson PM.** Nutritional supplements for weight gain. *Sports Science Exchange* 1998; **11**: 1–10.

**Costill DL, Dalsky G, Fink WJ.** Effects of caffeine ingestion on metabolism and exercise performance. *Med Sci Sports* 1978; **10**: 155–8.

**Delbeke F.** Nutritional supplements and doping. In: Peters C, T Schulz, H Michna (eds). *Biomedical Side Effects of Doping.* Bergisch Gladbach: Hansen, 2001, Pp 155–161.

**Dohm GL.** Protein as a fuel for endurance exercise. *Ex Sport Sci Rev* 1986; **14**: 143–73.

**Evans GW.** The effect of chromium picolinate on insulin controlled parameters in humans. *Int J Biosoc Med Res* 1989; **11**: 163–80.

**Geyer H, Marech-Engelke U, Reinhart U et al.** Positive dopingfalle mit norandrosteron durch verunreinigte nahrungserganzungsmittel *Dtsch Z Sportmed* 2000; **51**: 378–82.

**Geyer H, Henze M, Machnik M et al.** Health risks of nutritional supplements. In: Peters C, Schulz T, Michna H (eds). *Biomedical Side Effects of Doping.* Bergisch Gladbach: Hansen, 2001, Pp 141–53.

**Greenhaff PL.** Creatine and its application as an ergogenic aid. *Int J Sport Nutr* 1995; **5** (Suppl): S100–S110.

**Hargreaves M.** Carbohydrate and lipid requirements of soccer. *J Sports Sci* 1994; **12** (Suppl): S13–S16.

**Harris RC, Söderlund K, Hultman E.** Elevation of creatine in resting and exercised muscle of normal subjects by creatine supplementation. *Clin Sci* 1992; **83**: 367–74.

**Kanter M.** Free radicals and exercise: effects of nutritional antioxidant supplementation. *Exerc Sport Sci Rev* 1995; **23**: 375–97.

**Lang F, Busch GL, Volkl K.** The diversity of volume regulatory mechanisms. *Cell Physiol Biochem* 1998; **8**: 1–45.

**Lemon PWR.** Effect of exercise on protein requirements. *J Sports Sci* 1991; **9** (Special Issue) 53–70.

**Lemon PWR.** Do athletes need more dietary protein and amino acids? *Int J Sport Nutr* 1995; **5**: S39–S61.

**Lemon PWR.** Protein requirements of soccer. *J Sports Sci* 1994; **12** (Suppl): S17–S22.

**Low SY, Rennie MJ, Taylor PM.** Modulation of glycogen synthesis in rat skeletal muscle by changes in cell volume. *J Physiol Occup Physiol* 1996; **495**: 299–303.

**Low SY, Rennie MJ, Taylor PM.** Signalling elements involved in amino acid transport responses to altered muscle cell volume. *FASEB J* 1997; **11**: 1111–17.

# BIBLIOGRAPHY

**McNaughton L.** Sodium citrate and anaerobic performance: implications of dosage. *Eur J Appl Physiol Occup Physiol* 1990: **61**: 392–7.

**Maganaris CN, Maughan RJ.** Creatine supplementation enhances maximum voluntary isometric force and endurance capacity in resistance trained men. *Acta Physiol Scand* 1988; **163**: 279–87.

**Malm C, Svensson M, Sjöberg B et al.** Supplementation with ubiquinone-10 causes cellular damage during intense exercise. *Acta Physiol Scand* 1996: **157**: 511–12.

**Maughan RJ.** Creatine supplementation and exercise performance. *Int J Sport Nutr* 1995; **5**: 94–101.

**Maughan RJ, Shirreffs SM.** Fluid and electrolyte loss and replacement in exercise. In: Harries M, Williams C, Stanish WD, Micheli LL (eds).*Oxford Textbook of Sports Medicine.* 2nd Edn. Oxford: Oxford University Press, 1998, Pp. 97–113.

**Mertz W.** Chromium: history and nutritional importance. *Biol Trace Elem Res* 1992; **32**: 3–8.

**Mujika I, Padilla S**. Creatine supplementation as an ergogenic aid for sports performance in highly trained athletes: a critical review. *Int J Sports Med* 1997; **18**: 491–6.

**Newsholme EA**. Biochemical mechanisms to explain immunosuppression in well-trained and overtrained athletes. *Int J Sports Med* 1994; **15**(Suppl 3): S142–S147.

**Nieman DC, Nelson-Cannarella SL, Henson DA et al.** Immune response to exercise training and/or energy restriction in obese women. *Med Sci Sports Exerc* 1998; **30**: 679–86.

**Nissen S, Sharp R, Ray M et al.** Effect of leucine metabolite beta-hydroxy beta-methyl butyrate on muscle metabolism during resistance-exercise training. *J Appl Physiol* 1996; **81**: 2095–104.

**Poortmans JR, Auquier H, Renault V et al.** Effect of short-term creatine supplementation on renal responses in men. *Eur J Appl Physiol Occup Physiol* 1997; **76**: 566–7.

**Spriet LL.** Caffeine and performance. *Int J Sport Nutr* 1995; **5**: S84–S99.

**Spriet LL.** Ergogenic aids: recent advances and retreats. In Lamb DR, Murray D (eds) *Optimizing Sports Performance.* Carmel: Cooper Publishing, 1997, pp 185–238.

**Toler SM.** Creatine is an ergogen for anaerobic exercise. *Nutr Rev* 1997; **55**: 21–23.

**Vandenberghe K, Goris M, Van Hecke P et al**. Long-term creatine intake is beneficial to muscle performance during resistance training. *J Appl Physiol* 1997; **83**: 2055–63.

**Volek JS, Kraemer WJ, Bush JA et al.** Creatine supplementation enhances muscular performance during high-intensity resistance exercise. *J Am Dietetic Assoc* 1997; **97**: 765–70.

**Vukovich MD, Costill DL, Fink WJ.** Carnitine supplementation: effect on muscle carnitine and glycogen content during exercise. *Med Sci Sports Exerc* 1994; **26**: 1122–9.

**Wemple RD, Lamb DR, McKeever KH.** Caffeine vs caffeine-free sports drinks: effects on urine production at rest and during prolonged exercise. *Int J Sports Med* 1997; **18**: 40–46.

# BIBLIOGRAPHY

**Williams C.** Diet and sports performance. In: Harries M, Williams C, Stanish WD, Micheli LL (eds). *Oxford Textbook of Sports Medicine*, 2nd Edn. Oxford: Oxford University Press, 1998, Pp 77–97.

**Williams MH.** *Ergogenic Aids in Sport*. Champaign, IL: Human Kinetics, 1983.

**Williams MH, Branch JD.** Creatine supplementation and exercise performance: an update. *J Am Coll Nutr* 1988; **17**: 216–34.

## Chapter 8 – First aid

**Swenson C, Swärd L, Karlsson J.** Cryotherapy in sports medicine. *Scand J Med Sci Sports* 1996; **6**: 193–200.

**Thorsson O, Hamdal B, Lilja B et al.** The effect of external pressure on intramuscular blood flow at rest and after running. *Med Sci Sports Exerc* 1987; **19**: 469–73.

## Chapter 9 – Muscle injuries

**Garrett WE Jr.** Muscle strain injuries. *Am J Sports Med* 1996; **24** (Suppl): S2–8.

**Garrett WE Jr.** Muscle strain injuries: clinical and basic aspects. *Med Sci Sports Exerc* 1990; **22**: 436–43.

**Järvinen TA, Kaarianen M, Järvinen M et al.** Muscle strain injuries. *Curr Opin Rheumatol* 2000; **12**; 155–61.

**Lieber RL, Friden J.** Mechanisms of muscle injury after eccentric contraction. *J Sci Med Sport* 1999; **2**: 253–65.
**Lieber RL, Friden J.** Morphologic and mechanical basis of delayed onset muscle soreness. *J Am Acad Orthop Surg* 2002; **10**: 67–73.

**Peterson L, Renström P.** *Sports Injuries: Their Prevention and Treatment*. London: Martin Dunitz, 2001.

**Thorsson O, Lilja B, Nilsson P et al.** Immediate external compression in the management of an acute muscle injury. *Scand J Med Sci Sports* 1997; **7** 182–90.

## Chapter 10 – Head injuries

**Aubry M, Cantu R, Dvorak J et al for the Concussion in Sport Group.** Summary and agreement statement of the First International Conference on Concussion in Sport, Vienna 2001. Recommendations for the improvement of safety and health of athletes who may suffer concussive injuries. *Br J Sports Med* 2002; **36**: 6–10.

**Erlanger D, Saliba E, Barth J et al.** Monitoring resolution of postconcussion symptoms in athletes: Preliminary results of a web-based neuropsychological test protocol. *J Athl Train* 2001; **36**: 280–7.

# BIBLIOGRAPHY

Practice parameter: the management of concussion in sports (summary statement). Report of the Quality Standards Subcommittee. *Neurology* 1997; **48**:581–5.

**Kelly JP, Rosenberg JH**. Diagnosis and management of concussion in sports. *Neurology* 1997; **48**: 575–80.

**Kirkendall DT, Jordan SE, Garrett WE**. Heading and head injuries in soccer. *Sports Med* 2001; **31**: 369–86.

**McCrea M**. Standardized mental status assessment of sports concussion. *Clin J Sport Med* 2001; **11**: 176–81.

## Chapter 11 – Injuries to the upper extremities

**Bankart A**. Recurrent or habitual dislocation of the shoulder. *Br Med J* 1923; **2**: 1132–8.

**Culver JE, Anderson TE**. Fractures of the hand and wrist in the athlete. *Clin Sports Med* 1992; **11**: 101–28.

**Hovelius L**. Anterior dislocation of the shoulder. Thesis, University of Linköping, Sweden, 1982.

**Hovelius L**. Incidence of shoulder dislocation in Sweden. *Clin Orthop* 1982; **166**: 127–31.

**Ireland ML, Andrews JR**. Shoulder and elbow injuries in the young athlete. *Clin Sports Med* 1988; **7**: 473–94.

**Jobe FW, Pink M**. Classification and treatment of shoulder dysfunction in the overhead athlete. *J Orthop Sports Phys Ther* 1993; **18**: 427–32.

**Josefsson PO, Gentz CF, Johnell O, Wendeberg B**. Surgical versus non-surgical treatment of ligamentous injuries following dislocation of the elbow joint. A prospective randomized study. *J Bone Joint Surg Am* 1987; **69**: 605–8.

**Rockwood C, Matsen F**. *The Shoulder*. Philadelphia: WB Saunders, 1998.

**Stener B**. Displacement of the ruptured ulnar collateral ligament of the metacarpo-phalangeal joint of the thumb: a clinical and anatomical study. *J Bone Joint Surg Br* 1962; **44**: 869–72.

## Chapter 12 – Back injuries

**Andersson E, Swärd L, Thorstensson A**. Trunk muscle strength in athletes. *Med Sci Sports Exerc* 1988; **20**: 587–93.

**Hellström M, Jacobsson B, Swärd L, Peterson L**. Radiologic abnormalities of the thoraco-lumbar spine in athletes. *Acta Radiol* 1990; **31**: 127–32.

**Lundin O, Hellström M, Nilsson I, Swärd L**. Back pain and radiological changes in the thoraco-lumbar spine of athletes. A long-term follow-up. *Scand J Med Sci Sports* 2001; **11**: 103–9.

# BIBLIOGRAPHY

**Swärd L.** The thoracolumbar spine in young elite athletes. Current concepts on the effects of physical training. *Sports Med* 1992; **13**: 357–64.

**Swärd L, Hellström M, Jacobsson B, Karlsson L.** Vertebral ring apophysis injury in athletes. Is the etiology different in the thoracic and lumbar spine? *Am J Sports Med* 1993; **21**: 841–5.

**Swärd L, Hellström M, Jacobsson B et al.** Acute injury of the vertebral ring apophysis and intervertebral disc in adolescent gymnasts. *Spine* 1990; **15**: 144–8.

**Swärd L, Hellström M, Jacobsson B, Peterson L.** Back pain and radiologic changes in the thoraco-lumbar spine of athletes. *Spine* 1990; **15**: 124–9.

## Chapter 14 – Groin injuries

**Ekberg O, Persson NH, Abrahamsson P A et al.** Longstanding groin pain in athletes. A multidisciplinary approach. *Sports Med* 1988; **6**: 56–61.

**Ekstrand J, Hilding J.** The incidence and differential diagnosis of acute groin injuries in male soccer players. *Scand J Med Sci Sports* 1999; **9**: 98–103.

**Hackney RG.** The sports hernia: a cause of chronic groin pain. *Br J Sports Med* 1993; **27**: 58–62.

**Hölmich P, Uhrskou P, Ulnits L et al.** Effectiveness of active physical training as treatment for long- standing adductor-related groin pain in athletes: randomised trial. *Lancet* 1999; **353**: 439–43.

**Martens MA, Hansen L, Mulier JC.** Adductor tendinitis and musculus rectus abdominis tendopathy. *Am J Sports Med* 1987; **15**: 353–6.

**Renström P.** Groin injuries: a true challenge in orthopaedic sports medicine. *Sports Med Arthrosc Rev* 1997; **5**: 247–51.

**Roos HP, Renström PAFH.** Pain about the hip and pelvis. In Harries M, Williams C, Stanish W, Micheli L (eds) *Oxford Textbook of Sports Medicine*, 2nd Edn, Oxford: Oxford University Press, 1998, Pp. 911–24.

**Smedberg SG, Broome AE, Gullmo A, Roos H.** Herniography in athletes with groin pain. *Am J Surg* 1985; **149**: 378–82.

## Chapter 15 – Knee injuries

**Brittberg M, Lindahl A, Nilsson A et al.** Treatment of deep cartilage defects in the knee with autologous chondrocyte transplantation. *N Engl J Med* 1994; **331**: 889–95.

**Daniel DM, Fithian, DC.** Indications for ACL surgery. *Arthroscopy*, 1994;10:434–41.

**Daniel DM, Stone ML, Dobson BE et al.** Fate of the ACL-injured patient. A prospective outcome study. *Am J Sports Med* 1994; **22**: 632–44.

**Fox J, Del Pizzo W.** The patello-femoral joint. Edited, New York: McGraw-Hill, 1991.

# BIBLIOGRAPHY

**Johnson RJ, Beynnon BD, Nichols, CE, Renström PA.** The treatment of injuries of the anterior cruciate ligament. *J Bone Joint Surg Am* 1992; **74**: 140–51.

**Keller PM, Shelbourne, KD, McCarroll JR et al.** Nonoperatively treated isolated posterior cruciate ligament injuries. *Am J Sports Med* 1993; **21**: 132–6.

**Lohmander S, Roos H.** Knee ligament injury, surgery and osteoarthrosis. Truth or consequence. *Acta Orhop Scand* 1994; **65**: 605–9.

**Roos H, Adalberth T, Dahlberg L, Lohmander LS.** Osteoarthritis of the knee after injury to the anterior cruciate ligament or meniscus: the influence of time and age. *Osteoarthritis Cartilage* 1995; **3**: 261–7.

**Shelbourne KD, Patel DV.** Management of combined injuries of the anterior cruciate and medial collateral ligaments. *Instr Course Lect* 1996; **45**: 275–80.

**Werner S, Eriksson E.** Isokinetic quadriceps training in patients with patellofemoral pain syndrome. *Knee Surg Sports Traumatol Arthrosc* 1993; **1**: 162–8.

## Chapter 16 – Lower leg injuries

**Cetti R, Henriksen LO, Jacobsen KS.** A new treatment of ruptured Achilles tendons. A prospective randomized study. *Clin Orthop* 1994; **308**: 155–65.

**Ekenman I, Tsai-Felländer L, Westblad P et al.** A study of intrinsic factors in patients with stress fractures of the tibia. *Foot Ankle Int* 1996; **17**: 477–82.

**Kannus P, Jozsa L.** Histopathological changes preceding spontaneous rupture of a tendon. A controlled study of 891 patients. *J Bone Joint Surg Am* 1991; **73**: 1507–25.

**Matheson GO, Clement DB, McKenzie DC et al.** Stress fractures in athletes. A study of 320 cases. *Am J Sports Med* 1987; **15**: 46–58.

**Nistor L.** On the treatment of Achilles tendon rupture. Thesis. University of Gothenburg, Sweden, 1979.

**Sölveborn SA, Moberg A.** Immediate free ankle motion after surgical repair of acute Achilles tendon ruptures. *Am J Sports Med* 1994; **22**: 607–10.

**Styf J.** Diagnosis of exercise-induced pain in the anterior aspect of the lower leg. *Am J Sports Med* 1988; **16**: 165–9.

## Chapter 17 – Ankle injuries

**Broström L.** Sprained ankles. A pathologic, artrographic, and clinical investigation. Thesis, Stockholm University, 1966.

**Ekstrand J, Tropp H.** The incidence of ankle sprains in soccer. *Foot Ankle* 1990; **11**: 41–4.

**Karlsson J.** Chronic lateral instability of the ankle joint. A clinical, radiological and experimental study. Thesis , Gothenburg University, Sweden, 1989.

# BIBLIOGRAPHY

**Karlsson J, Bergsten T, Lansinger O, Peterson L.** Reconstruction of the lateral ligaments of the ankle for chronic lateral instability. *J Bone Joint Surg Am* 1988; **70**: 581–8.

**Leandersson J, Wredmark T.** Treatment of acute ankle sprain. *Acta Orthop Scand* 1995; **66**: 529-31.

**Löfvenberg R, Kärrholm J, Sundelin G, Ahlgren O.** Prolonged reaction time in patients with chronic lateral instability of the ankle. *Am J Sports Med* 1995; **23**: 414–7.

**Tropp H.** Functional instability of the ankle joint. Thesis. Linköping University, Sweden,1985.

## Chapter 18 – Injuries to the foot

**Bennell KL, Malcolm SA, Thomas SA et al.** The incidence and distribution of stress fractures in competitive track and field athletes. A twelve-month prospective study. *Am J Sports Med* 1996; **24**: 211–7.

**Ferkel RD, Karzel RP, Del Pizzo W et al.** Arthroscopic treatment of anterolateral impingement of the ankle. *Am J Sports Med* 1991; **19**: 440–6.

**Johnson K** (ed). The Foot and Ankle. Master Techniques in Orthopaedic Surgery. New York; Raven Press, 1994.

**Orava S, Karpakka J, Hulkko A, Takala T.** Stress avulsion fracture of the tarsal navicular. An uncommon sports-related overuse injury. *Am J Sports Med* 1991; **19**: 392–5.

**Rodeo SA, O'Brien S, Warren RF et al.** Turf-toe: an analysis of metatarsophalangeal joint sprains in professional football players. *Am J Sports Med* 1990; **18**: 280–5.

**Turan I, Rivero-Melian C, Guntner P, Rolf, C.** Tarsal tunnel syndrome. Outcome of surgery in longstanding cases. *Clin Orthop* 1997; **343**: 151–6.

**Van Hal ME, Keene JS, Lange TA, Clancy WG Jr.** Stress fractures of the great toe sesamoids. *Am J Sports Med* 1982; **10**: 122–8.

## Chapter 19 – Post-injury functional testing for return to competitive play

**Hawkins RD, Hulse MA, Wilkinson C et al.** The association football medical research programme: an audit of injuries in professional football. *Br J Sports Med* 2001; 35: 43–7.

## Chapter 20 – Football-specific injury rehabilitation

**Ekstrand J.** Soccer injuries and their prevention. Thesis, Linköping University, Sweden, 1982.

**Leaman AM, Simpson DE.** Treatment of sprained ankles by physiotherapists at professional soccer clubs. *Arch Emerg Med* 1988; **5**: 177–9.

**Leandersson J, Wredmark T.** Treatment of acute ankle sprain. *Acta Orthop Scand* 1995; **66**: 529–31.

# BIBLIOGRAPHY

**Lephart SM, Pincivero DM, Giraldo JL, Fu FH.** The role of proprioception in the management and rehabilitation of athletic injuries. *Am J Sports Med* 1997; **25**: 130–7.

**Peterson L, Renström P.** *Sports Injuries: Their Prevention and Treatment.* London: Martin Dunitz, 2001.

**Thomee R.** A comprehensive treatment approach for patellofemoral pain syndrome in young women. *Phys Ther* 1997; **77**: 1690–703.

**Tropp H.** Functional instability of the ankle joint. Thesis , Linköping University, Sweden,1985.

**Tropp H, Askling C, Gillquist J.** Prevention of ankle sprains. *Am J Sports Med* 1985; **13**: 259–62.

## Chapter 21 – Illness and medication

**Fletcher G.** Cardiovascular response to exercise, American Heart Association Monograph series. Edited, Mount Kisco, NY: Futura publishing Company, 1994.

**Gotshall RW.** Exercise-induced bronchoconstriction. *Drugs* 2002; **62**: 1725–39.

**Harries M, Micheli L, Stanish W, Williams C. (Eds)** *Oxford Textbook of Sports Medicine.* Oxford: Oxford University Press, 1996.

**Pedersen BK, Rohde T, Zacho M.** Immunity in athletes. *J Sports Med Phys Fitness* 1996; **36**: 236–45.

**Pelliccia A, Di Paolo FM, Maron BJ.** The athlete's heart: remodeling, electrocardiogram and preparticipation screening. *Cardiol Rev* 2002; **10**: 85–90.

**Sallis R.** *ACSM's Essentials of Sports Medicine.* St Louis, Missouri: Mosby-Year Book, 1997.

**Thompson P.** *Exercise and Sports Cardiology.* New York: McGraw-Hill, 2001.

**Williams CC, Bernhardt DT.** Syncope in athletes. *Sports Med* 1995; **19**: 223–34.

## Chapter 22 – Late sequelae of football – osteoarthrosis

**Adalberth T, Roos H, Lauren M et al.** Magnetic resonance imaging, scintigraphy, and arthroscopic evaluation of traumatic hemarthrosis of the knee. *Am J Sports Med* 1997; **25**: 231–7.

**Arendt E, Dick R.** Knee injury patterns among men and women in collegiate basketball and soccer. NCAA data and review of literature. *Am J Sports Med* 1995; **23**: 694–701.

**Kujala UM, Kettunen J, Paananen H et al.** Knee osteoarthritis in former runners, soccer players, weight lifters, and shooters. *Arthritis Rheum* 1995; **38**: 539–46.

**Lindberg H, Roos H, Gärdsell, P.** Prevalence of coxarthrosis in former soccer players. 286 players compared with matched controls. *Acta Orthop Scand* 1993; **64**: 165–7.

# BIBLIOGRAPHY

**Roos H.** Are there long-term sequelae from soccer? *Clin Sports Med* 1998; **17**: 819–31, viii.

**Roos H, Lauren M, Adalberth T et al.** Knee osteoarthritis after meniscectomy: prevalence of radiographic changes after twenty-one years, compared with matched controls. *Arthritis Rheum* 1998; **41**: 687–93.

**Roos H, Lindberg H, Gärdsell P et al.** The prevalence of gonarthrosis and its relation to meniscectomy in former soccer players. *Am J Sports Med* 1994; **22**: 219–22.

**Roos H, Ornell M, Gärdsell P et al.** Soccer after anterior cruciate ligament injury – an incompatible combination? A national survey of incidence and risk factors and a 7- year follow-up of 310 players [see comments]. *Acta Orthop Scand* 1995; **66**: 107–12.

**Sandmark H, Vingard E.** Sports and risk for severe osteoarthrosis of the knee. *Scand J Med Sci Sports* 1999; **9**: 279–84.

**Turner AP, Barlow JH, Heathcote-Elliott C.** Long term health impact of playing professional football in the United Kingdom. *Br J Sports Med* 2000; **34**: 332–6.

## Chapter 23 – Children and Football

**Betz M, Klimt F.** [Requirements and risk profile of soccer-playing children. Orthopedic aspects]. *Schweiz Z Sportmed* 1992; **40**: 169–73.

**Junge A, Chomiak, J, Dvorak J.** Incidence of football injuries in youth players. Comparison of players from two European regions. *Am J Sports Med* 2000; **28** (Suppl): S47–50.

**Junge A, Dvorak J, Chomiak J et al.** Medical history and physical findings in football players of different ages and skill levels. *Am J Sports Med* 2000; **28** (Suppl): S16–21.

**Lipp EJ.** Athletic physeal injury in children and adolescents. *Orthop Nurs* 1998; **17**: 17–22.

**Metzl JD, Micheli LJ.** Youth soccer: an epidemiologic perspective. *Clin Sports Med* 1998; **17**: 663–73, v.

**Micheli LJ, Ireland ML.** Prevention and management of calcaneal apophysitis in children: an overuse syndrome. *J Pediatr Orthop* 1987; **7**: 34–8.

**Micheli LJ, Metzl, JD, Di Canzio J, Zurakowski D.** Anterior cruciate ligament reconstructive surgery in adolescent soccer and basketball players. *Clin J Sports Med* 1999; **9**: 138–41.

**Peterson L, Junge A, Chomiak J et al.** Incidence of football injuries and complaints in different age groups and skill-level groups. *Am J Sports Med* 2000; **28**(Suppl): S51–7.

**Peterson L, Renström P.** *Sports Injuries: Their Prevention and Treatment.* London: Martin Dunitz, 2001.

**Saris WH.** Habitual physical activity in children: methodology and findings in health and disease. *Med Sci Sports Exerc* 1986; **18**: 253–63.

**Schmidt-Olsen S, Jörgensen U, Kaalund S, Sörensen J.** Injuries among young soccer players. *Am J Sports Med* 1991; **19**: 273–5.

# BIBLIOGRAPHY

## Chapter 24 – Specific aspects of women's football

**Davis JA, Brewer J.** Applied physiology of female soccer players. *Sports Med* 1993; **16**: 180–9.

**Good L, Odensten M, Gillquist J.** Intercondylar notch measurements with special reference to anterior cruciate ligament surgery. *Clin Orthop* 1991; **263**: 185–9.

**Huston LJ, Wojtys EM.** Neuromuscular performance characteristics in elite female athletes. *Am J Sports Med* 1996; **24**: 427–36.

**Jones BH, Bovee MW, Harris JM 3rd, Cowan DN.** Intrinsic risk factors for exercise-related injuries among male and female army trainees. *Am J Sports Med* 1993; **21**: 705–10.

**Möller-Nielsen J, Hammar M.** Women's soccer injuries in relation to the menstrual cycle and oral contraceptive use. *Med Sci Sports Exerc* 1989; **21**: 126–9.

**Östenberg A, Roos E, Ekdahl C, Roos H.** Isokinetic knee extensor strength and functional performance in healthy female soccer players. *Scand J Med Sci Sports* 1998; **8**: 257–64.

**Östenberg A, Roos H.** Injury risk factors in female European football. A prospective study of 123 players during one season. *Scand J Med Sci Sports* 2000; **10**: 279–85.

**Söderman K, Alfredson H, Pietilä, T, Werner, S.** Risk factors for leg injuries in female soccer players: a prospective investigation during one out-door season. *Knee Surg Sports Traumatol Arthrosc,* 2001; **9**: 313–21.

**Traina SM, Bromberg DF.** ACL injury patterns in women. *Orthopedics* 1997; **20**: 545–9; quiz 550–1.

## Chapter 25 – The role of the referee

**Castagna C, Abt G, D'Ottavio S.** Relation between fitness tests and match performance in elite Italian soccer referees. *J Strength Cond Res* 2002; **16**: 231–5.

**Eissmann H-J.** The referee. In: Ekblom, B (ed) *Handbook of Sports Medicine and Science: Soccer.* Oxford: Blackwell Scientific, 1994.

**Ekstrand J.** Soccer injuries and their prevention. Thesis, Linköping University, Sweden,1982.

**FIFA.** The laws of the game. 2002.

**Hawkins RD, Fuller CW.** Risk assessment in professional football: an examination of accidents and incidents in the 1994 World Cup finals. *Br J Sports Med* 1996; **30**: 165–70.

**Inklaar H.** The epidemiology of soccer injuries in a new perspective. Thesis, University of Utrecht, 1995.

# BIBLIOGRAPHY

### Chapter 26 – Travelling abroad with a team

**Reid DC.** *Sports Injury Assessment and Rehabilitation*. New York: Churchill Livingstone, 1992.

**Reilly T, Atkinson G, Waterhouse J.** Travel fatigue and jet-lag. *J Sports Sci* 1997; **15**: 365–9.

**Waterhouse J, Edwards B, Nevill A et al.** Identifying some determinants of "jet lag" and its symptoms: a study of athletes and other travellers. *Br J Sports Med* 2002; **36**: 54–60.

# INDEX

## A

A-active movement, 'on field'
assessment 200
A-ask 198
   abdominal injuries
   diagnosis 283–4
   injury mechanism 281
   prognosis 285
   treatment 284
abdominal wall weakness ('sportsman's
hernia')
   diagnosis 298
   injury mechanism 297
   treatment/prognosis 298
abdominal weakness 109
'accident susceptibility' 57
'accident-prone people' 57
Achilles' tendon
   damage 49, 346
      6–12 months for improved
      condition 59
      complete rupture
         diagnosis 347
         injury mechanism 346
         treatment/prognosis 348
      overuse injury and tendon
      attachment 349–50
                  injury mechanism 350
                  prognosis 352
                  treatment 351–2
      partial rupture, examples 349
      Thompson's test, complete
      rupture 347
   'stressing' activities 407–8, 410
aching joints see arthrosis
acromioclavicular joint dislocation
   injury mechanism 249
   symptoms and signs 250
   treatment and prognosis 250
acute ligament damage, injury
mechanism 362
acute treatment (1–2 days)
   pressure/cold 416
   raising/avoiding strain 416
acute/sub acute phases, of
rehabilitation 418
acyl groups transfer, carnitine role,
across mitochondrial membrane 180
adductor longus muscle 290
adductor tenotomy see hip adductor
muscle, division surgery

adenosine diphosphate 146
adenosine triphosphate (ATP) 146
adequate management control,
absence 24
aerobic function, fat and carbohydrate
(and protein) breakdown 148
aerobic working capacity, in
women 494–5
aggressive playing style 74–5
agility training (stretching) 88–9, 427–31
   effects 427
alcohol 26
alternative treatments 213–15
amenorrhoea (absence of
menstruation) 498
amino acids 149
   enter pool, synthesise new proteins 187
anabolic agents 188
anabolic steroids 531
anaemia 169
anaerobic function, equation 146
anatomical postural abnormalities 48–9
ankle
   with bent knee, bending capacity
   test 113
   deltoid ligament 370
      and plantar fascia 362
   function instability 103–4
   inside of ankle, ligament damage 370
   with knee straight, bending capacity
   measurement 113
   ligament damage 363
      diagnosis and injury mechanism 371
      treatment and prognosis 371
ankle calcification 70–1
ankle examination 103–5
ankle fracture 345
ankle injuries 361–80
   diagnosis 363
   prognosis 366
   rehabilitation progress
   report 365
   treatment 364
ankle kick, force maximisation and
length 131
ankle lateral ligament complex,
'stressing' activities 410
ankle ligaments 361
ankle orthosis 86
ankle protectors 86
ankle sprain, shooting-leg 99

ankle taping, prophylaxis against
injury 85
annulus fibrosus 272
anorexia
   over training 482
   signs 502
anorexia nervosa 501–2
anterior cruciate ligament (ACL) 43
   damage 309
      anterior drawer test 312
      injury mechanism/diagnosis 311
   damage assessment, Lachman drawer
   test 312
   function reinforcement by
   hamstring 506
   injury risk 6–7
   reinforced function in women 506
   treatment/prognosis 315
anterior cruciate ligament damage 466–7
anterior drawer test, anterior cruciate
ligament damage 312
anterior and posterior cruciate ligaments
rupture 309
anterior and posterior thigh muscles 88
anterior talofibular ligament 361–2, 374
   increased anterior drawer
   movement 364
anterior thigh muscle
(quadriceps)
   muscle damage 417
   rehabilitation schedule 418
anterior thigh muscles
   intramuscular bleeding
   signs 417
   testing 114
anterior thigh (quadriceps)
   exercise 428
   flexibility exercise 428
anterior tibial bone spurs 373
anterior/posterior cruciate
ligament rupture 309
anti-inflammatory drug
therapy 355, 357
antibiotic therapy 333, 453
antioxidant nutrients 192
antioxidant supplementation, regular
training, benefit not experienced 192
Apley's test, meniscus damage, of knee
joint 322–3
apophysis, heel pain 491
apophysitis, definition 382

arginine 188
arthrofibrosis, cicatrization of joint
capsule 315
arthroscopy 313, 315, 373, 378
    damaged interior meniscus in the knee,
    with flap rupture 314
    definition 467
    as diagnosis aid, knee injuries 314
arthrosis 463–73
    facts 472
    following knee injuries 466
    joints most often affected 465
    as loss of cartilage, with joint
    cartilage's normal function 464
    risk factors 465
    treatment 464–5
arthrosis reduction, knee injuries 472
arthrotomy, definition 467
asthma 13
asthma attack, causes 457–8
asthma (common), treatment 458
asthma and exercise-included
asthma 457–60
asthma problems
    avoidance
        medicine 460
        non-pharmacological 459–60
asthma and sport 458
asthma in sport, triggers 459
athletes in competition, limited intake of
caffeine 183
athlete's foot 455
athlete's heart 460
    exercise effects 461


B

back injuries 267–80
    anatomy and develop-
    ment 267–9
    emergency treatment 269
back problems 302
badly injured player, mental
symptoms 82
balance and coordination training 104
balance test, stabilometry method 104–5
balance training
    balance board 425
    balancing board 423
        bouncing ball 424
    knee bends on one leg using step
    platform 425
    post-ankle injury 423
    post-knee injury, soft mat 424
    stand on injured foot, receive passes

    and kick back with good foot 424
balancing board training, calf muscle
strength 87
ball speed increase, methods 131
ball/foot speed, in kick 132
Bankart injury 244–5
basic movements 121
basic training 77
    increase, 10–15 % pa 60
bee pollen 193
beep test, running speed, route
example 158
beta-hydroxy beta-methyl butyrate
(HMB) 190
bicarbonate 182–3
    adverse gastrointestinal effects 182–3
biceps femoris 218
bicipital femoral tendon damage
    injury mechanism/symptoms 335–6
    treatment/prognosis 336
big toe
    wear (hallux rigidus)
        arthrosis, reduced movement and
        pain 391
        injury mechanism/diagnosis 390
        treatment and prognosis 390–1
biomechanics of football 121–37
biomechanics and skill in football 126–9
bleeding
    different types 220
    smaller muscle rupture 211
bleeding from under toe nail, pain reduction method 287–8
blood haemoglobin concentration
(Hb level) 495–6
blood pressure 13, 209
bloody extravasation, haemarthrosis 312
body temperature 152–3
    and exertion load 152
body tissues, adapt to training principle 67
body of vertebrae and adjacent
nerves 268
boots suitability, fitness training 90–1
boron 193
boys vs. girls, av. increase in height per
year 494–5
Brazilian free kick equation 131
breathing or heartbeat impedence, team
personnel first aid training 29
bronchitis 453
'brute force' 478
bulimia nervosa (compulsive eating) 503
    signs 502
burn-out signs 79

bursa 243
bursa inflammation 302
bursitis 350
    of the knee joint 333
    symptoms and signs 253
    treatment and prognosis 253
bursitis ('snapping hip') 302


C

caffeine 183–6, 195
    5mg/kg dose, performance increase
    without positive doping result 186
    actions on the body 183–4
    as diuretic 184
    free fatty acids levels 185
    side-effects 184
caffeine doses, effects 186
caffeine effects, on performance 184–5
caffeine use, ethical
issues 185–6
caffeine withdrawal, symptoms 184
calcaneofibular ligament 361, 374
calcification of the bleeding in a
muscle 227
calf muscle rupture
    aponeurosis 352
    diagnosis 353
    injury mechanism 352
    treatment and prognosis 353
calf muscles
    balancing board training stretch 87
    (long and short) (gastrocnemius and
    soleus) stretch 431
cancerous tumour 302
carbohydrate burning 149
carbohydrates, anaerobic breakdown 147
carbohydrates (sugar) 149
carnitin 170
carnitine 180–1, 195
carnitine presence, red meat and dairy
product diet 181
central fatigue, during long-term
exertion 168
cervical spine
    fractures 275–6
    muscle and ligament damage
        diagnosis 270
        injury mechanism 270–1
        symptoms and signs 270
        treatment 270–1
change of activity frequency, by
player 152
cheekbone fractures 239
chest abdominal and skin injuries 281–9

chest injuries
  injury mechanism and diagnosis 281–2
  prognosis 282–3
  symptoms 281
  treatment 282
chest and lumbar region
  muscle and ligament injuries 271
    injury mechanism 271
    prognosis 272
    symptoms and treatment 271–2
children and football 475–91
'chin lift' 207
'chondromalacia patellae' *see*
patella-femoral pain
chromium picolinate, insulin
potentiation 189–90
chronic ankle problems, differential
diagnosis 374
chronic compartment syndrome
(chronically high tissue pressure)
  injury mechanism 356
  symptoms 356–7
  treatment and prognosis 357–8
chronic groin pain 302
chronic ligament instability
anatomical reconstruction 368–9
    diagnosis 367
    injury mechanism 367
    ligament mechanism 367
    treatment and prognosis 368–70
chrysin 195
cicatrization of joint capsule,
arthrofibrosis 315
clavicle fracture, as common childhood
injury 485
clinical fitness vs functional fitness 405
clinical/functional assessment protocol,
fitness testing procedure,
assessment/prediction making 404
club management and coaches, injury
prevention role 24
coaches 75
'cold' clinical assessment 404–5
collagen development remodelling,
within the limits of discomfort 224
collar bone
  fractures 243–4
    injury mechanism 243
    prognosis 244
    symptoms and signs 244
    treatment 244
collateral ligament damage,
treatment 310–11
compartment syndrome 343, 356–7

competitive match, time of injury 21
compressive dressing, injured area
covering foam pad, covered by elastic
board 418
computerized tomography (CAT) scan
236–7, 274, 276, 331
concentric muscle force 143
concentric strength training 422
'concept of injury', defined 1–9
concussion 229–39
  classification 232
  consequences 236
  definition 231
  differing definitions 231
  grade II, definition 234
  grades 1-III, treatment schedules 235
  player positioning 234–5
  common signs 231
  suitable observation
  period 232
  symptoms, early signs/common
  signs 231
concussion rehabilitation, balance and
coordination 234
Concussion in Sport Group 235
congenital excessive mobility, in joints,
risk-factor 49
contusion, definition 415
contusion injuries 222
  point of impact 218
coordination, definition 54
coordination training 87, 106–7, 422–3
  injury prevention 54
coordination and weight training, using a
Body-Bow 426
cortisone therapy 295
coxa plana (Perthes disease) 487
cramp 228
creatine 175–80, 195
  metabolic role 175–6
  as supplementation and muscle CP
  concentration 176
creatine and body mass 178–9
creatine kinase (CK) reaction 176
creatine and muscle
strength 177–8
creatine phosphate (CP) 175
  as 'quick charge' 146
creatine and phosphate
(PCr) 147
creatine supplementation
  effects, exercise performance 177
  health concerns 179–80
  and muscle CP concentration 1767

cruciate and collateral ligament damage,
in the child knee 488
cruciate ligament
  damage
    arthrosis increased risk 468
    rehabilitation progress report 317
  increased injury risk, reasons
  considered 505
cruciate ligament injury 99, 107
  risk reduction 106–7
cruciate ligament surgery, two
techniques 316
cruciate lower attachment to the tibia,
and fragment of loose bone 489
cystitis, lower urinary tract infection 453

**D**

daily recommended calorie intake,
men/women 163
deltoid ligament 436
diabetes (diabetes mellitus) 13
  background and symptoms 443–5
  blood sugar 447
  too high/too low 445
  blood sugar level check method, urine
  stick 447
  conditions for sporting activity 446–7
  diabetic coma 444
  in footballers 446
  insulin 448
  insulin coma 444
  mealtimes 447
  physical activity benefits 445
  strategy for good sugar control, during
  activity 447–8
  treatment 445
diet analysis 27
diet and energy sources 164–5
diet and fluid intake 94
diet intake analysis vs. energy
consumption 27
disease and medication 443–62
distension, definition 415
distension injuries, muscle rupture 217–18
distension rupture 417
diurnal rhythm 521–3
division and playing position, age
distribution demographics 16–17
doping 529–35
  accidental doping 530
  alcohol and marijuana 532
  banned techniques 532
  classes of banned substances 529–32
  diuretic medicines 531

erythropoietin (EPO) 532
facts 535
heart medicine 533
local anaesthetics and cortisone 533
natural remedies 530
restricted pharmaceutical classes 532–3
stimulants 530–1
strong analgesics 531
testing process 533–4
doping offence, caffeine intake 183
doping regulations 12, 26
dorsal extension 378
drinks during training and matches 167
drop finger
injury mechanism 265
prognosis 265
symptoms and signs 265
treatment 265
drug-free football 535
drugs testing 175
Duoderm, complete blister cover 288
dynamic strength training,
example 421–2

E
early mobilization, muscular
regeneration/reconstruction 223
eccentric muscle force 143
elasticity, jump test 160–1
elbow fracture (supracondylar fracture of
the humerus) 486
elbow injuries 251–65
symptoms and signs 252
treatment and prognosis 252
electrocardiograph (ECG), heart's
electrical activity 156
emergency attention, basic rules 216
emergency measures, medical check
list 34
endurance training 151–2, 187–8
energy balance and nutritional
requirements 164
energy production decrease, protein
oxidation contribution 188
energy renewal with oxygen access 148–9
energy systems, different 145–6
energy transfer efficiency, the harder the
shot 130
ephedrine
cough medicine associated 451
herbal remedy, common
ingredient 193, 195
epilepsy 206
ergogenic aids 173

exercise machine, injured leg, strength
training 420
exercise-included asthma,
avoidance/treatment 458–9
exotic supplements 192–3
external feedback system 126
external force, examples 128
external strain, equation 128

F
FA's professional player, audit of injuries
research study 407
fasciotomy 357–8
definition 355
fast/slow muscle fibres 144–5
fats burning 148
Federation of International Football
Associations (FIFA) 1, 509
female training physiology 494–5
femur fracture 487
fibre re-orientation, stretching 224
final decision, after varying stages of
rehabilitation 395–6
finger
ligament injuries
injury mechanism 262
symptoms 262
treatment 263
two-finger dressing, injured
stabilizing 263
finger joint
dislocation
injury mechanism 263–4
joint reduction, and tape support 264
symptoms and signs 264
treatment and prognosis 264
drop finger extensor tendon torn
away 264
first aid 197–216
'VALTAPS' 197
first aid bag 29
first aid training, team personnel 29
fitness, development 476–7
fitness components, examples 399
fitness testing
assessment 411
functional testing 395
'similar profile' players and goalkeeper 410
fitness testing procedure:making assess-
ment/predictions 412
'fitness to play' assessment, clinical
assessment 404
fitness training 94

Fixomull self-adhesive/elastic
material 439–40
as skin protection 440
fluids, sugary drinks and endurance
increase 166
follow-up and check results, weak points
elimination 119
food, nourishment and eating
disorders 501–3
food and food supplements 27–8
food poisoning 456
foot
functional units 381
shock absorption function,
assessment 103
foot injuries 381–94
football activities during matches and
training during an entire season 122–3
football activity and injuries, Swedish
Super League, 1-year period 2
football boots, requirement criteria 91
football boots, injury risk vs. jogging
shoes 70
football and demands of the game awareness, by medical practitioner 398
football kick, interplay between muscles,
phases 1–4 132–3
football medicine
division of responsibilities 35–7
example 37
football medicine services 76
football training, medical
aspects 76
football-related arthrosis,
prevention 471–3
football-specific injury
rehabilitation 415–41
footballer's ankle
anterior joint surfaces build-up of
bone 378
injury mechanism 377
mobility reduction and
pain 378
prognosis 379
symptoms and signs 378
treatment 378
force, kicking a ball, factors which
influence 128
force bodily influences 127–8
force creation, bent torso, muscle contraction, hip bent, stretched knee 135
forward leaning side position, ensuring
open air passage 206
fractures of cervical spine

diagnosis 276
injury mechanisms 275–6
prognosis 276
treatment 276
free substitution, player injury and
immediate substitution 93
functional profiles
advantages 401
assessments 401
functional assessments 400
measurements, player's functional
ability, post-injury lay off 400
as progress/regression assessment 399
test example 402
functional testing 407
ill-advised with dysfunctional
player 403
key rules 402
and performance, factors for
consideration 397
performance factors, to be considered
in advance 397
functional testing event,
progression 406–8
fungal infection of the
nails 455
fungal infection of skin 455

G
gastrocnemius muscles, 'stressing'
activities 407–8
gastroenteritis 456
general health, supplements which may
improve 190
ginseng 193
giving advice
feedback for the individual player 117
feedback for the team 118
glandular fever (infectious
mononucleosis) 456–7
glutamine 191
glycogen
muscle and liver 149
content change 154
depletion 155
glycogen synthesis, stimulation 179
'golden hour', expression 204
groin, examination 107–8
groin discomfort, strain or overuse 110
groin fungus 455
groin injuries
desensitization test 295
symptoms and diagnosis 290–90
groin muscles (adductors)

long groin muscle stretch 430
provocation tests 293
short groin muscles
stretch 429
groin pain
clinical/objective diagnosis 303–5
criteria for diagnosis 305
examination and treatment 303–4
growing and maturation or training
effects 476
guarana 195

H
haemarthrosis 312
haematoma, evaluation of bleeding,
24/48 hour 221
haemoglobin values 156
haemorrhaging, types 237
haemorrhaging in the
brain 237–9
Haglund's disease
calcaneus strain
diagnosis/treatment 383
injury mechanism 382–3
prognosis 383
hamstring muscles, 'stressing'
activities 407–9
hamstrings (H) 53
hand hygiene 28
hand and wrist injuries 255–62
hanging arm technique, dislocated
shoulder setting 246
head injuries 229–40
epidural bleeding 238
subdural bleeding 239
head injury, evaluation test 240
heading action, catapult comparison 136
heading the ball, injury
risk 134–6
heading technique 134–6
heart rate 151
during match 153–4
heel pain, apophysis 491
hepatitis A (epidemic hepatitis), and B
(serum hepatitis) 520
herniography 303, 305
high blood pressure (hypertension) 461
and football 462
physical activity recommendations 462
high training/match quotient and greater
success 64
higher level of play, greater risk of
injury 60–1
hip, examination 107

hip adductor muscle
division surgery 294
'stressing' activities 407–8, 409
hip flexor (gluteus muscles), hip rotator
stretch 431
hip flexor (iliopsoas), hip stretch 429
hip joint
bending capacity test 112
compression test 108
and groin, coordination and weight
training 426
outward angling measurement 111
pain 301–2
rotation test 107–8
stretching capacity 112
hip joint (coxitis), inflammation 487
histidine 188
hormones/contraceptive pill 95
HQ quotient 53

I
ilioinguinal and iliohypogastric nerve
course 295
iliopsoas muscle 290
impaired healing process 212
increased pronation, postural defect 48
individual technique training,
methodology 124–6
indoor play, as increased injury risk 74
infection, avoidance of spreading 451
infection of cuts 454–5
infection examples 451–7
infection risk, precautions 30
infections, stomach and intestines 456
infections in footballers
athlete's proneness to illness? 449–50
background 449
high temperature 450
return to playing 450–1
inflammation, five signs 197
inflatable supports, early stage of
rehabilitation, time spent reduction on
sick level 366
influenza 47
infringements and injuries 92–3
inguinal hernia
diagnosis 297
herniography, as diagnostic method 299
injury mechanism 296
treatment and prognosis 297
injured player
health when accident happened 205
medication taking on regular basis 205
past history 205

previous illness or injuries of
significance 205
injuries in children, growth zone
damage 484
injuries and illnesses, for medical record
inclusion 99
injury
  avoidance 23
  competitive match, time of injury 21
  cooling, pain alleviation 214
  defined 2
  degree of seriousness 4
  elevated position, swelling
  reduction 213–14
  emergency attention, basic rules 216
  localization and degree of
  seriousness 5
  mechanism of injuries 20
  medication as treatment 215–16
  methods of treatment 213–15
  pressure bandages 214–15
  preventative policies 23
  prevention work 4
  rest, as recovery aid 213
  training vs. match
    distribution across season 18
    location/nature of injuries 18–19
  types 4
injury analysis, accidental injury
variation 62
injury assessment
  clinical/functional assessment
  protocol 404–6
  on pitch, treatment off the pitch
  514–16
injury audit, professional football 16
injury audit analysis 16–17
injury audit recommendations 21–2
injury distribution, across season 7–8
injury grades, examples 202
injury or illness
  assessment 29
  emergency measures 29–30
injury and illness, measurement
prevention 12–28
injury incidence increase, just before and
during menstruation 497
injury incidence reduction, women as
contraceptive pill users 497
injury incident, playing activity 17
injury mechanism 230
injury prevention 39–119
  anatomical factors 48–9
  bodily constitution and state of

health 46–7
  equipment 89–92
  football factors 47–8
    skill technique 47
    training 47–8
  goalkeeper/collateral ligament
  rupture 261
  internal factors 45–7
    age 45
    gender 45–6
  mental factors 56–7
  methods 77–119
  muscle prioritization and injury
  susceptibility 88–9
  team discussion
    pre-season 15
injury prevention measures 44
injury pronation, and the well-trained
player 62
injury risk
  driving rain 73
  facts 3
  foot and ground friction 72
  heading the ball 134–6
  increase
    with indoor play 74
    player change of style 74
  increase/decrease 4
  match won vs. match lost 8–9
  per 1000 hours activity 3
  post menstruation 95
  water-logged pitch 73
injury severity, absence days from
training/playing 17–18
injury sign, loss of function 200
inner feedback support, for game
movements 125–6
insole types, examples 92
insoles, shock absorption reduction 91–2
insulin, diabetes medicine 206
intense pain, as symptom of
over-training 78
intensive training, delayed puberty
link 482
intercondylar notch, as factor of susceptibility to cruciate ligament damage 506
intermuscular bleeding 219–20
intermuscular (dispersed)
haemorrhaging 416
internal bleeding, different types 219
'internal blood transfusion' 207–8
internal forces 128
International Football Association
Board 510

International Olympic Committee's
(IOC) medical council, banned
substances/procedures 529
Internet neuropsychological
post-concussion test 235
intramuscular bleeding 219
intramuscular (contained)
haemorrhaging 416
intramuscular glycogen stores, depletion
180
inversion test, inward twisting
measurement, relation to the lower leg 364
inward twisting increase anterior fibular
ligament, and anterior calcaneofibular
ligament damage 364
iron in food, sources 496
iron intake excess, more harm than
good 191
iron mineral 169
  deficiency 170
iron status value 156
isokinetic equipment, measuring
apparatus, examples 51
isolated ligament damage, prognosis 311

**J**
Janda test, mobility measuring 110–11
'jaw thrust' 207
Jefferson's fracture 275
jet-lag
  alleviation measures 522–3
  symptoms 521
joint cartilage
  great strain, long term arthrosis
  link 470
  normal function, with loss of cartilage,
  as arthrosis 464
joint and muscle flexibility 479
joint play, joint capsule and ligaments as
limitation 507
joint stability 50
Jones' fracture, foot injury, 5th
metatarsal 388
jump test, and elasticity 160–1
jumper's knee, take-off leg 99
jumping 137
jumping exercises, variations 426

**K**
kick, biomechanics 129–3
kick speed, equation 132
knee and cruciate ligaments 308
knee flexion exercises, using barbell 421
knee injuries 307–4

arthroscopy as diagnosis
aid 314
increased risk, among women 505
injury risk, higher level player greater
risk 473
ligament injuries, injury
mechanisms 308–9
prevention methods 105
treatment, arthrosis development
risk 468–9
knee joint
anatomy 307
bending capacity, outer ankle bone
measuring device 112
bone growth zones 483
lateral meniscus damage 322
meniscus damage
injury mechanism 321
symptoms and signs 321
reduction in joint space moderate/
pronounced wear 465
knee joint and thigh muscles,
coordination and weight training 426
knee ligament damage, women's
football 46
knee protectors 87
knees examination 105–7

L
L-look, injured site 198
Lachman drawer test, anterior cruciate
ligament (ACL), damage diagnosis 312
lactic acid 176
concentration 154
formation 147–8
and training 478
laparoscopy, surgical procedure 297
Lasègué's test 274–5
lateral collateral ligament
damage 309
with fragment of bone breakage 309
lateral ligaments of ankle, 'stressing'
activities 407–8
Leukotape P tape 439
ligament injuries, diagnosis 309–10
lightning strike, risk level 73
'listen to body signals' 79
long peroneal tendon 374
loose cartilage fragments in the knee
(osteochondritis) 488
low body fat, female sex hormone
decline 500–1
lower leg fractures 343–6
ankle fracture 345

injury mechanism/diagnosis 344
prognosis 345–6
spiral fracture of tibia and fibula 343
splinter (comminuted) fractures 344
treatment 344–6
lower leg injuries 343–60
lower level of play, injury risk during
training 61
lower urinary tract infection, cystitis 453
lymphadenitis 454
lymphangitis 454
lysine 188

M
McMurray's test
meniscus damage
of knee joint 322–3
examination findings 322–3
magnesium 193
magnetic responance imaging (MRI)
223, 274, 276, 303, 373
Achilles' tendon, injury diagnosis 350
patella-femoral pain (PFP) 331
posterior cruciate ligament, injury
assessment 318
manganese 193
match frequency 65
match-time training 521–3
matches, travel time change and climate,
mental preparations 66
maxillary bone fractures 239
meals in conjunction with matches 165–6
mechanical energy, equation 145–6
mechanical instability, ankle mobility
increase 103
medial collateral knee ligament,
'stressing' activities 407–8
medial collateral ligament
damage 309
displacement test 310
medial ligament of knee, 'stressing'
activities 409
medial tibia syndrome 357
medical condition
foot arch, as shock absober 102
general condition, assessment 101
mirror box examination 101
muscle weakness (atrophy) 102
spine 101
medical documentation, and patient
confidentiality 98
medical examination, necessity 14
medical examination record, example 100
medical fees 22

medical and fitness and conditioning
staff 26
medical information 26
medical record, medication, diet,
allergies, vaccinations 99
medical service 75–6, 94
for team 11–37
medical treatment plan 205–10
medication doping alcohol and
smoking 26
medicine service team 31–2
medilla malleolus 393
meniscus damage 467–8, 488
arthrosis risk 467–8
treatment and prognosis 323–4
types 320
meniscus ganglion, definition 323
menstrual disturbances 498
development and possible
consequences 500
menstruation cycle 496
menstruation disturbances
development of, significant factors 498
inadequate energy intake 500
menstruation postponement, under
medical consultation 497
mental 'burn out' 65
mental preparations, matches travel time
change and climate 66
mental training 56, 95–6
methandienone 195
methionine 188
mitochondrion
capacity 152
energy renewal in muscle 148
fatty acids transportation 180
mobility 51
mobility measuring 110
mobility test 110
Morton's metatarsalgia (neuroma)
injury mechanism/diagnosis 392–3
treatment/prognosis 393
mouth-to-mouth resuscitation 208
mouth/throat, alien material,
examples 206
movement patterns 141–2
muscle activation results, resistance
movement affected 142
muscle activity, in football kick 132–3
muscle carnitine levels, supplementation
effects 181
muscle energy renewal, mechanical
energy conversion 152
muscle fibre

regeneration 220
types 144–5
muscle glycogen synthesis 188
muscle injuries 217–28
complications 227
healing, factors influencing 220–1
treatment 221–6
muscle injury, different types 415
muscle (or group of muscles), as
agonist/antagonist 132
muscle pain, in players 110
muscle ruptures
(acute injuries)
diagnosis/treatment 291
prognosis 291
surgical indications 225
(chronic injuries – overuse)
diagnosis/treatment 292
mechanisms 291–2
prognosis 292
in lower extremities, typology 415
recovery potential 223
rehabilitation progress report 225
muscle soreness 228
muscle strength 51, 142–5
imbalance, example 53
muscle tightness, range of flexibility
measurement and limit values 113
muscle tissue construction, and
proteins 166–7
muscles' speed 478
muscular bleeding 416
muscular regeneration/reconstruction,
early mobilization association 223
muscular stiffness 51

N
nandrolone 194–5
nerve desensitization 304
nerve impulses, central nervous system
(CNS) via spine to muscles 124
neuropeptides, signalling substances 168
neurotomy, nerve removal 295
Newton metres (Nm), torque
measurement 53
non-steroid anti-inflammatory drugs
(NSAID) 215–16
nucleus pulposus 268, 272
'nutraceuticals' 174
nutrition and football 163–71
nutrition strategy 174
nutritional supplements 173–95
and muscle mass increase 186–90
overuse 173–4

O
obesity, increased injury risk 46
oestrogen
positive effects on bone 499
examples 499
oestrogen supplement, positive influence
on bone mass 500
'on field' recognition testing,
'VALTAPS' 202
one leg hop test, thigh muscle
strength 114
open airway, method 207
optimal training, highly developed
intuition 63
ornithine 188
os trigonum 376–7
ankle joint bent forward, pain
associated 376
diagnosis 377
injury mechanism 376
treatment and prognosis 377
Osgood-Schlatter's disease
in childhood 489
injury mechanism/diagnosis 339
patellar tendon's attachment
fragmentation to tibia 339
treatment/prognosis 339–40
ossification 227
osteitis pubis see pubic bone,
inflammation
osteoarthrosis, as late sequelae of
football 463–73
osteochondritis dissecans
ankle injury
detached cartilage-covered bone
fragment 325
mechanism 324
prognosis 326
symptoms and signs/treatment 325–6
osteochrondral injury 379
osteophytes 70–1
over training syndrome 64
'over-matching', physical tiredness
manifestation 65
over-training 63–4, 481–2
avoidance 78
over-training symptoms, remedy
examples 79
overuse injuries
Haglund's disease 484–5
Osgood-Schlatter's
disease 484
ovulation failure 499
oxidative metabolism 187

oxteochondritis dissecans
diagnosis 380
injury mechanism 379
prognosis 380
treatment 380
oxygen absorption capacity,
maximisation, defined 150
oxygen consumption in muscle, as
parallel, to exertion increase 151
oxygen transportation system 150

P
P-passive movement testing, player
demonstration of good range of active
movement 200–1
pain assessment
and impaired healing process 210
visual analogue scale 78–9
pain-related scoliosis 272
pangamic acid 193
paracetamol 215
passing water, pain 302
patella dislocation 326
in childhood 490
diagnosis 328
injury mechanism 327–8
prognosis 330
treatment and prognosis 329
patella instability, apprehension test 329
patellar attachment, Q angle, dislocation
risk patella 327
patellar tendon rupture (jumper's knee)
injury mechanism/diagnosis 337–8
treatment/prognosis 338
patellar tendon's attachment to patella,
partial rupture 337
patellar-femoral pain (PFP)
bursitis
excessive loading 332
injury mechanism 332
symptoms 332
patello-femoral pain (PFP)
crepitation 331
diagnosis 331
injury mechanism 330–1
prognosis 332
symptoms and signs 331
in teenage years 490
treatment and prognosis 332–3
periostitis 49
in older adolescents 490
recurrent injury risk reduction 90
periostitis (medial tibia syndrome)
diagnosis 354–5

injury mechanism 354
treatment and prognosis 355
peroneal tendon
dislocation 374–6
diagnosis 375
injury mechanism 375
treatment and prognosis 375–6
personal medical register, by player 13
phenyalanine 188
physical fatigue, and neuropeptides 168
physical performance capacity
factors dictating 157
testing 156–61
physical profile, football
game 139–41
physical/functional fitness aspects 400
physiological profile, of
player 155–6
physiological strain, during match 153–5
physiological testing, composition 156–61
physiology 139–61
physiotherapy 303
planning for season 77–80
plantar fasciitis (calcaneal spur)
diagnosis 384–5
injury mechanism 384
treatment/prognosis 385
plantar flexion 376
'plastic stretch, ' shape retention, after
elongated stress release 224
player, state of health awareness 12–13
player activities, examples 141
player health, management's perception,
as whole club role 25
player movement profile 139–40
player position/functional profile 398–9
player test results and specific player,
results, as data protected 118
player's shot, leans away from ball,
leverage extension in shooting leg 130
players and staff, integrated approach on
health 25
player's study, during match 141
playing tactics 74–5
playing and training surface,
significance 122
pneumonia 453
polio viral disease 519–20
popliteal tendon inflammation
diagnosis/treatment 335
injury mechanism/symptoms 334
prognosis 335
popular drinks, caffeine content 183
post-injury functional testing

aims 397
for return, to competitive play
395–413
post-injury or illness measures,
rehabilitation and return 30–2
post-injury rehabilitation 80–4
posterior cruciate ligament injury
injury mechanism/diagnosis 318
posterior drawer test 319
treatment/prognosis 319
posterior drawer test, posterior cruciate
ligament injury 319
posterior talofibular ligament 361
posterior thigh (hamstrings), stretching
exercise 428
postural defect, compensation 49
'pre-competition functional testing' 395
pre-menstrual tension (PMT), injury risk
increase 46
pre-season friendlies 80
pre-season medical examination
procedure and contact 98–103
reasons and value 96–7
precision of movement, influenced by
player's skill 129
pregnancy 503–5
post pregnancy training, positive
effects 504–5
training during pregnancy
general advice 504
negative effects 503–4
positive effects 503–4
pressure and pain, increased 212
preventative measures
medical check list 33
in practice 96–7
previous injuries
player record 100
review 98
professional football
player importance to club 23
risk management 22–3
Profile of Mood States (POMS) 56,
115–16
pronation, defined 48
pronation increase, foot arch collapse 48
prostate gland inflammation 302
prostatitis see prostate gland
inflammation
protein
and amino acids 187–9
requirement 166–8
protein burning 149
pubic bone

inflammation
diagnosis 299
injury mechanism 298
treatment and prognosis 300
pulse monitoring 28
purpose, defined 129

Q
Q-angle 327–8, 331
quadriceps (Q) 53
complex, 'stressing' activities 409
quadriceps tendinosis
(inverted jumper's knee) 338
quality of movement equation 129

R
radius fractures
lower
injury mechanism 255
prognosis 256
symptoms and signs 255–6
treatment 256
range of motion, training 419
reaction forces, example 127
recovery, endurance development 67
rectus femoris muscle 290
'stressing' activities 407–8, 409
recurring accidents, and lack of
rehabilitation 55
Red Cross's A-E
A-open airway 206
B-breathing 207
C-blood circulating and bleeding 207
D-Has the brain been affected? 209
E-examine systematically 209–10
Red Cross's ABC rule, A-E ensures
systematic action 205
red meat and dairy product diet, carnitine
presence 181
referee 75
blood infections transmission 511
boots and stud size deregulation,
safety regulation '...danger to him or
herself or another player' 512
and direct sending-off
rule 513
and disciplinary action 514
and Laws of Game 510
player assessment, and faking an
injury 516
responsibilities, injury prevention
during match 516–17
role 509–17
and rule 1 – pitch 510

and rule 2 – ball 510
and rule 4 players' equipment 510, 512
rule 5 – referee's authority 512
rule 12 – unlawful play and unsuitable
contact 512–14
rules application, as game safeguard
509, 514–17
rules enforcement, risk of injury
510–14
referred pain 274
reflex controlled muscle contraction 145
rehabilitation
    after earlier injuries 106
    basic principle 80–1
    coaches interest and commitment 83
    cooperation between player, coach and
    medical team 83
    key to successful 82
    as normalization 82
rehabilitation aims 418
    examples 55–6
rehabilitation measures, medical check
list 34
rehabilitation phase, dynamic strength
training, example 421
rehabilitation plan 81
rehabilitation process, testing in
stages 395
rehabilitation and return, after injury or
illness measures 30–2
relative muscle weakness 108
repetitions, definition 425
repetitive injury, avoidance 55
respiratory passages
    infection 451–3
    viral cold 451–2
respiratory tract, bacterial infection 452
return to play 413
risk factors, risk of injury
connected 41–2
risk management, professional
football 22–3
royal jelly 193
rules 92–3
runner's knee 43
    injury mechanism/diagnosis 340
    or jumper's knee 41
    pain lower outer femur, tendon
    irritation, sliding tendon over bone 341
    treatment and prognosis 340
running, jogging 422
rupture of muscle 217–18
    bleeding, back of thigh 218
    recovery potential 223

S
S-strength testing 201
scaphoid fractures
    arthrosis 258
    injury mechanism 256
    (navicular) bone 257
    symptoms and signs 256
    treatment 258
scar tissue
    development 220
    'plastic' properties 224
Scheuermann's disease
    diagnosis 278
    injury mechanism 278
    treatment and prognosis 278–9
Schmorl's node 274
sciatica 273
scintigraphy (isotopic)
scan 257
screw studs, enable less shock
absorbtion 71
second impacy syndrome 237
serious injuries and illness, football
context 203–10
serious injury, action points 210
sesamoid bone
        fracture 840
        diagnosis/treatment 389–90
        prognosis 390
shin pads, requirement criteria 89–90
shock absorption, training shoes 70
shooting leg 99
short peroneal tendon 374
    over outer ankle bone dislocation 374
shoulder
    muscles, tendons and ligaments 242
    skeletal structure 241–65
shoulder dislocation 486
    injury mechanism 244
    symptoms and signs 245–7
    treatment and prognosis 246
shoulder instability
    recurrent 247–9
        injury mechanism 247
        symptoms and signs 247
        treatment and prognosis 248
skill equation 126
skin infections 454
skin injuries
    diagnosis 285–6
    normal stitches vs. surgical staples 286
    prognosis 287
    treatment 286–7
skull fractures 239

slight injuries 210–15
slipped discs 302
    diagnosis 274
    injury mechanism 272–3
    treatment and prognosis 274–5
smoking 26
sonography, lower leg injuries 350
special training for children 475
speed creation, motion of player
extremities 129
speed test, from standing position 160
spinal cord 269
spinal cord damage with paralysis 273
spine, soft parts injuries 270–4
splinter (comminuted) fractures, lower
leg injuries 344
spondylolsis-spondylolisthesis 302
    diagnosis 280
    injury mechanism 279
    treatment and prognosis 280
spondylolysis, defects in vertebral
arches 302
sports combining 68
sports injuries, in children 483
sports injury, types 40–4
'sportsman's hernia' see abdominal wall
weakness
sprained ankles, children vs. adults 491
stability testing, under anaesthetic 318
stabilometry method, data analysis,
body's tendency to lean to one side 104
stamina increase 478
standing on one leg eyes closed
(SOLEC) test 104–5
statis muscle force 143
status after earlier injury 55–6
stomach infection, avoidance 525–6
straight-leg lift, as diagnosis aid 295
strain 110
    as external factor 57–60
strain and arthrosis 469–70
strain and capacity 44
strain injury risk, different surfaces 73
strain and occasions of strain,
correlation 57–8
stress fracture
    diagnosis 300, 359
    foot injury
        injury mechanism/diagnosis 386–7
    treatment and prognosis 387
    groin injuries, treatment and
    prognosis 301
    Jones' fracture
        injury mechanism/diagnosis 388

treatment/prognosis 388–9
lower leg injuries
    diagnosis 359
    fibula 359
    injury mechanism 358–9
    tibia 359
    treatment/prognosis 360
menstrual disturbances 499
overuse during training 499
stress fracture syndrome, lower leg
injuries 357
stress fracture to second metatarsal 386
stretch fracture, causal examples 499
studded boots, concentration of load 70–1
studs, length and number, knee and ankle
injury risk 72
subdural bleeding 239
supplements, energy metabolism
influence 175
supplements and drug
tests 193–5
supports, examples 86–7
supraspinatus tendon 243
swelling, original bleeding, as indirect
cause 211–12
symphysitis see pubic bone,
inflammation
syndesmosis, provocation 373
syndesmosis rupture
    ankle injury
        diagnosis 372
        injury mechanism 372
        treatment and prognosis 372–3

**T**

T-touch, injured part exposure, and
palpation 198
take-off leg, uneven distribution between
legs 99
tape bandage see ankle protector
taping 432–41
    Achilles' tendon
        'anchor' application 439
        'anchors' 438
        two ends of tape 439
    ankle joint
        'anchors' 433, 436
        'figure-of-eight' 435
        'heel-lock' 435–6
        'horseshoes' 435
        inside ligaments
        (medial ligaments) 436
        outside ligaments
        (lateral ligaments) 434

'stirrups' 434
basic principles 432–3
during rehabilitation 85
of the foot arch 437–8
    indications 438
heel and foot 'anchors' 437
heel and foot 'fan' 437
heel and foot 'strips' applied, at right
angles to previous ones 438
ligaments between scapula and
clavicle 440–1
pressure-relieving, patellar
tendon 439–40
preventative value
    recurrence risk reduction 84–5
    and rehabilitation use 84–5
to relieve pressure on joint between
scapula and clavicle
(acromioclavicular) 441
tarsal tunnel syndrome
    injury mechanism/diagnosis 393–4
    treatment and prognosis 394
team doctor 13
team feedback, from medical
examination results 118
team personnel, first aid training 29
technique training 478–81
tendinosis 350
    partial rupture 337
tendon and muscle injuries 290
test course, beep test, with running
speed 158–9
test timing 411–13
testosterone 195, 478, 531
tetanus and diphtheria vaccinations 519
thigh muscle, knee and hip joint, using
slide board 427
thigh muscle strength
    measurement
        by isokinetic equipment 52
        isokinetic technique 54
    one leg hop to test 114
thigh muscles, anterior and posterior 88
thoracic and lumbar spine fractures
    diagnosis 277
    injury mechanism 277
    prognosis 277
    treatment 277
throw-in, types 136
thrower's elbow
    injury mechanism 254
    prognosis 254
    symptoms and signs 254
    treatment 254

thumb
    collateral ligament injury 260
    ligament rupture in the thumb, injury
    mechanism 259
    symptoms and signs 260
    treatment 260–1
tiredness
    as muscle injury risk factor 144
    and neuropeptides 168
tissue strength
    reduction 58–9
        poor state of health 46
'toe kick, ' equation 131
tonsillitis 453
total loss approach principle 23
training 13–15
    after an injury 31
    individual's technique
    significance 123
    overseas 15
    team vs. injured player 159–60
training camps 68
    over-training association 78
training for children 481
'training dose' determination 61
training effects 13–15
    children and adults, relative
    differences 477
training effects and immobilization,
body tissue
strength 58
training increase, brings success 61–72
training shoes, shock absorption 70
training and success, correlation 61
training time, different tissue effects 59
training in water 420
training/match quotient 66
    and injuries correlation 65
trapped nerves, foot injuries 392–4
trapped nerves ('entrapment')
    groin area 294
        diagnosis/treatment 295
        prognosis 296
traveller's diarrhoea 456
travelling abroad with
team 519–28
    check list 528
    climate, fluids and sunbathing 524–5
    diet and the 'framework' menu 525
    getting medical help while
    abroad 527–8
    hotel kitchen, standards of
    hygiene 527
    location and accommodation 523–4

*Tribulus terrestris* 195
tuberosity of tibia see patellar
attachment
turf toe
   injury mechanism/diagnosis 391–2
   treatment/prognosis 392

**U**

UEFA training/match quotient 66
ultrasonography 223, 303, 373
Union of European Football
Associations (UEFA) 1
upper respiratory tract infections
(URTI) 191
urinary tract infections 453–4
urine test 302

**V**

V-vision – see the injury occur 198
vaccinations, club's medical director
responsibility 519
'VALTAPS' term, assessment procedure
197–202
vanadium 193
variation in performance, menstruation,
example 496
vascular problems and sport, exercise
problems 460–2
vegetarians, creatine phosphate (PCr)
lower level 147
vertebra and adjoining nerves 268
visual analogue scale (VAS)
classification, pain assessment 78–9, 419
vitamins and minerals 169–71

**W**

warming up 88
   and cooling down, significance 15
water retention 178–9
wear and tear, injury examples 14
wedge surgery osteotomy 464
weight training 478
whiplash injury 269
Wingate test, anaerobic capacity 157
women players
   increased injury, risk post-
   menstruation 95
   using contraceptive pills, fewer
   accidental injuries, association 95
women's football, specific aspects
493–508
wrist instability
   injury mechanism 258
   symptoms and signs 259

   treatment and prognosis 259
wrist and lower arm fracture, in
childhood 487

**Z**

zinc 193, 195